Surgical Short Cases
for the
MRCS
Clinical Examination

Catherine Parchment Smith
BSc(Hons) MBChB(Hons) MRCS(Eng)

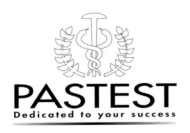

PASTEST
Dedicated to your success

© 2002 PasTest Ltd
Egerton Court
Parkgate Estate
Knutsford
Cheshire WA16 8DX

Telephone: 01565 752000

First published 2002
Reprinted 2003
Reprinted 2005

ISBN: 1 901198 44 8

A catalogue record for this book is available from the British Library.
The information contained within this book was obtained by the author from reliable sources. However, while every effort has been made to ensure its accuracy, no responsibility for loss, damage or injury occasioned to any person acting or refraining from action as a result of information contained herein can be accepted by the publisher or author.

Every effort has been made to contact holders of copyright to obtain permission to reproduce copyright material. However, if any have been inadvertently overlooked, the publisher will be pleased to make the necessary arrangements at the first opportunity.

PasTest Revision Books and Intensive Courses
PasTest has been established in the field of postgraduate medical education since 1972, providing revision books and intensive study courses for doctors preparing for their professional examinations. Books and courses are available for the following specialities:

MRCP Part 1 and Part 2, MRCPCH Part 1 and Part 2, MRCOG, DRCOG, MRCGP, MRCPsych, DCH, FRCA, MRCS and PLAB.

For further details contact:

**PasTest Ltd, Freepost, Knutsford, Cheshire, WA16 7BR
Tel: 01565 752000   Fax: 01565 650264
Email: enquiries@pastest.co.uk   Web site: www. pastest.co.uk**

Typeset by Saxon Graphics Ltd, Derby
Printed by Gutenberg Press Limited, Malta
Illustrations: Raymond Evans, The Unit of Art in Medicine, University of Manchester

CONTENTS

FOREWORD

The curriculum for each of the examinations marking the milestones during Basic and Higher Surgical Training has altered in very many ways with the changes in training introduced by Sir Kenneth Calman. In addition, the recently introduced examinations for the Membership of the Royal College of Surgeons represent a significant departure from the former 'Primary' and 'Second Part' Fellowship examinations of yesteryear.

Many trainees (and trainers) are becoming aware, and possibly concerned that the reduction in the number of hours, and the introduction of shift work limits their opportunities to gain sufficient experience of common surgical and orthopaedic conditions before the stresses of being examined on them in a clinical examination.

This book contains all the necessary equipment that a candidate will need to pass the clinical part of the MRCS examination, with authoritative, yet informally presented clinical information on the various conditions likely to be encountered. Also included are statistics on the most likely patients to be seen by a candidate in each of the examination bays, and advice on the best way of approaching the patients (and also the examiners) on the day.

The layout of the book also allows the candidate to study the many detailed essential notes on the surgical and orthopaedic conditions described, aided by a large selection of appropriate illustrations on the page opposite.

Having studied this book carefully, I regard it as excellent preparation for the MRCS examination, and thoroughly recommend it.

I only wish that a similar book had been available when I was studying for the FRCS!

Jonathan D. Harrison DM FRCS
Consultant General Surgeon

ACKNOWLEDGEMENTS

To my husband, Jon, who tells me I deserve to have it all.
To my mother, Judy, who makes it possible for us to have it all.
To my children Isabel and Benjamin, who are the reason for it all.

I would also like to thank the people who helped me with this book, including Ritchie Chalmers, Heather Harford and Rebecca Hunter. Jon Harrison, apart from being a lovely man, excellent surgeon and top boss, is also a pedant obsessed with Latin and Greek terminology, eponyms, spelling and grammar. He kindly put these idiosyncrasies to good use by reading over this manuscript, for which I am grateful. Thanks also to Sue Harrison and Cathy Dickens at PasTest who put up with my irritating perfectionism with patient good humour (most of the time!). For their continued support, love to my family especially Holly who had a big year, and friends, especially Cath Hernon, best mate and godmother extraordinnaire.

Finally, to my father, Ronnie Parchment. Thank you for always being so proud of me.

Thanks also go to the knowledgeable David Crabbe

Cathy Parchment Smith

PERMISSIONS

Images on the following pages have been reproduced by kind permission of The Wellcome Photographic Library, London.
Chapter 2: pages 44, 45(B), 46, 47(R) 49(BL&R), 50, 54, 55(R), 58(R), 61, 63(T), 64(BR), 67(BL), 68(L), 69(T), 71(R), 73, 79, 93(TR&B), 99, 101(L), 103(R), 106(R), 107, 109(R), 110, 115(BL&R), 121, 127, 128.
Chapter 3: 158, 195(TR), 197(B), 213, 225, 236.
Chapter 4: 281, 283, 285, 289, 291, 293(BL&R), 295(TR), 307, 311, 319, 325(TR), 327.
Chapter 5: 357(L), 361, 363(B), 365(L), 369, 371, 372, 375, 381, 383, 385(C), 387(L), 388(L), 413, 417, 420, 422, 425(T).

Illustrations on the following pages have been reproduced by kind permission of Oxford Medical Illustration at the John Radcliffe Hospital.
Chapter 2: 45(T), 59, 60, 93(TL) 97, 295(TL,BL&R), 297(B), 298(L), 359(L),

Images on the following pages have been reproduced by kind permission of Biophoto Associates.
Chapter 3: 195(BL).
Chapter 5: 385(R).

The following figures in this book have been reproduced from *The New Aird's Companion in Surgical Studies,* Burnand K et al., 2nd ed., 1998 by kind permission of the publisher Churchill Livingstone.

Fig. 11.18	Page 317 **(see page 313T)**
Fig. 16.6a	Page 259 **(see page 106)**
Fig. 17.3	Page 305 **(see page 305)**
Fig. 17.20	Page 318 **(see page 313B)**
Fig. 17.71, 17.7	Page 369 **(see page 329)**
Fig. 19.6	Page 419 **(see page 325B)**
Fig. 25.13	Page 607 **(see page 123L)**
Fig. 31a,b,c	Page 741 **(see page 421)**
Fig. 49.5	Page 1356 **(see page 376)**
Fig. 49.11	Page 1360 **(see page 384)**

The following figures in this book have been reproduced from *Concise System of Orthopaedics,* Apley 2nd ed., 1994 by kind permission of Elsevier Science Limited.

Fig. 19.21	Page 192 **(see page 183)**
Fig. 19.22	Page 191 **(see page 183)**
Fig. 19.24	Page 193 **(see page 181T)**
Fig. 20.15	Page 206 **(see page 189)**
Fig. 21.8	Page 216 **(see page 201)**
Fig. 24.8	Page 250 **(see page 247)**
Fig. 24.10	Page 251 **(see page 215R)**
Fig. 24.13	Page 254 **(see page 215L)**
Fig. 30.4	Page 320 **(see page 184)**
Figs. 30.6, 30.6c	Page 321 **(see page 186)**

The following figures in this book have been reproduced from *Clinical Signs*, Hayes C and Bell D, new edition, 1996 by kind permission of the publisher Churchill Livingstone.

Figs. 87, 88, 89, 90 Page 60 **(see page 399)**
Fig. 93   Page 62 **(see page 397)**
Fig. 104   Page 72 **(see page 429BR)**

The following figures in this book have been reproduced from *Orthopaedics*, Hooper 2nd ed., 1997 by kind permission of the publisher Churchill Livingstone.

Fig. 127   Page 84 **(see page 216)**
Fig. 169   Page 116 **(see page 138)**
Figs 171, 172   Page 118 **(see page 217)**
Figs. 184, 185   Page 128 **(see page 187)**
Figs. 218, 219   Page 152 **(see page 224)**

The following figures in this book have been reproduced from *Surgery*, Corson J and Williamson R, 1st ed., 1991 by kind permission of the publisher Mosby.

Page 7.30.7 **(see page 418)**
Fig. 6.7   Page 4.6.5 **(see page 315)**
Fig. 7.28   Page 3.7.16 **(see page 393)**
Fig. 18.6b   Page 4.18.3 **(see page 299)**
Figs. 18.8, 18.9 Page 4.18.4 **(see page 299)**
Figs. 18.10, 18,11 Page 4.18.5 **(see page 301)**

The following figures in this book have been reproduced from *Clinical Anatomy for Medical Students*, R Snell, 6th ed., 2000 by kind permission of the publisher Lippincott Williams & Williams.

Fig. 3.27   Page 106 **(see page 278)**
Fig. 10.11   Page 527 **(see page 260)**
Fig. 10.18   Page 536 **(see page 292)**

The following figures in this book have been reproduced from *ABC of Colorectal Diseases*, Jones D J, 2nd ed., 1999 by kind permission of the publisher BMJ Books.

Fig. 20.2   Page 76 **(see page 388)**

The following figures in this book have been reproduced from *ABC of Breast Disease*, Dixon, 1st ed., 1997 by kind permission of the publisher BMJ Books.

Page 32 **(see page 114)**
Page 35 **(see page 111**
Page 65 **(see page 116)**
Page 67 **(see page 117)**

The following figures in this book have been reproduced from *ABC Urology*, Dawson C and Whitfield H, 1st ed., 1997 by kind permission of the publisher BMJ Books.

Page 14 **(see page 377)**

The following figure has been reproduced from *Oxford Handbook of Acute Medicine*, edited by Remrakha P S, and Moore K P, 1997, by kind permission of the publisher Oxford University Press.
Insertion of a chest drain Page 87 **(see page 415)**

The following figures in this book have been reproduced from *Picture Tests in Surgery*, Stiff et al, 1ˢᵗ ed., 1996 by kind permission of the publisher Churchill Livingstone.

Fig. 29A	Page 17 **(see page 119)**
Fig. 54B	Page 35 **(see page 101R)**
Fig. 82B	Page 54 **(see page 357R)**
Fig. 86	Page 57 **(see page 105R)**
Figs. 94A & B	Page 63 **(see page 367)**
Fig. C	Page 70 **(see page 287)**
Fig. 107	Page 74 **(see page 363T)**
Fig. 141	Page 95 **(see page 377B)**

The following figures in this book have been reproduced from *An Introduction to the Symptoms and Signs of Surgical Disease*, N Browse, 3ʳᵈ ed., (Arnold, 1997) by kind permission of the publisher Hodder Headline.

Fig. 2.7 A & B	Page 39 **(see page 69)**
Fig. 3.4D	Page 77 **(see page 57R)**
Fig. 3.5	Page 79 **(see page 63B)**
Fig. 3.8A	Page 83 **(see page 58L)**
Fig. 11.12	Page 258 **(see page 105L)**
Fig. 11.5	Page 260 **(see page 103L)**
Fig. 13.1	Page 311 **(see page 373)**
Fig. 16.19	Page 391 **(see page 405)**

The following figures in this bookhave been reproduced from *An Aid to the MRCP Short Cases*, Ryder R E J et al, 1ˢᵗ edition, 1991, by kind permission of the publisher Blackwell Science Ltd.

Fig. 3.4	Page 141 **(see page 317)**
Fig. 3.15a	Page 91 **(see page 321)**
Fig. 3.66a, b	Page 195 **(see page 427)**
Fig. 3.82	Page 221 **(see page 423)**

The following figures in this book have been reproduced from *Clinical Anatomy*, Ellis H, by kind permission of the publisher Blackwell Science Ltd

Fig. 178a, b	Page 262 **(see page 309)**
Figs. 190	Page 287 **(see page 92)**

The following figures have been reproduced from *Spot diagnosis in General Surgery*, Ellis H, 2nd ed., by kind permission of the publisher Blackwell Science Ltd.

Fig. 14 **(see page 296R)**
Fig. 30 **(see page 209B)**
Fig. 32 **(see page 218)**
Fig. 37 **(see page 127L)**
Fig. 79 **(see page 397L)**
Fig. 85 **(see page 411)**
Fig. 86 **(see page 409)**
Fig. 101 **(see page 385L)**
Fig. 102 **(see page 379)**
Figs. a, b Page 107 **(see page 91)**

The following figures have been reproduced from Practice Exercise Therapy, Hollis M, 1998, Blackwell Science Ltd

Fig. 10.5b   Page 135 **(see page 252C)**
Fig. 10.6a   Page 137 **(see page 252R)**

The following figure in this book has been reproduced from *Practical Fracture Treatment*, McRae R, 2nd ed., 1989 by kind permission of the publisher Churchill Livingstone.

Fig. 9   Page 171 **(see page 236TL)**

CHAPTER ONE
INTRODUCTION

A   The MRCS/AFRCS examination

From January 2004 an intercollegiate MRCS examination will replace the individual College MRCS/AFRCS examinations. The new intercollegiate MCQ papers will differ in format from the old examination. The first paper will be entirely on the applied basic sciences and the second paper will be devoted to clinical problem solving.

In 1997, the old Fellowship of the Royal College of Surgeons (FRCS) was replaced as part of the restructuring of surgical training in Britain. At the time of writing this book, the new exams were called:

Membership of the Royal College of Surgeons of England MRCS (Eng)
Membership of the Royal College of Surgeons of Edinburgh MRCS (Ed)[1]
Membership of the Royal College of Surgeons of Glasgow MRCS (Glas)
Associate Fellowship of the Royal College of Surgeons in Ireland AFRCS (I)

Although the old Fellowship examination sittings continued past the date of introduction of the new exams, trainees who began their Basic Surgical Training in or after August 1996 are expected to take one of these new exams to mark the end of their basic surgical training and to become eligible for higher specialist surgical training.

Bear in mind that each of the Royal Colleges has slightly different regulations and requirements, and that these regulations may change from year to year. It is important that no basic surgical trainee should rely on information from published revision guides (including this one!) or from clinical advisors without confirming it directly with the college at which the examination is to be taken. This should be done early in your basic training to ensure that the jobs you are planning to do qualify you to take the examinations. You should also check just before your examination to make sure there have been no important changes in the regulations.

---

[1] This was previously known as the Associate Fellowship of the Royal College of Surgeons of Edinburgh AFRCS(Ed).

Full details of the dates, regulations, syllabus, eligibility requirements and application forms for these examinations, the individual examination offices should be contacted:

Examinations Department
Royal College of Surgeons of England
35/43 Lincoln's Inn Fields
London WC2A 3PN
Tel 0207 405 3474
www.rcseng.ac.uk

Examinations Department
Royal College of Surgeons of Edin.
Nicolson Street
Edinburgh EH8 9DW
Tel 0131 527 1600
www.rcsed.ac.uk

Examinations Department
Royal College of Surgeons of Glasgow
232–242 St. Vincent Street
Glasgow G2 5RQ
Tel 0141 2216072
www.rcpsglasg.ac.uk

Examinations Department
Royal College of Surgeons in Ireland
123 St Stephen's Green
Dublin 2
Tel 003531 4022224
www.rcsi.ie

THE MRCS (ENG) EXAMINATION[2]

Until December 2002 this examination consists of four sections in the following order:

- MCQ 1 (Core Modules 1–5)
- MCQ 2 (System Modules A-E)
- Clinicals
- Vivas

From December 2002 the clinical and viva sections of the MRCS are reversed and candidates will now be required to pass the viva before attempting the clinical section. The order will therefore be:

- MCQ 1 (Core Modules 1–5)
- MCQ 2 (System Modules A-E)
- Vivas
- Clinical

Candidates who have already attempted the clinical section by the end of May 2002 will have the opportunity to complete the examination under the old system (see website www.rcseng.ac.uk for details).

To be eligible for the MRCS (Eng) Diploma candidates must
- possess a primary medical qualification that is acceptable to the United Kingdom General Medical Council for **full** or **limited** registration.
- have satisfactorily completed 24 months of mandatory clinical training or the equivalent in approved flexible training.
- have satisfactorily completed the mandatory Basic Surgical Skills course.
- hold an authenticated logbook of this training.
- provide three satisfactory assessments of their performance of approved basic surgical training posts.
- have passed all sections of the MRCS Diploma examination.
- have been engaged in acquiring professional knowledge and training for at least 36 months since obtaining the primary qualification required above.
- have complied with all the regulations.
- have signed, in the presence of an officer of the college, a declaration of compliance with the Ordinances of the College.

---

[2] Some of the information in this section is from the Royal College of Surgeons website May 2002.

The mandatory clinical training involves two years spent in clinically approved posts. These must include:

- Twelve months made up of two **Category 1** posts (specialties in which a significant proportion of the work will be spent with surgical emergencies requiring the general care of the patient and care of the critically ill) e.g. general surgery, trauma and orthopaedics, or accident and emergency.
- No more than six months should be spent in any one Category 1 speciality.
- Twelve months spent in **Category 2** posts. This may consist of two six-month posts or of more posts of three or four months' duration if the latter form part of a suitable rotation speciality.
- Overall, trainees must train in at least three separate CCST surgical specialties.
- No more than six months should be spent in one specialty.
- Anatomy demonstrating posts are not recognised as part of the clinical training but trainees can take the MCQ examinations during a demonstrating post provided they are in an approved BST rotation.
- The Basic Surgical Skills course is compulsory.
- The Advanced Trauma Life Support course (ATLS) and the Care of the Critically Ill Surgical Patient Course (CCrISP) are recommended but not compulsory.

The Clinical Examination Requirements
- Until October 2002, both MCQ papers must have been passed to take the English Clinical Examination, but these can be from the Royal College of Surgeons of Glasgow, Edinburgh, Ireland or England.
- From December 2002, the viva section of the MRCS (Eng) must also be taken before the clinical.
- Both MCQ papers must have been passed at the same college.
- Candidates must have completed 20 months in approved posts (see above) before December 2002, 22 months after December 2002.
- Logbooks must be brought to the clinical examination.
- Candidates must successfully complete the MRCS (Eng) examination within two years of the date of their first attempt at the Clinical section (before December 2002), and within two years of the date of their first attempt at the viva section after December 2002.
- They may apply for an extension if there are valid extenuating circumstances (e.g. illness, maternity leave, armed service assignments, flexible training or part-time posts).

The MRCS (Eng) Clinical Examination Structure and Marking Scheme
Up to October 2002, the Clinical section will last for one hour and be based upon a mixture of short cases in the form of four clinical bays and a communications skills bay. The titles of the bays are:

Bay 1: Superficial Lesions
Bay 2: Musculoskeletal and Neurology
Bay 3: Circulatory and Lymphatic
Bay 4: Trunk (Abdomen and Respiratory)
Bay 5: Communication Skills

All candidates are examined for 10 minutes in each bay.
The assessment of communication skills is derived from all surgical specialties and is relevant to the whole syllabus. All five bays are equally weighted.

From October 2002 the Communication Skills Test will be part of the viva examination and will not be included in the clinical examination. The test will be expanded and will include a written component. Further details should be obtained from the college. The MRCS (Eng) Clinical Examination will be undergoing significant changes at the end of 2002. The first of the new clinical examinations will be held in January 2003 and the format had not been finalised at the time of this edition going to press.
It is understood that the new examination

a) will not include a Communication Skills bay (this will be included in the viva as explained above).
b) will still include the four clinical bays which are covered in this book. The bays will have the same sort of cases and require the same examination techniques described in this book.
c) may include some modified stations, for example an Objective Structured Clinical Examination (OSCE) is being considered for inclusion in the Superficial Lesions bay.
d) will have a different marking scheme to that currently in use.

The Royal Colleges are continually updating and reformatting the examinations. Before each sitting candidates are advised to contact the relevant college to confirm the format of the examination.

MRCS (ED) EXAMINATION

At the time of writing this consisted of four sections:

- MCQ 1 (Sections 1–9 Principles of Surgery in General)
- MCQ 2 (Sections 10–19 Systematic Surgery)
- Orals
- Clinical

The eligibility and Clinical training regulations are broadly similar to those for the Royal College of Surgeons of England but should be checked by sending for the most recent set of regulations from the college. Important differences include:

- Candidates must have passed the oral section of the MRCS (Edin) exam before they are eligible to take the Clinicals.
- Dates of the examinations tend to be different, enabling candidates to attempt the exam at different colleges within a few weeks or months of each other. Send to the relevant colleges for their examination timetable. As the examinations are interchangeable, it may be worth selecting the college which fit in best with your personal study timetable, study leave, courses etc.
- Don't forget that although you can take your MCQs at any college, both MCQ papers must have been passed at the same college. Similarly, both the clinicals and the vivas should be passed at the same college, although this need not be the same college at which the MCQs were passed.
- The clinical examination structure is completely different from the English college's 'Clinical bays' structure.

The Clinical examination is held in a surgical ward setting. It lasts for 40 minutes with two examiners who are experienced surgeons and each examiner will question you for 20 minutes. You will be expected to demonstrate your ability to take concise, accurate and relevant history, to demonstrate the appropriate physical signs and to give a differential diagnosis. You may be asked to give a very brief opinion on the appropriate management of the case. During the clinical examination you will be shown at least five cases from different surgical specialities[3].

---

[3] Notes to candidates for the MRCS (Ed) Examination, sent out in January 2000.

MRCS (GLAS) EXAMINATION

At the time of writing this consisted of four sections:

- MCQ 1 (Sections 1–9 Principles of Surgery in General)
- MCQ 2 (Sections 10–19 Systematic Surgery)
- Orals
- Clinical

The eligibility and Clinical training regulations are broadly similar to those for the Royal College of Surgeons of England but should be checked by sending for the most recent set of regulations from the cozllege. Important differences include:

- Candidates must have passed the oral section of the MRCS (Glas) examination before they are eligible to take the Clinicals.
- Dates of the examinations tend to be different, enabling candidates to attempt the exam at different colleges within a few weeks or months of each other. Send to the relevant college for their examination timetable. As the examinations are partly interchangeable, it may be worth selecting the colleges which fit in best with your personal study timetable, study leave, courses etc.
- Don't forget that although you can take your MCQs at any college, both MCQ papers must have been passed at the same college. Similarly, both the clinicals and the vivas should be passed at the same college, although this need not be the same college at which the MCQs were passed.
- The clinical exam structure for the MRCS (Glas) is completely different to the English college's 'Clinical Bays' structure.

The examination will last at least 40 minutes and will consist of a 'ward round' situation with a minimum of four patients from a variety of surgical specialties. The object of the examination will be to ensure that the candidate is able to elicit a concise history to demonstrate clinical findings and to appreciate, and attach the significance to clinical symptoms and signs. The candidate will be expected to communicate effectively with the patients and to discuss the clinical findings and the appropriate management with the examiners[4].

---

[4] Information from the Royal College of Surgeons (Glas) website.

AFRCS(I) EXAMINATION

This consists of three sections:

- Part 1: MCQ 1 (Basic Sciences) and MCQ 2 (Clinical Surgery)
- Part 2: Orals
- Part 3: Clinical

The eligibility and Clinical training regulations are broadly similar to those for the Royal College of Surgeons of England but should be checked by sending for the most recent set of regulations from the college. Important differences include:

- At the time of writing, the Irish examination was still called the Associate Fellowship, not the Membership of the Royal College of Surgeons.
- The MCQs consist of two papers, Basic Sciences (a negatively marked 1½ hour paper) and Clinical Surgery (a non-negatively marked 1 hour paper). As of January 2002 the format was undergoing change, candidates are advised to contact the college for further details.
- Candidates must have passed the oral section of the AFRCS(I) examination before they are eligible to take the Clinical.
- Dates of the examinations tend to be different, enabling candidates to attempt the examination at different colleges within a few weeks or months of each other. Send to the relevant colleges for their exam timetable. As the exams are partly interchangeable, it may be worth selecting the college which fits in best with your personal study timetable, study leave, courses etc.
- Don't forget that although you can take your MCQs at any college, both MCQ papers must have been passed at the same college. Similarly, both the clinicals and the vivas should be passed at the same college, although this need not be the same college at which the MCQs were passed.
- The clinical examination structure for the Irish College is undergoing changes.
- Up to January 2002, the clinical examination lasted for about one hour, based on three to five short cases and a history taking case lasting about 20 minutes in which the examiners watched you ask the patients some questions[5].
- From January 2002 the college has undergoing significant changes to the format of the clinical exam. The examination will still be called the Associate Fellowship rather than the Membership, but the format will be more in line with the clinical component of the English MRCS.

The new Clinical section[6] will last approximately one hour and be based upon a mixture of short cases in the form of four clinical bays and a communication skills bay.

---

[5] Information given out by the examinations office in January 2000. The 1998 Basic surgical training and examinations document sent out by the Royal College at that time states that the clinical exam lasts for about an hour and is based on a minimum of five short cases, but according to the Examinations office this is not invariably the case.

[6] Information from the Royal College website May 2002.

The titles of the bays are:

Bay 1: Superficial Lesions
Bay 2: Musculoskeletal and Neurology
Bay 3: Vascular
Bay 4: Abdominal and GI
Bay 5: History taking and Communication skills

Further details should be obtained from the college.

B How to prepare for the clinicals

The clinical exams are all about **preparation** and **presentation.**

Preparation

> 'Only one short case came up in my exam which I had not prepared a
> revision card for, and the examiners admitted that they did not know
> what that lump was either! All the other cases were predictable[7].'

There are very few surprises in the clinical exam. Most medical students could list
the 20 cases most likely to come up in a surgical clinical exam, and you are
unlikely to fail the whole exam on one rare case about which you are unsure. Far
more people fail because they have not adequately prepared for the cases they
know they are going to see. The best way to prepare is therefore:

- Make a list of all the common cases for each bay.
- Plan a systematic examination schedule for each of the common clinical
  examinations.
- Make a note of basic facts, sensible observations and (brief!) principles of
  investigation and management about each short case you are likely to see.
- Practise, practise, practise performing the examinations and discussing the
  cases until it is second nature.

Luckily for you, I have done the first three steps for you in this book. All you have
to do now is practise!

Once you have read through a chapter of this book, it is best to practise in groups
of three. One takes the role of the examiner, one the candidate and the third (who
need not be medical – ask your boyfriend/girlfriend or mum!) the patient. Try to
make the conditions as realistic as possible, with a bed, a chair and a mock
'serious' exam atmosphere. If you are too embarrassed to perform confidently in
these conditions you will flounder in the real thing, so the more unnatural it feels,
the more you need to make yourself do it. Studying on your own will not
compensate for practising these examinations out loud with mock patients.

---

[7] Quote from a candidate questioned in our survey.

You will need the summary cards for each examination, which are provided in this book. The 'candidate' should simply go through each of the examinations in turn with the 'examiner' marking against the summary cards as each bit is completed. After the examination, the examiner should give constructive criticism and point out which bits were missed. You can then change roles. Try to get into the habit of greeting the 'patient' and being polite and professional each time. It will then come naturally to you in the exam. To begin with don't worry how long it takes you for each case, just try to be thorough and do not rush.

After you have each gone through the basic examinations often enough to feel proficient, try to get slick. Each examination should take no longer than 90 seconds. This allows you four cases in a ten-minute bay with a minute's discussion for each case.

Finally, when you know the examinations and are getting 'slick', try to reproduce mock cases. This is best done in pairs with both of you revising for the examination. The 'patient' selects a case from the book in secret, and as the 'candidate' goes through the examination, the 'patient' reproduces or tells the 'candidate' the signs and asks the diagnosis at the end. There then follows a short discussion about the condition, investigations and management.

If you follow this scheme you will be amazed how relieved you feel in the real examination when the standard cases come up for which you are well prepared. They form the vast majority of the examination, and your competence and confidence will impress the examiners and carry you through the inevitable tricky or obscure case for which you can never be fully prepared.

Presentation

Be smart

Be professional

Be kind

Be keen

Be smart

Girls should wear a smart suit or a dress and jacket. Trousers as part of a smart suit are acceptable (this is the 21st century, after all!) but canvas or denim clothes, T-shirt or sweatshirt material tops, are NOT. Keep the colours neutral: grey, navy or black (you are not going to a wedding). Keep jewellery, loud nail varnish, peep toe shoes, micro miniskirts and cleavage to a minimum. Make sure your shoes are clean and comfortable. Avoid sandals, back-less slip-on shoes or trainers (however trendy or expensive).

Men should traditionally wear a grey suit with a white shirt and smart tie although smart navy and black suits will only be frowned upon by the most traditional of examiners. Do not wear cotton, linen or canvas suits. Do not wear jewellery apart from a watch and wedding ring and keep away from loud or novelty ties – the only point you'll make is at your own expense. Cut your hair and shave. Wear black leather lace-up shoes that are clean and avoid suede, loafers or shoes with buckles or bars. If your dad thinks you look scruffy, so will the examiner so take his advice.

It is not traditional to wear a white coat and it is embarrassing if you are the only one doing so.

Look at yourself in a mirror. Could you be mistaken for a senior registrar or consultant? If so, you have the right look.

Be professional

Pretend you are in clinic. Look the examiners in the eye. Do not mumble or mutter. They do not often want to waste time shaking your hand, so unless a hand is offered, a polite smile, nod and 'Good morning' is the correct response to their introduction. The right tone to strike is friendly, efficient and businesslike. Do not delay, but do not be too panicked and rushed. When they give their instructions, however vague, try to assess what they want in your head, turn to greet the patient and proceed promptly with the most relevant examination. If you do it firmly, without pause and talk through your examination confidently it will seem that you have taken control of the patient and the situation, and they are less likely to interrupt or get exasperated. If they do interrupt, however, stop immediately, address their question and then continue with your examination when they are satisfied. If they seem to be trying to guide you in another direction, take the hint and move on to a more suitable examination. If they ask you to 'skip that bit' or 'only examine this bit' you must be flexible and change your routine. You will soon find the thread again if you have practised the examinations as already described. When you have finished the examination, or they have stopped you, move away from the patient, look at the examiners and be prepared to discuss it with them. Struggling for answers while still hunched over the bewildered patient does not give a good impression.

Be kind

Depending on your response to stress you will be either nervous and flustered or arrogant and over-confident. Neither of these predisposes to a likeable, friendly, natural demeanour (which is what you should be striving for). Make sure you smile at the examiners and patient and greet each patient, however briefly. You may not have time to introduce yourself to each patient, but a quick 'hellodo you mind?' with a reassuring smile as you start the examination is important. Be gentle but firm. Act like a doctor. Never hurt the patient, and if there is any sign of discomfort, apologise immediately with 'I'm sorry, was that tender? I'll be more gentle' acknowledging the fact. Ignoring it or continuing with a painful or distressing examination will automatically fail you the exam. It is far harder to fail a nice candidate whose performance borders on the adequate than an unpleasant character who produced the same standard of performance.

Be keen

The examiners want to see an enthusiastic surgical trainee who is doing their best to put on a good performance for them. Being laid back, demoralised or arrogant will count against you immediately. The hardest part of this examination (and the vivas) is to keep persevering brightly and politely when all seems to be going wrong. Don't let one poor case or disastrous bay put you off – many a candidate has moped their way to failure after a minor setback that probably would not have cost them the examination. Avoid the downward spiral! Take a deep breath and attack the next case anew. Don't get surly and recalcitrant. Listen attentively to the examiner's questions, nod in agreement and look fascinated if they make a point. Try to give some kind of intelligent response to each question even if you don't know the exact answer. A good guess or a relevant bit of information is better than an 'I don't know' and stimulates discussion. 'I haven't seen anything like this case before, but it looks like descriptions I have read of severe long-standing lymphoedema.' 'I can't think what this lump is but I have seen similar cases in my cardiothoracic job when they developed vein harvest seromas.' 'This lady has no signs in her hands, but from the history I would be looking for splinter haemmorhages, colour changes, finger pulp wasting and loss of pulses.' These were all sentences I came up with when completely stumped in my clinical exam. Give them something, and they may give you a mark. Give them nothing, and they couldn't pass you even if they wanted to.

C   What to take to the examination

You must bring your up-to-date log book with all the relevant sections signed. Other than this a stethoscope is really all you need – everything else should be provided for you but if you have deep pockets it would be worth taking:

A tourniquet for varicose vein examination
A disposable pin for neurological examination
A tape measure for leg length in the orthopaedic examination
A piece of card for the ulnar nerve examination

However, don't overload yourself with bulging pockets jangling with equipment you may not need and could not find in a hurry. A tendon hammer is useful, but too big to carry around, so if they want you to use one they will probably have one available.

D   Survey of past candidates

When I set out to write this book, I wanted to concentrate on those cases that came up most often. One way to do this was using an 'exit poll' of candidates who had sat the examination and ask them to list the cases they had seen. With the help of PasTest and the many candidates who filled in questionnaires, we gathered enough data to give us a reasonable picture of the MRCS clinical examination.

Candidates who had sat the MRCS or AFRCS examination supplied details of every case seen within the last three years, be it in England, Scotland or Ireland. Here I have analysed the results to indicate the frequency of each case and to give an indication of how often things come up and what kind of questions candidates get asked. This is not a scientifically selected group, but it is a substantial one and I think the results will be helpful to those of you who have not yet sat the examination. These are, after all, real experiences of the actual examination, not just what the book's author thinks should be included! The aim is to give you an idea of what to expect, show you which cases to focus on, and to help you see the relevance of the cases and the background information in this book.

Each case was counted separately, even if they occurred on the same patient. For the purposes of analysis, I have grouped together similar cases even if they occurred in different bays (e.g. lipomas occurred in both the Superficial Lesions bay and the Abdomen bay but I have counted them all as 'Superficial Lesion' cases). In addition, when these candidates were examined some of the colleges had no bay system at all and the candidates were led from one unrelated short case to the next. Be aware, therefore, that in the examination the DVT you expected to see in the Circulatory bay may crop up in the Orthopaedics bay. Do not let this throw you; what you have learned will apply, no matter which bay the cases turn up in.

Details about the questionnaire results for each bay will be found in the relevant chapter. You will see that the most common five cases in each bay account for the vast majority of the exam. If you have time, it would be ideal to work through all the cases in this book. If you have left your revision too late my advice is to concentrate on getting these top five examinations in each bay really slick and spend less time on the less frequently seen cases.

SUMMARY OF SUPERFICIAL LESIONS BAY CASES

Total of 132 cases.
2.5 Superficial Lesion cases seen in the average examination.
Top 5 cases account for 85/132 = 64.4% of cases in this bay.

TOP 5 CASES

Lipoma	**22**	(16.7%)
Skin cancer	**22**	(16.7%)
Thyroid	**17**	(12.9%)
Breast	**14**	(10.6%)
Salivary glands	**10**	(7.6%)

Sebaceous cyst	**8**	(6%)
Thyroglossal cyst	**7**	(5.3%)
Neck lumps	**7**	(5.3%)
Neurofibromata	**6**	(4.5%)
Tracheostomy	**4**	(3%)
Histiocytoma	**2**	(1.5%)
Dermoid cyst	**2**	
Haemangioma	**2**	
Benign papilloma	**1**	(<1%)
Cervical rib	**1**	
Hypertrophic scar	**1**	
Keratoacanthoma	**1**	
Branchial cyst	**1**	
Seborrhoic keratosis	**1**	
Pharyngeal pouch	**1**	
Laryngectomy	**1**	
Seroma of vein harvest scar on leg	**1**	

SUMMARY OF ORTHOPAEDICS AND NEUROLOGY BAY CASES

Total of 152 cases.
2.9 Orthopaedic and Neurology cases seen in the average examination.
Top 5 cases account for 98/152 = 64.5% of cases in this bay.

TOP 5 CASES

Dupuytren's contracture	**26**	(17.1%)
Hip	**21**	(13.8%)
Knee	**20**	(13.2%)
Rheumatoid hand	**17**	(11.2%)
Great toe	**14**	(9.2%)

Upper limb neurology	**8**	(5.3%)
Carpal tunnel	**7**	(4.6%)
Wrist	**7**	
External fixators	**6**	(3.9%)
Ganglion	**6**	
Shoulder	**3**	(2%)
Elbow	**3**	
Trigger finger	**2**	(1.3%)
Ankylosing spondylitis	**2**	
Paget's disease	**2**	
Gout	**1**	(<1%)
Winged scapula	**1**	
Ankle	**1**	
Ingrowing toenail	**1**	
Lower limb neurology	**1**	
Bone Graft	**1**	
Exostosis	**1**	
Osteochondrosarcoma of chest wall	**1**	

SUMMARY OF CIRCULATORY BAY CASES

Total of 122 cases.
2.3 Circulatory System cases seen in the average examination.
Top 5 cases account for 97/122 = 79.5% of cases in this bay.

TOP 5 CASES

Venous disease of legs	**32**	(26.2%)
Ischaemic leg (excluding diabetic leg)	**29**	(23.8%)
Aneurysms	**15**	(12.3%)
Arteriovenous fistula	**12**	(9.8%)
Diabetic feet	**9**	(7.4%)

Venous disease of upper body	**5**	(4.1%)
Upper limb ischaemia	**4**	(3.3%)
Carotid disease	**3**	(2.5%)
Lymphoedema	**3**	
Raynauds	**3**	
Hyperhidrosis	**3**	
Deep vein thrombosis	**3**	
Osler Weber Rendu syndrome	**1**	(<1%)

SUMMARY OF TRUNK BAY CASES

Total of 128 cases.
2.5 Abdominal and Respiratory System cases seen in the average examination.
Top 5 cases account for 84/128 = 65.6% of cases in this bay.

TOP 5 CASES

Groin hernias	**25**	(19.5%)
Scrotum	**17**	(13.3%)
Stomas	**16**	(12.5%)
Hernias (other than groin)	**15**	(11.7%)
Liver disease	**11**	(8.6%)

Splenomegaly	**10**	(7.8%)
Palpable kidney	**9**	(7%)
Abdominal mass (not liver, kidney or spleen)	**7**	(5.5%)
Thoracic cases	**5**	(3.9%)
Fistulas	**3**	(2.3%)
Abdominal scars	**3**	
Bladder	**2**	(1.6%
Peutz Jeghers syndrome	**2**	
Pilonidal sinus	**1**	(<1%)
Peyronie's disease	**1**	
Ovarian cancer	**1**	

SUMMARY OF COMMUNICATION SKILLS BAY CASES

Total of 52 cases.
1 communication bay case seen in every MRCS (Eng) examination.
At the time these candidates sat the examination some colleges did not include this bay.

Explain to a relative...	**32**	(61.5%)
Consent a patient	**13**	(25%)
Breaking bad news	**4**	(7.7%)
Investigate presenting complaint	**2**	(3.8%)
Dealing with complaint	**1**	(1.9%)

HELPFUL HINTS FROM PAST CANDIDATES

What were the examiners like?
Well mannered, gave very specific instructions.
Expected a management plan as well as a diagnosis.
Like consultants in an outpatient clinic.
Friendly and patient.
Not much feedback – I felt like saying 'Am I doing OK?!!'
The orthopaedic examiners were unreasonable and grumpy but the rest were fair and civil.
Mostly OK but I let one horrible pair demoralise me.
Very varied; some friendly, some stony.
Very pushy in the orthopaedics bay!
One examiner was quite sarcastic. When I said I was sure he was right about something, he said 'of course I'm right, I'm the examiner!'
Stern and aggressive.

What did you think of the exam overall?
Very fair (most common response).
The bay system means you know what you will see.
Very rushed!
Stressful!
Pot luck!
A demanding day!
Easy to pass, easy to fail!
Nerve-racking!

What would you do differently if you had to do the clinical again?
Practise on real patients on the ward under exam conditions (most common response).
Learn the background anatomy for common cases.
Practise, practise, practise!
Go through 'proper' examinations in the clinic and on the wards, not taking shortcuts but doing 'mock exams'.
More reading, especially of orthopaedics.
Go round the wards with other SHOs and practise.
Treat the examination with a bit more respect – it's not just medical school finals.
I should have done a course, practised more, broken up with some of my girlfriends.

What was your biggest mistake?
Not being 'slick' enough with my examinations.
Speaking without thinking.
I got harassed when they interrupted my systematic examination.
Not saying enough!
Getting flustered over stoma types when I KNOW THEM!
Rushing.
Giving up on answers too easily and saying 'I don't know' instead of trying to give a reasonable attempt.
Talking nonsense – like saying the word 'shin' to an orthopaedic surgeon!
Getting stressed – calmness is the key to success!
Not being prepared for it.

What did you do most successfully?
Started by giving my 'inspection' findings thoroughly and clearly.
They seemed to like that I was polite to them and the patients.
I got the answers right!
My examinations were all done in a logical manner; inspect, palpate etc.
Played along with the actor in the clinical bay – holding her hand etc.
Stuck to the basics.
My good interaction with the patients saved the day.
I passed!

What is your one main bit of advice to future candidates?

Do not rush – be systematic.

Do a course – it's all about technique!

Be positive and confident – you are probably doing better than you think!

Try to think before you speak – everyone I knew came out with at least one embarrassingly stupid comment!

Talk through your examinations.

Stay calm – it's quite fast so you need to keep cool!

Have ready common causes of common cases such as Dupuytren's and carpal tunnel syndrome.

Stick to routines – anxiety makes you forget it all!

Practice examinations on each other.

Relax! It's all luck.

Start with the basics – keep it simple, stupid!

The London examination goes very quickly so keep your cool!

Don't get disheartened even if it seems to have gone pear-shaped!

Stick to the principles and don't worry if you haven't seen anything like it before (like my Peutz-Jeghers!) just keep to a systematic approach.

Don't worry about the examiners – concentrate on the patients.

Focus only on what the examiners want you to discuss.

Good luck and stay calm!

Thanks to Ritchie Chalmers, Senior House Officer in Surgery at Harrogate, for her assistance with this section.

CHAPTER TWO

CLINICAL BAY 1
SUPERFICIAL LESIONS

CONTENTS

SUPERFICIAL LESIONS

A   The Bay

In the MRCS (Eng) examination the superficial lesions or 'lumps and bumps' bay currently lasts 10 minutes. This will be extended to 15 minutes after December 2002 (see pg 5 for details of the changes). During this time candidates are expected to see 3–4 patients. For each patient a potential 5 marks can be achieved, 3 for the clinical approach and 2 for the discussion and investigations. The MRCS (Eng) syllabus gives the following guidelines on this bay:

'Aim: to determine the ability of a candidate to identify palpable or superficial lumps including skin lesions. Candidates are expected to be able to describe the morphology and anatomy of the lesion with accuracy. The candidate may be asked to describe its layer of origin if appropriate e.g: 'demonstrate why the lesion is arising from the skin/subcutaneous tissue/thyroid.' The examiner will explore the differential diagnosis including the use of simple investigations that might be used to assist in making the diagnosis. Principles of treatment only will be expected, not details. One examiner will lead the candidate around the bay and ask the questions. The second examiner will make notes and both agree on what marks are allocated.'

EXAMINATION OF A LUMP

Introduction and SITE
'Hello, my name is Dr Parchment Smith. Could I have a look at that please? Is it tender at all[1]? I'm just going to describe it to the examiners.'
To the examiners:
'There is a non- tender lump on the right shoulder.'
Feel its SIZE[2], SHAPE[3], SURFACE[4] and EDGES[5]
'It is about 3 cm in diameter, hemispherical in shape, with a lobulated surface and diffuse edges.'
Test for CONSISTENCY[6] now, doing a definite test of FLUCTUANCE[7], hold still for PULSATILITY[8] and pressing it into the underlying structures for COMPRESSABILITY[9] and REDUCIBILITY[10].
'It is soft, fluctuant, non-pulsatile, non-compressible and non-reducible.'

---

[1] If the pathology is obvious, go immediately to the spot diagnosis description described in the 'Cases' section of this chapter. If you are not sure what it is, or the examiners indicate that they want a full examination, or your diagnosis is questioned, go through this logical description of the lesion.
[2] Think in 3 dimensions: width, length and depth or thickness?
[3] Think in 3 dimensions: 'hemispherical' not 'circular?'
[4] Smooth or irregular?
[5] Clearly defined or diffuse?
[6] **Consistency** includes stony hard (not indentable), rubbery (hard to firm but slightly squashable), spongy (soft and squashable with some resilience) and soft (squashable with no resilience).
[7] **Fluctuation** can only be elicited by feeling at least two other areas of the lump while pressing on a third. If two areas on opposite aspects of the lump bulge out when a third area is pressed in, the lump fluctuates and contains fluid. This is best achieved by holding two opposite edges of the lump, e.g. between finger and thumb of one hand, and pressing on the surface of the lump with the finger of the other. Note that lipomas often show fluctance due to the low density of fat, although not strictly a fluid.
[8] Lumps may be **pulsatile** because they lie adjacent to an artery. Aneurysms and vascular malformations tend to be **expansile** i.e. a finger placed on either side of the lump will be forced apart with each pulsation.
[9] Some fluid filled lumps can be **compressed** until they disappear and then reform when the compressing hand is removed (e.g. venous malformations). This is not the same as **reducibility** – technically, the reducible lump will not spontaneously reappear after reduction but has to have a force such as gravity or coughing exerted upon it.
[10] **Reducibility** is a feature of herniae. The lump will be felt to move to another place when it is gently compressed. If you ask the patient to cough, the lump will return, expanding as it does so (**cough impulse**).

Assess LAYER OF ORIGIN[11], FIXITY[12], and TETHERING[13]. Move the skin. Does the lump move with the skin[14], or does the skin move over the lump[15]? Does the skin pucker when the lump under it is moved[16]? Move the lump in the direction of the fibres of the underlying muscle.

To the patient:

'Tense that muscle against my hand.'

Provide the appropriate resistance, e.g. pushing the elbow down in the case of a shoulder lump, and move the lump in the direction of the muscle fibres and at right angles to them. Does the lump become immovable when the muscle is tensed? Does the lump become less easy to feel[17]?

To the examiners:

'The lump lies superficial to the muscle, and the skin moves easily over it. It therefore arises from the subcutaneous tissues and is not tethered or fixed.'

Inspect and feel the OVERLYING[18] and SURROUNDING[19] skin.

To the examiners:

'The overlying and surrounding skin is normal; not red, discoloured, inflamed or warm.'

Feel for the LOCAL LYMPH NODES[20].

To the patient:

'I'm just going to feel in your armpit/groin. Have you noticed any lumps or bumps here yourself?'

---

[11] It is important to determine the relationship of the lump to deep (usually muscle) and superficial (usually skin) tissues.

[12] Attachment to deeper structures can be difficult to decide. If there is an organ in the vicinity of the lump, moving the organ (deep breaths in a liver mass, swallowing in a thyroid lump, sticking out tongue in a thyroglossal cyst) will help decide if the lump is fixed to it.

[13] If the lump is tethered to the skin, the skin will pucker when you try to move the skin over the lump. This is a bad sign in breast lumps that only tend to invade the skin if malignant.

[14] This suggests the lump arises from the skin e.g. sebaceous cyst, basal cell carcinoma.

[15] This suggests the lump arises from the subcutaneous tissue or deeper and is not tethered to the skin.

[16] This suggests tethering to the skin.

[17] These features indicate that the lump is tethered to, lies within or deep to the muscle. If tensing the muscle makes no difference to mobility, or makes the lump more prominent, the lump probably lies superficial to the muscle.

[18] Is the lump ulcerating through the skin, causing excoriation, or does it have increased vasculature? Is there pus or fluid pointing?

[19] The surrounding skin may show evidence of ischaemia (which would make any planned excision more problematic), venous insufficiency, oedema (e.g. peau d'orange in breast cancer) or inflammation.

[20] This is advised in all but the most straightforward and obvious benign lumps that may be accepted as a spot diagnosis (see individual cases later in this chapter).

Closing comments.

To the examiners:

'A full examination of a lump[21] **traditionally includes transillumination, listening for a bruit and examining the distal arterial and nerve supply, but in this case I think the diagnosis is...'**

---

[21] Any of these examinations should be carried out if there is an obvious indication (e.g., feel for pulses in an obviously ischaemic foot with a ?malignant melanoma (this is relevant for post op healing). Transilluminate testicular or obviously fluid-filled lumps. Listen for a bruit over pulsatile or vascular compressible lumps. However, do not go through the motions brainlessly and automatically. You will look very stupid listening for a bruit over a squamous cell carcinoma, or trying to transilluminate it!

EXAMINATION OF THE THYROID

This very common case was seen by nearly one third of the candidates we surveyed. It can be approached in one of three ways depending on what the examiners ask. Decide immediately which one of the following to do:

Is it an examination of a thyroid lump?

If you are told to 'examine this patient's thyroid gland' or 'examine this neck lump' in a patient with an obvious thyroid lump, you should carry out the 'examination of the thyroid lump' (see pg opposite).

Is it an examination of a neck lump of unknown origin?

'Examine this patient's neck' in the lumps and bumps bay means something different from the same instruction in the Orthopaedics and Neurology bay (see pg 155). If it is not obvious where the lump arises from (or indeed, you cannot see a lump) then you should carry out the examination of a neck lump (see pg 37).

Is it a general thyroid status examination?

If you are told to 'examine this patient's thyroid status' or asked 'is this lady euthyroid?' or, after you have examined the neck lump the examiners ask you 'can you tell if she is hyper/hypo/euthyroid?' you should follow the examination scheme for examination of thyroid status (see pg 35).

EXAMINATION OF A THYROID LUMP

'Hello, my name is Dr Parchment Smith. Would you mind if I examined your neck? Could you sit on a chair away from the wall with the buttons of your blouse undone (in a lady)/your shirt off (in a man). Do you mind if I talk about you to the examiners as I go along?'
Stand back, your hands behind your back and look from in front.
To the examiners:
'On INSPECTION, there is a swelling, more prominent on the right, in the anterior triangle of the neck.'
Hand the patient a glass of water (which should be available).
To the patient:
'Could you take a sip and hold it in your mouth until I ask you to swallow?'
Step back again.
'Could you look up slightly? Now swallow please.'
To the examiners:
'The lump moves with swallowing.'
To the patient:
'Could you stick out your tongue[22]?'
To the examiners:
'It does not move on sticking out the tongue. I would now like to PALPATE the lump.'
Move to behind the chair.
'Just point out the area which concerns you[23]. Ah, I see, there on the right? Is it tender at all? I'll be gentle then.'
Place one hand flat against the abnormal (e.g. right) lobe of the thyroid, pushing it gently towards the midline. This will make the left side more prominent and allow you to examine this normal side first. Keep the right hand still, and gently palpate the left side in a few brief but systematic movements, trying to feel the upper, lower, medial and lateral borders and the surface.

---

[22] This is to exclude a thyroglossal cyst (see pg 93).

[23] It is sometimes impossible to see the lump, and asking the patient will save a lot of embarrassing fumbling around, but is a risky tactic. Asking outright might be construed as cheating by some examiners, but few could object if you combine it with an enquiry about whether the lump is tender (as your motive is then avoiding any undue distress). If you have reservations about this approach, go with your conscience and do not try to ask, as cheating results in an automatic fail.

To the examiners:

'I am now palpating the left lobe of the thyroid.'

To the patient:

'Swallow please[24]. And now the right side. Swallow again!'

To the examiners:

'There is a swelling on the right lobe of the thyroid. It feels firm but not craggy and is not tethered to the overlying skin. It is non-tender, about 2 cm in diameter, round with a smooth surface. It is not pulsatile or reducible. The overlying skin is normal. I would now like to examine the LYMPH NODES in the neck[25].'

Feel the eight groups of neck nodes quickly; parotid, mastoid, occipital, superficial cervical, deep cervical, submandibular, submental and anterior cervical (see pg 38).

Stand back and say to the examiners:

'There is no enlargement of the regional lymph nodes clinically. If this were a diffusely enlarged thyroid rather than a prominent lump I would PERCUSS for retrosternal extension and AUSCULTATE for a Graves' bruit. To complete my examination I would like to formally assess this patient's THYROID STATUS[26].'

---

[24] The thyroid gland and any lumps arising from the thyroid move on swallowing but not on sticking out the tongue.

[25] The thyroid drains chiefly into the deep cervical lymph nodes along the internal jugular vein, but one would be concerned about any palpable nodes in a neck with a thyroid swelling as thyroid cancer can metastasise via the lymphatics.

[26] See pg opposite.

EXAMINATION OF THYROID STATUS[27]

'Hello, my name is Dr Parchment Smith. Would you mind if I examined you?
Could you sit on a chair away from the wall with the buttons of your blouse
undone (in a lady)/your shirt off (in a man). Do you mind if I talk about you to
the examiners as I go along?'

Stand back and look.

'On GENERAL INSPECTION this lady looks comfortable at rest. I am looking for
signs of hyperthyroidism such as tremor, restlessness, wasting, signs of
hypothyroidism such as myxoedema facies, a dull aspect or periorbital puffiness.
In addition I am looking for goitre or scars in the neck. Can I start with your
HANDS please?'

Take her hands, look at them, feel the pulse.

'In a hyperthyroid patient I would look for sweaty, warm palms with a
tachycardic or irregular pulse. I would also look for acropachy. In the
hypothyroid the hands are dry, cool and pale with rough, inelastic skin and non-
pitting puffiness. Do you get any tingling or numbness in the hands[28]? She might
be bradycardic. Now I would like to look at the FACE. Just look ahead please.'

Look at it from in front.

To the examiners:

'In Graves' disease I would expect exophthalmos, lid retraction and signs of
corneal irritation.

To the patient:

'Can you follow my finger with your eyes please, keeping your head still.'

Move your finger up and then down.

---

[27] **Causes of hypothyroidism** (details on pg 86)
   1. Iatrogenic (90%)
   2. Primary idiopathic myxoedema
   3. Hashimoto's disease

Causes of hyperthyroidism (details on pg 88)
   1. Graves' disease
   2. Toxic multinodular goitre
   3. Toxic solitary adenomas

[28] Carpal tunnel syndrome is associated with hypothyroidism.

To the examiners:

'There is no lid lag. In a hypothyroid lady I would look for thinning, dry, brittle hair, loss of the outer third of the eyebrows and a sallow complexion. Now I would like to examine the NECK for a goitre or thyroid lump.'

Carry out thyroid lump examination (see pg 33).

'Finally I would like to check ANKLE REFLEXES[29] and ask the patient some QUESTIONS[30].'

---

[29] Hypothyroid patients have **slow relaxing reflexes**, best demonstrated if you ask the patient to stand next to a chair and put one knee on it, supporting herself on the back of the chair and allowing the foot to hang off the chair. A tap on the Achilles tendon should show the gastrocnemius plantar flexion reflex that would be brisk in a hyperthyroid patient, but the foot would be slow to return to the normal position in the hypothyroid patient. Because this is quite awkward to do, just offer to do it in the exam, but make sure you practice it so that if they call your bluff you can perform it smoothly. The normal patellar tendon reflex that is more easily done in a sitting position has the confounding effect of gravity pulling the leg back into position.

[30] **Questions to elicit abnormal thyroid status**

'Are you on any medication for your thyroid?'

'Have you had any thyroid operations or radiotherapy to the neck in the past?'

'Do you prefer a warm (hypo) or cold (hyper) room?'

'Have you lost (hyper) or gained (hypo) weight recently?'

'How are your bowels? (diarrhoea in hyper, constipation in hypo)'

'How is your appetite? (increased in hyper)'

'Have you become more anxious (hyper)/depressed (hypo?)'

'Have you suffered palpitations or angina? (hyper)'

'Have your periods changed?(either)'

'Have you noticed any changes in your face/appearance?'

'Are you being treated for anaemia/diabetes?' (associated autoimmune diseases).

Diseases associated with hypothyroidism: depression, carpal tunnel syndrome, dementia (myxoedema madness).

EXAMINATION OF A NECK LUMP

'Hello, my name is Dr Parchment Smith. Would you mind if I examined your neck? Could you sit on a chair away from the wall with the buttons of your blouse undone (in a lady)/your shirt off (in a man). Do you mind if I talk about you to the examiners as I go along?'

Stand back, your hands behind your back and look from in front.

'On GENERAL INSPECTION, I am looking for any evidence of myxoedema, hyperthyroidism or plethoric facies[31]. Looking at the neck, I can/cannot see any neck lump (say where and how big if you can).'

Offer the patient a drink.

'Could you take a sip and hold it in your mouth until I ask you to swallow?'

Step back again.

'Could you look up slightly? Now SWALLOW please.'

To the examiners:

'The lump moves/does not move with swallowing/there is no lump seen on swallowing.'

To the patient:

'Could you STICK OUT YOUR TONGUE[32]?'

To the examiners:

'The lump moves/does not move with extending the tongue/there is no lump seen on extending the tongue. I am now going to PALPATE the neck from behind. Is the neck tender anywhere? Have you noticed any swellings or lumps yourself? Right, I'll be gentle.'

If you identify a thyroid lump proceed with the thyroid lump examination (see pg 33). If you feel a lump elsewhere, palpate it feeling for and describing its tenderness, site, size, shape, surface, edges, composition, consistency, fluctuance, pulsatility[33], compressibility, reducibility, layer of origin, fixity, tethering, overlying and surrounding skin as described in examination of a lump (see pg 29).

---

[31] Due to superior vena cava obstruction (commonly due to lymphadenopathy)

[32] This is to exclude thyroglossal cyst (see pg 93)

[33] If a lump is pulsatile it should be auscultated for a bruit, and gently compressed to see if it shows compressibility.

'I am now going to examine the LYMPH NODES[34] **the parotid, mastoid, occipital, superficial cervical, deep cervical, submandibular, submental and anterior cervical. My differential diagnosis is…**[35]**.'**

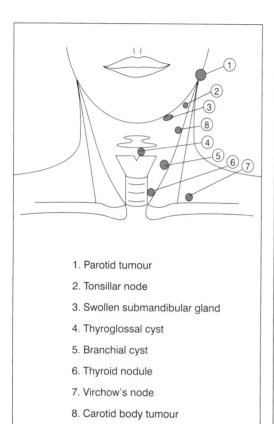

1. Parotid tumour

2. Tonsillar node

3. Swollen submandibular gland

4. Thyroglossal cyst

5. Branchial cyst

6. Thyroid nodule

7. Virchow's node

8. Carotid body tumour

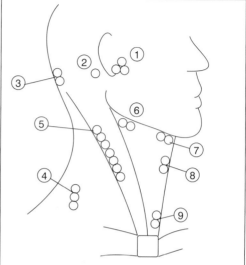

1. Parotid (scalp, face, parotid gland)
2. Mastoid (scalp, auricle)
3. Occipital (scalp)
4. Superficial cervical (along external Jugular vein) (breast, lung, viscera, face, parotid)
5. Deep cervical (along internal Jugular vein) (all neck nodes ultimately drain to here)
6. Submandibular (tongue)
7. Submental (antrum and floor of mouth, lips)
8. Anterior cervical (oesophagus, front of neck)
9. Tracheal (thyroid)

Differential diagnosis of a lump in the neck

Lymph nodes of the head and neck

---

[34] Lymph nodes are felt as subcutaneous swellings.
Enlarged lymph nodes may be:
- Separate – reactive hyperplasia
- Infective mononucleosis (glandular fever)
- Lymphoma
- Matted – neoplastic (metastatic or lymphoma), tuberculous
- Mobile – a good sign
- Fixed – to skin or deep tissues (more worrying)
- Rubbery – Hodgkin's
- Hard – neoplastic

If enlarged lymph nodes are felt, you should at least offer to examine the axillae, groins, spleen and liver.
[35] See figures (above) for sites and causes of a lump in the neck.

EXAMINATION OF THE BREAST[36]

'Hello, my name is Dr Parchment Smith. Would you mind if I examined your breasts? Please sit at 45° with your shirt off, hands on your hips. Do you mind if I talk to the examiners as I go along?'
Stand back, hands behind your back, and inspect.
To the examiners:
'On INITIAL INSPECTION the patient looks generally well, with no evidence of weight loss, jaundice, shortness of breath or pallor. Looking at the BREASTS I am looking for asymmetry in size or shape, skin changes such as redness, puckering, peau d'orange, nodules or ulcers. In the NIPPLES AND AREOLAE I am looking for retraction, destruction, asymmetry and discharge. Inspection of the AXILLAE AND ARMS may show swelling, nodes, veins or wasting of muscles. Finally I am looking for any signs of PREVIOUS TREATMENT such as mastectomy, scarring, radiation burns, telangiectasia, hair loss, lymphoedema or ink marks.'
To the patient:
'Could you RAISE YOUR ARMS slowly over your head please? This enables me to look under the breasts[37] and at the axillae, and can draw attention to asymmetry or tethering. Thank you, put your hands BEHIND YOUR HEAD and lean back. Now I would like to PALPATE THE BREASTS. Are they tender at all? Have you noticed any lumps yourself[38]? I'll start my examination on the side with no lump.'
Palpate the breast with the flat of your fingers.

---

[36] **Causes of a breast lump**
95% will be one of:
> Carcinoma of the breast (26%) (see pg 109).
> Localised area of fibroadenosis -benign breast change (36%) (see pg 112).
> Cyst (15%) (see pg 112).
> Fibroadenoma (13%) (see pg 113).

The rest will be fat necrosis, other cysts (cystadenoma, galactocoele, chronic abscess, retention cyst of glands of Montgomery), infections and inflammation, swelling arising from the chest wall (TB or tumour of a rib, lipoma, thrombosis of superficial veins also known as Mondor's disease).

[37] You may have to lift a large or pendulous breast gently with the back of your hand to see the whole underside and inframammary fold.

[38] As anyone who has done a breast clinic can testify, finding a small breast lump is hard enough with the patient pointing it out, never mind when you don't even know which breast it is in. If the breast lump is large, ulcerating or obvious then you don't have to ask, otherwise, consider prompting the patient as above. Bear in mind that you run the risk of an examiner taking a dim view of this, or even considering it cheating. You could justify it as carrying out the examination as you would in a clinic, but it is a personal decision, and you must be happy in your own mind that you do not consider it cheating.

To the examiners:

'I am feeling for abnormalities in all four quadrants, the centre, the nipple and the axillary tail. Most lumps occur in the upper outer quadrant. Now I would like to FEEL THE AXILLA.

To the patient:

Relax your arm, let me take your elbow.'

Holding the patient's forearm with your non-palpating hand, support the elbow and lift it to shoulder height. Ensuring the patient's arm is relaxed, systematically examine the four walls of the axilla (lateral, medial, anterior, posterior) and gently into the apex.

'Now I would like to PALPATE THE BREAST WITH THE LUMP [39]**.'**

To the examiners:

'There is a small, non-tender lump in the upper outer quadrant of the left breast. It is about 2 cm in diameter, round and irregular in shape with a craggy surface and indistinct edges. It is stony hard, not fluctuant, not pulsatile, compressible or reducible. It is tethered to the skin but does not appear to be fixed to the chest wall. It appears to arise from the subcutaneous breast tissue. The overlying skin is not warm or red and is intact. The surrounding skin is healthy. I would just like to ASSESS FIXITY more thoroughly before moving on to the axilla.'

Make sure patient's hands are still on her hips.

To the patient:

'Relax your arms.'

Take the lump between your fingers and move it gently in the line of pectoralis major fibres, then at right angles to this plane.

To the patient:

'Now press your fists into your hips, tensing your chest muscles.'

Repeat the movement of the lump, noting if contraction of pectoralis major significantly restricts the movement of the lump.

---

[39] Examine it in the same way, identifying the lump and examining it as for the examination of a lump (see pg 29).

To the examiners:

'Clinically, the lump does not appear to be fixed to the chest wall. Now I would like to examine THIS AXILLA. Relax your arm and let me take your elbow.'
Repeat the axillary examination as above. Feel the supraclavicular area on both sides. Stand up and turn to the examiners.

'To complete my examination I would like to CHECK FOR NIPPLE DISCHARGE[40], LISTEN TO THE CHEST and EXAMINE THE ABDOMEN for liver enlargement[41].'

---

[40] In the clinical setting you would have asked about nipple discharge in the history. If it was a feature, you would try to express the discharge pressing on each quadrant in turn to determine which quadrant the discharge is from, also looking for whether the discharge is expressed from a single duct or multiple ducts, and the nature of the discharge.

Causes of nipple discharge:

Physiological (2/3 of all discharge)

Duct ectasia (watery, cheesy, often more than one duct, may be bloodstained)

Duct papilloma (single duct, bloody)

Epithelial hyperplasia (occasionally bloodstained, usually single duct)

Galactorrhoea (?pregnant ?prolactin levels)

Carcinoma (single duct discharge, watery, serous or bloody, usually associated with palpable mass)

[41] In order to look for signs of lung or liver metastases.

EXAMINATION OF A PAROTID LUMP

If asked to examine a subcutaneous lump at the angle of the jaw the chances are that this is arising from the parotid gland[42]. Alternatively you may be asked directly to examine the parotid gland.

'Hello, my name is Dr Parchment Smith. Would you mind if I took a look at this lump?'

To the examiners

'On INITIAL INSPECTION there is an obvious swelling visible over the angle of the right jaw.'

To the patient:

'Is it tender at all? Can I feel it?'

PALPATE it feeling for and describing its tenderness, site, size, shape, surface, edges, composition, consistency, fluctuance, pulsatility, compressibility, reducibility, layer of origin, fixity, tethering, overlying and surrounding skin as described in examination of a lump (see pg xx). Mention also if the rest of the gland is enlarged or feels normal. The findings will depend on the pathology (see individual cases of parotid on pages 118–125).

---

[42] <u>**Lumps arising from the parotid gland include**</u>:
1. **Benign pleomorphic adenomas** (3/4 of all parotid adenomas). Contain epithelial and mesothelial stroma. Occur in middle-aged men and women as a slow growing painless lump. (see case pg 119)
2. **Benign monomorphic adenomas** (1/4 of parotid adenomas). No sign of stroma. Includes Adenolymphoma, *also known as* Warthin's tumour that contains epithelial and lymphoid tissue.
Together adenomas account for 90% of salivary gland neoplasms
3. **Intermediately malignant tumours** (such as acinic cell tumours, mucoepidermoid tumours)
4. **Carcinomas** (adenocarcinomas, squamous cell carcinomas, undifferentiated carcinomas) very malignant with local invasion along nerve sheaths, sinuses, blood vessels, into base of skull. Also widespread metastases (see pg 123).

<u>A lump at the angle of the jaw not arising from the parotid could be</u>:
Arising from the skin: sebaceous cyst, basal cell carcinoma, squamous cell carcinoma, malignant melanoma.
Subcutaneous: lipoma, dermoid cyst, lymphoma or a metastatic deposit from an extraparotid primary.
<u>A generally enlarged parotid gland is caused by</u> (details on pg 124):
- Chronic parotitis
- Mikulicz's syndrome
- Sjögren's syndrome
- Drugs
- Sialadenosis
- Acute parotitis

'I would now like to examine the LYMPH NODES... the parotid, mastoid, occipital, superficial cervical, deep cervical, submandibular, submental and anterior cervical. Have you noticed any other lumps or sores on your scalp sir[43]? I would now like to take a look INSIDE THE MOUTH. Is there a glove and pen torch available?'

Look inside the mouth.

'Open wide! Lift your tongue please? Move it to the left... to the right... thank you. There are no obvious ulcers or tonsillar swellings in the mouth[44]. Can I just feel the inside of your cheek with my gloved finger, sir[45]? I can't feel a stone in the parotid duct.'

Withdraw your finger and take off the glove.

'Let me just take another look at your FACE sir. There are no obvious lesions on the face. Could you show me your teeth please sir, like this... now raise your eyebrows like this... and scrunch your eyes tight closed. The FACIAL NERVE seems intact[46].'

Stand up and face the examiner and give your diagnosis (see cases: pleomorphic adenoma pg 119, parotid carcinoma pg 123, chronic parotitis pg 125).

---

[43] Be aware that the lump over the angle of the jaw could itself be an enlarged lymph node secondary to a malignant lesion elsewhere. Parotid lymph nodes typically drain from the scalp, face and parotid gland.

[44] Malignancies here can drain to neck nodes causing lumps in the parotid area.

[45] Gently slide the index finger into the side of the mouth that the lump is on. With the other, ungloved hand, feel the lump from the outside. The parotid gland cannot be palpated bimanually because it lies behind the anterior edge of the masseter muscle and the vertical ramus of the mandible. A pleomorphic adenoma in the deep part of the parotid can push the tonsil and the pillar of the fauces towards the midline. From the inside feel for the parotid duct which drains opposite the second upper molar tooth. A stone will feel sharp or like a piece of grit on the inner cheek.

[46] Facial nerve infiltration is a sign of malignancy so carcinoma of the parotid gland should be suspected.

C   The Cases

Lipoma
Top Five Case: seen by 42.3% of candidates surveyed. Accounted for 16.7% of the cases in this bay.

[47] **Definition**: lipomata are hamartomas (overgrowth of cell types normally found in that organ). A lipoma is a cluster of mature fat cells that have become overactive and distended with fat.

Presentation: patients usually present because it is unsightly, inconvenient, or they are worried about the diagnosis.

Treatment: simple excision under LA or GA due to cosmetic reasons, or if unduly large or suspicious of a liposarcoma.

Liposarcoma: does not arise from lipoma but *de novo* from different sites, deeper tissues and in the retroperitoneum. Tend to affect older patients. Firmer and more vascular than lipomata. Need urgent excision.

Lipomatosis: a condition of multiple contiguous lipomata causing enlargement and distortion of the subcutaneous tissues. Usually occurs in the buttocks, occasionally the neck (see below).

[48] Common sites, but can occur anywhere where there is fat. Tend not to occur on the palm, sole of the foot or the scalp because in these areas the fat is contained within dense fibrous septa.

[49] Can be of any size.

[50] Lipomata are roughly spherical but are usually compressed between skin and deep fascia so become discoid or hemispherical.

[51] Although the soft fat in a lipoma is not liquid, it can be jelly-like and larger lipomata may fluctuate. Most small lipomata are soft and yielding but do not truly fluctuate like a fluid-filled cyst would.

[52] Subcutaneous lipomata are not usually attached to superficial or deep structures and can be moved freely in all directions. Some lipomata, however, arise from the fat within muscles (intramuscular lipomas), are fixed to the muscle and, unlike the usual lipoma, become less prominent on contracting the muscle rather than more prominent.

[53] May be stretched and translucent with visible veins. There may be a scar or previous excision as recurrence is common.

[54] Lipomata rarely transilluminate unless they are extremely large and prominent. There is no fluid thrill; no bruit and they are dull to percussion. They rarely disrupt the distal circulation, venous drainage or neurology, although an extremely large intramuscular lipoma may do.

[55] People with one lipoma may have others. **Dercum's disease** is a familial syndrome of multiple lipomata.

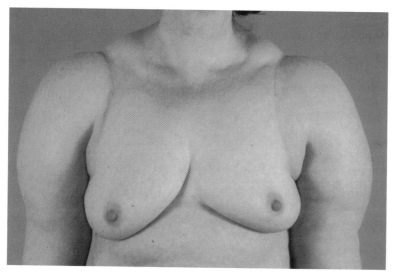

Diffuse lipomatosis over the neck and shoulder

44

LIPOMA[47]

Carry out examination of lump, (see pg 29).

'There is (in this adult of any age) a non-tender lump on the back/shoulder/neck/trunk/forearms[48]. It is 4 cm in diameter[49], hemispherical in shape[50] with a lobulated smooth surface. The edges are also lobulated and slip away from the fingers (the slip sign). It is soft and fluctuant/but does not fluctuate[51], non-pulsatile, non-compressible and non-reducible. The skin moves over it and it appears/does not appear to be fixed to the deep tissues[52], as it becomes less distinct/more distinct on contraction of the underlying muscle. The overlying skin is normal[53] and the regional lymph nodes are not enlarged[54]. This is a lipoma. I would like to ask if the patient has noticed any others[55].

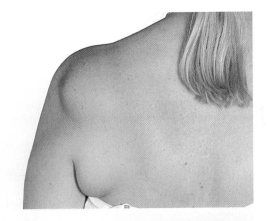

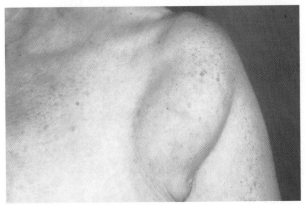

Lipoma on the shoulder

45

Basal call carcinoma

Skin cancer was a Top Five Case: seen by nearly one third of candidates surveyed. Basal cell carcinoma alone accounted for 11.4% of cases in this bay and was seen by over 1 in 4 candidates surveyed.

[56] **Definition**: common slow growing malignant epidermal tumour that rarely metastasises

Epidemiology: most common skin cancer. Seen on the face of middle-aged or elderly fair people. Twice as likely in males than females.

Aetiology: sunlight, X-rays, arsenic, immunosuppressed patients, basal cell naevus syndrome (dominantly inherited, associated with multiple BCCs), people with inherited defects such as xeroderma pigmentosum

Pathology:

Macroscopically: raised rolled (not everted) edges. Pearly nodules with visible fine blood vessels. Slow growing over years with central ulceration and scabbing.

Several variations:

Multifocal: emerge from epidermis and spread over several cm

Nodular lesions: grow deep into dermis as cords and islands.

Flesh coloured: commonest

Scarring, cystic or pigmented (less common)

Microscopically, solid sheets of uniform, darkly staining cells arising from the basal layers of the skin. Histologically similar to basal cell layer of epidermis. NO prickle cells, NO epithelial pearls (seen in squamous cell carcinoma)

Spread: slow but steady local infiltration and destruction of surrounding tissues including skull, face, nose and eye. Hence the term 'rodent ulcer'. Lymphatic and haematological spread are extremely rare.

Treatment: excision has low recurrence rate if adequate. If advanced, extensive or invading nearby structures, radiotherapy gives good results. The prognosis is good.

[57] May arise on any part of the skin including the anal margin, but 90% occur on the face above a line joining the angle of the mouth to the external auditory meatus. They are especially common around the eye, nasolabial folds and hairline of the scalp.

[58] Most patients present while the lesion is small, but if neglected they can become bigger and erode large areas of the face (see above)

[59] Of dried serum and epithelial cells, which bleeds slightly if picked off

[60] Differential diagnosis: squamous cell carcinoma (shorter history, everted edge see pg 49)

Keratoacanthoma (short history, deep, scabby slough see pg 73)

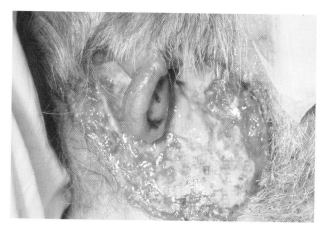
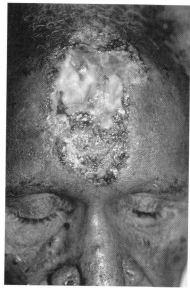

Basal cell carcinoma or rodent ulcer showing extensive tissue destruction

BASAL CELL CARCINOMA[56]

Examination of an ulcer (see pg 274).

There is (in this fair-skinned middle-aged or elderly man) a small non-tender nodule just under the lateral aspect of the right eye[57]. The lesion is one centimetre in diameter[58], round with a rolled, pearly edge that is not everted and a necrotic, ulcerated centre. The base (or centre) of the ulcer is covered with a shallow sloughy coat[59]. The lesion is confined to the skin and is freely moveable over the deep structures and the surrounding skin is normal/shows signs of sun damage. The regional lymph nodes are not enlarged. This is a basal cell carcinoma[60].

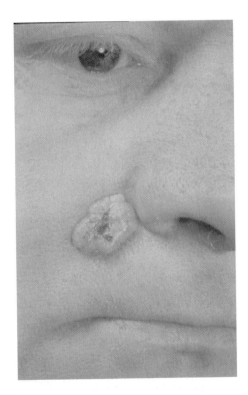

Basal cell carcinoma

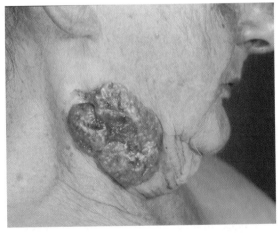

Large basal cell carcinoma showing typical rolled pearly edge

Squamous cell carcinoma (SCC)

Skin cancer was a Top Five Case: SCC alone was a common case seen by more than 1 in 20 candidates surveyed.

[61] **Definition**: common invasive malignant epidermal tumour with a low but significant potential for metastasis.

Epidemiology: very common. Usually in elderly male especially in sun exposed areas i.e. face and back of hands. More common in men than women.

Aetiology: predisposing factors include:

- Exposure to sunshine or irradiation
- Carcinogens (pitch, tar, soot, betel nuts, papilloma virus)
- Lupus vulgaris
- Immunosuppressive drugs
- Chronic ulceration e.g. **Marjolin's ulcer** which is malignant change in a long-standing scar, ulcer or sinus (typically chronic varicose ulcer, unhealed burn, sinus of chronic osteomyelitis). Marjolin's ulcer tends to be slow growing, painless and tends to spread to the lymphatics later than classical SCCs. The edge is not always raised and everted. Other features may be masked by the pre-existing ulcer/scar. Unusual nodules or changes in a chronic non-healing ulcer or scar should be viewed with suspicion and biopsied early. Despite being less invasive and slower growing than a spontaneous squamous cell carcinoma it should be treated as vigorously.
- Premalignant conditions e.g. 1) **Bowen's disease** 'carcinoma *in situ*' – a premalignant intraepidermal carcinoma. Appears as a slow growing thickened brown or pink well-defined plaque. Flat papular clusters covered with crusts, it can look like eczema, and can occur on any part of the body especially the trunk. It is not usually associated with sun damage. A small proportion progress to squamous cell carcinoma. Microscopically it is full thickness dysplasia of the epidermis. **Erythroplasia of Queyrat** is Bowen's disease of the glans penis. Treatment is excision with a minimum 0.5 cm margin.
- Premalignant conditions e.g. (2): **Solar keratosis** 'squamous cell carcinoma *in situ*' resulting from solar damage to the skin and hyperkeratosis of the skin. Usually found in old weather beaten men (e.g. farmers) on the backs of fingers and hands, face and helix of the ears. The skin is usually yellow, grey or brown crusty patches from which arises a protruding plaque of horny skin. 25% progress to squamous cell carcinoma if untreated. Histologically there is hyperkeratosis and epidermal dysplasia. Unlike Bowen's disease there is dermal collagen damage. The treatment is excision, shaving, cryotherapy or topical application of 5FU chemotherapy. Developing tethering, fixity or regional enlarged lymph nodes are worrying features.

Pathology of squamous cell carcinoma: macroscopically a typical carcinomatous ulcer with raised everted edges and a central scab. '*In situ*' squamous cell carcinoma is where the lesion has not invaded through the basement membrane of the dermo-epidermal junction. Microscopically solid columns of epithelial cells growing into dermis with epithelial pearls of central keratin surrounded by prickle cells

Spread: local infiltration and lymphatics. Rarely haematological

Clinical: hyperkeratotic and crusty on sun damaged skin e.g. pinna. Ulcerating if on lips or genitals. Friable or papilliferous varieties may occur.

Treatment: surgical excision as for basal cell carcinoma with a wider margin required in less well-differentiated lesion. Surgical block dissection or radiotherapy or both treat regional node spread.

Prognosis: the local recurrence rate is twice that of basal cell carcinoma. Metastasis to local lymph nodes occurs in 5–10% of SCCs if left untreated – less in those arising in sun damaged skin (0.5%) and more in tumours arising in mucosal surfaces, irradiated areas or Marjolin's ulcers (see above).

[62] It can occur on any part of the skin but is more common in sun exposed areas.

[63] Tendons, muscle and bone can be exposed in advanced, deep lesions.

[64] Advanced tumours may be fixed to underlying structures and immobile.

[65] Although it should be assumed that these are metastatic until proved otherwise, in one third of patients with palpable lymph nodes they are reactive due to secondary infection of the ulcer.

[66] Differential diagnoses include: basal cell carcinoma (see pg 47 : raised, pearly but not everted edge, slow growing, lymph nodes hardly ever involved), keratoacanthoma (see pg 73, no bleeding, history of spontaneous regression), malignant melanoma (see pg 51), solar keratosis (see pg 72) pyogenic granuloma (see pg 60, short history, soft red nodule covered with epithelium.) and infected seborrhoeic wart (see pg 68).

SQUAMOUS CELL CARCINOMA[61]

Examination of an ulcer (see pg 274).

'There is (in this middle-aged or elderly, fair skinned patient), an ulcer on the right cheek[62]. It is 2 cm in diameter and irregularly round in shape. It is a few millimetres deep, penetrating the skin to the subcutaneous fat, and has an everted edge. The base is covered in necrotic slough, dried serum and blood and there is pale, unhealthy granulation tissue. No underlying structures are evident beneath the subcutaneous fat[63]. The ulcer is confined to the skin and moves freely with it over the underlying muscles and bones[64]. The local lymph nodes (say which ones) are enlarged[65]. The surrounding tissues look normal apart from some adjacent inflammation. This is a squamous cell carcinoma[66].'

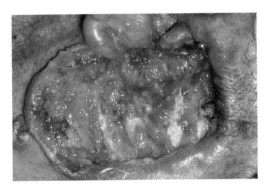

Ulcerating squamous cell carcinoma of the face showing tissue destruction and everted edges

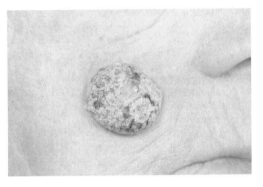

Raised squamous cell carcinoma on the face

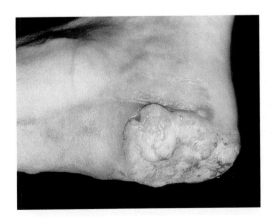

Marjolin's ulcer – a squamous cell carcinoma arising in a long-standing ulcer of the heel

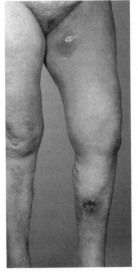

Marjolin's ulcer – malignant change in a long-standing ulcer showing involvement of the draining lymph nodes

Malignant melanoma

Skin cancer is a Top Five Case: Malignant melanoma alone was a common case seen by over 1 in 20 of candidates surveyed.

[67] True malignant melanomas are usually treated so quickly and associated with such anxiety that they are not common examination cases, but it is so important that almost any suspicious skin lesion is likely to lead to a discussion about melanoma, and it is important to know the principles of pathology and management.

[68] The majority of malignant melanomata are found on the limbs, head, neck and trunk. Trunk melanomata are found more often in men, and lower limb melanomata in women.

[69] They may be any colour from pale pinkish brown (amelanotic melanoma) to black.

[70] Nowadays patients are quite aware of risks and usually present while their enlarging moles are quite small.

[71] This is the commonest presentation of malignant melanoma, but there are four common clinical types that differ significantly in appearance.

1. **Superficial spreading melanoma**: This is the most common type. It may occur on any part of the body, is usually palpable but thin with an irregular edge and a variegated colour.

2. **Nodular melanoma**: Thick, protruding, with a smooth surface and regular outline. May become ulcerated and bleeding.

3. **Lentigo maligna melanoma**: This is a malignant melanoma arising in a Hutchinson's lentigo. The malignant areas are thicker than the surrounding pigmented skin, usually darker in colour but seldom ulcerate.

4. **Acral lentiginous melanoma** (including subungual melanoma). This is a rare type but can present as a chronic paronychia or subungual haematoma. It is an irregular expanding area of brown or black pigmentation on the palm, sole or beneath a nail. This is the commonest type in black patients.

[72] **Management of regional lymph nodes**: If no clinical lymph nodes are detectable only certain subgroups are thought suitable for elective lymph node dissection (see Specialist referral, pg 52). If node involvement is suspected clinically, surgical clearance after FNA confirmation is indicated. Chemotherapy is generally used only for metastatic disease and radiotherapy only for certain types of melanoma (e.g. desmoplastic tumours). Regular follow-up is advisable, especially for thicker melanomas (at least 5 years) and recurrent disease.

[73] For metastatic spread. Lungs, liver and brain are the commonest blood-borne sites.

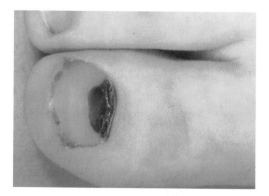 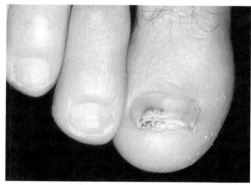

Subungual melanomas. These do not grow out with the nail. This characteristic is useful to elicit in the history, but diagnosis by biopsy should not be delayed in order to observe

MALIGNANT MELANOMA[67]

Examination of a lump (see pg 29).

'There is (in this fair-skinned adult) a non-tender lump on the right arm[68]. It is purple-black in colour[69] about 2 cm in diameter[70], roughly hemispherical with an ulcerated, friable surface and irregular edges with surrounding satellite nodules. The primary tumour has a firm, solid consistence. Small satellite nodules feel hard[71]. The lump is not fluctuant, compressible, pulsatile or reducible. It arises from the skin and is not fixed to the deeper structures. The surrounding skin shows satellite nodules but is otherwise normal. The regional lymph nodes are/are not enlarged[72]. I would be concerned to exclude a malignant melanoma in this patient, and a complete examination would include listening to the chest and examining the liver[73].'

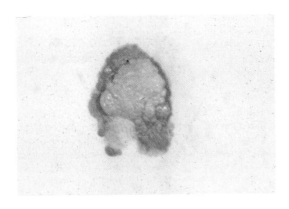

Superficial spreading melanoma

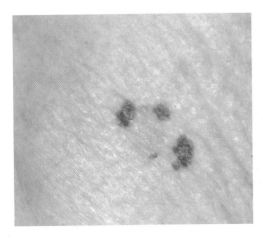

Lentigo maligna

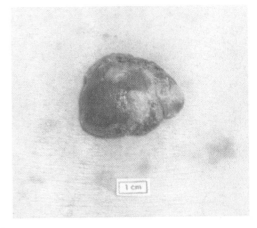

Nodular malignant melanoma

51

Malignant melanoma continued

[74] **Definition**: malignant melanoma is an increasingly common invasive malignant epidermal tumour of melanocytes with significant metastatic potential.

Epidemiology: 10/100,000 in UK, 42/100,000 in Australia. Mostly cutaneous but also occur in mucous membrane of nose, mouth, anus, conjunctiva, choroid and pigmented layer of retina. Rare in coloured races, increasing in white people. Black people tend to get them on the non-pigmented sole of the feet.

Aetiology: sunlight (both UVA and UVB implicated). Childhood exposure is linked with future development of melanoma. Sun beds and tanning lamps carry a potential risk.

Inheritance of multiple primary melanomas accounts for a small number of cases. 2% of all melanomas have a significant family history, and mutations on chromosome 1,6,9,10 and 11 have been implicated. Overall, however, familial melanoma is rare.

Congenital giant naevi (>20 cm maximum diameter at term) have an increased risk of malignant change, which may occur in the first ten years of life. Risks and benefits of excision versus observation are a difficult clinical decision. See fig pg 55.

Pathology: half of malignant melanoma cases arise *de novo* in previously clear skin. Half arise in pre-existent junctional naevi from the melanoblasts in the basal layer of the epidermis (originating from neural crest cells embryologically). Some melanoblasts contain no pigment but all have a positive DOPA reaction (converting dihydroxyphenylalanine – DOPA – into melanin). Horizontal melanoma grows radially. Vertical melanoma grows into the dermis and is associated with metastasis. May cease to grow or regress naturally due to immune response. Antibodies may be seen early in disease but not in metastatic disease.

Signs of malignant change in a naevus:

1. Increase or irregularity in size or pigmentation
2. Bleeding or ulceration
3. Itching, pain or altered sensation
4. Spread of pigment from the edge of the tumour
5. Formation of daughter nodules
6. Lymph nodes/distant metastases

Diagnosis of a suspicious skin lesion: any changing or new lesion not diagnosed clinically should be referred for a specialist opinion, or an **excision biopsy** should be performed for histopathological examination. The excision biopsy should always involve complete excision of the lesion, including full thickness of the skin with a **2 mm** lateral clearance margin. Incomplete, wedge or **incision biopsies** may be tempting in large lesions in cosmetically difficult areas but should **never** be carried out by a non-specialist because they may miss malignant foci in the lesion and because important diagnostic features involving the margins of the lesion are not available to the pathologist in these specimens.

Specialist referral: if the histology turns out to be malignant melanoma, specialist opinion should be sought for several reasons:

1. The scar must be excised with adequate margins (see opposite) which may need reconstructive surgery.
2. Lymph node dissection may be necessary (e.g. in clinically node-positive patients and in some clinically node negative patients such as men with intermediate thickness lesions of the trunk, or young patients with 1–2mm thick tumours)
3. Radiotherapy may be required (e.g. in desmoplastic melanomas)
4. Appropriate follow-up and management of any recurrence must be arranged.

Histopathology reporting of malignant melanoma:
The four essential components of the report (apart from patient details and site) are:
1. Diagnosis of melanoma
2. Maximum tumour thickness according to Breslow's method to the nearest 0.1 mm
3. Completeness of excision
4. Microscopic margins of excision.
Other useful information includes histological classification, level of invasion (Clark), vascular invasion, lymphocytic infiltration, horizontal or vertical growth, predominant cell type.

Classification:
A modified version of the American Joint Committee on Cancer/Union Internationale Contre le Cancer (AJCC/UICC) staging system is the most widely used.

	AJCC staging	
	pT_x	Primary tumour cannot be assessed
	pT_0	No evidence of primary tumour
Clark level I	pT_{IS}	Melanoma in situ (intraepidermal)
Clark level II	pT_1	<0.75 mm and invades the papillary dermis
Clark level III	pT_2	0.75–1.5 mm thick and/or invades to papillary/reticular dermis interface
Clark level IV	pT_3	1.5–4 mm thick and/or invades reticular dermis
	pT_{3a}	1.5–3 mm thick
	pT_{3b}	3–4 mm
	pT_4	>4 mm

Staging by the TNM system:

Stage I	pT_1/T_2	N_0	M_0
Stage II	pT_3/T_4	N_0	M_0
Stage III	Any p_T	N_{1-2}	M_0
Stage IV	Any p_T	any N	M_1

Treatment:
Excision margins depends on the maximum tumour thickness according to Breslow's method (available from the histology report). Remember an excision biopsy is inadequate for melanoma, as its margins are 2 mm, so the scar must be excised.

Melanoma in situ	5 mm margin
0.1–1.5 mm thick (pT1–2)	10 mm margin
1.6–4 mm thick (pT3)	10–20 mm margin
>4 mm thick (pT4)	20–30 mm margin

Historically very wide margins (up to 5 cm) were recommended, and the evidence is still controversial. This protocol is considered acceptable by John Keenly, Chairman of the Regional Cancer Organisation Expert Tumour Panel on Skin Cancer, Consultant plastic surgeon at Frenchay Hospital, Bristol (Ref: *Surgery* March 1999 Vol 17: 3 pg 68–72).

Prognosis: this relates most closely with Breslow thickness, nodal involvement and metastasis. Few patients with three or more nodes or disseminated disease survive 5 years.

Tumour thickness(mm)	approx 10 year survival
<0.76	>95%
1.5–2.5	70%
4–7.99	50%
>8	30%

Other prognostic factors include anatomical site (trunk and scalp worse prognosis than peripheral lesion) and type of growth (superficial spreading better than penetrating, ulcerating lesion).

Benign naevus

[75] There are several pathologies causing a **brown blemish** on the skin.

1. **Freckle**: normal number of melanocytes in their normal position, each producing excess melanin.

2. **Lentigo**: increased number of melanocytes in their normal position, each producing normal quantities of melanin.

3. **Mole/pigmented naevus**: increased number of melanocytes in abnormal clusters at the dermo-epidermal junction producing normal or excess quantities of melanin.

There are four microscopic **types of pigmented naevus**:

  a) <u>Intradermal melanoma or naevus</u>: common mole. Light or dark, flat or warty. Hairy mole is nearly always intradermal. Found everywhere except palm of hand, sole of foot or scrotal skin.

  b) <u>Compound melanoma or naevus</u>: clinically indistinguishable from intradermal naevus but histologically it has junctional elements which make it potentially malignant.

  c) <u>Juvenile melanoma</u>: melanomas before puberty are relatively unusual. Microscopically they may be indistinguishable from malignant melanoma but usually pursue benign course.

  d) <u>Junctional melanoma</u> or naevus: pigmented variably light brown to black. Flat, smooth, hairless. May occur anywhere, including (unlike intradermal) palm, sole and genitalia. Histologically, naevus cells seen in basal layers of epidermis as well as in dermis. Only a small percentage of junctional naevi undergo malignant change, but it is from this group that the vast majority of malignant melanomas arise.

4. **Dysplastic naevus**: as above with nuclear abnormalities but no invasion

5. **Malignant melanoma**: a mole with signs of abnormal and excessive multiplication or invasion of adjacent tissues (see pg 51).

6. **Café au lait patches**: see neurofibromatosis (see pg 59).

7. **Circumoral moles** of Peutz-Jeghers syndrome (see pg 423).

There are several **clinical** varieties of mole:

1. **Hairy mole**: always intradermal naevi. Contains sebaceous glands which may become infected. (See fig below.)

2. **Non-hairy mole**: may be intradermal, junctional or compound naevi.

3. **Blue naevus**: uncommon mole deep in the dermis with smooth overlying skin. Seen in children.

4. **Hutchinson lentigo**: a large area of pigmentation. Commonly appears in the over 60 years on the face and neck and slowly growing. Mainly smooth, but may develop rough areas of junctional activity which are at increased risk of malignant change.

5. **Congenital giant naevus** (see pg 55).

Treatment: most Caucasians have 15–20 moles. They do not need excision unless they are disfiguring, a nuisance in some way (e.g. catching on clothes) premalignant (e.g. Hutchinson lentigo, congenital giant naevus) or develop any suspicious changes (see malignant melanoma, pg 51).

[76] Signs of malignant change in a mole.

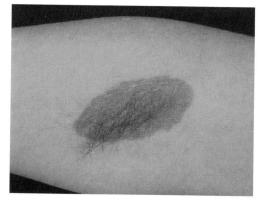

Hairy naevus

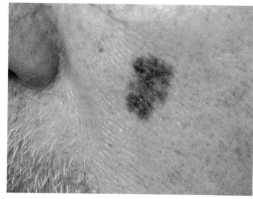

Hutchinson's lentigo

BENIGN NAEVUS[75]

Examination of a lump (see pg 29).

'There is (in this patient of any age) a small well demarcated brown pigmented lump on the right cheek. It is hemispherical, 3 mm in diameter with a slightly wrinkled surface and well-defined edges. It is soft, arises from the skin and is not deeply fixed. There is no evidence of excoriation, ulceration, variation of pigmentation, satellite nodules or extension of pigmentation beyond the edge of the lesion[76].

The surrounding skin and draining lymph nodes are normal. This looks like a benign naevus but I would like to know if the patient has experienced enlargement or change in sensation of this lesion in recent weeks or months.'

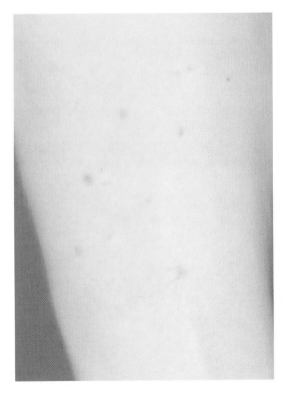

Benign naevi on the forearm

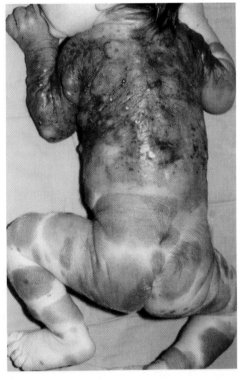

Congenital giant naevus

Sebaceous cyst/epidermal cyst

Very common case: seen by over 1 in 10 of the candidates surveyed.

[77] Also known as: epidermoid cysts, epidermal cysts, trichilemmal cysts, pilar cysts. They occur in all age groups but are rare in children. They are slow growing and usually asymptomatic apart from being unsightly or catching on the hairbrush when on the scalp, apart from when they get infected when they become suddenly enlarged, red, painful and can discharge offensive purulent contents. There are two main types (neither derived from sebaceous glands):

1. Epidermal cysts

Pathology: Arises from infundibular portion of hair follicles. Histologically comprises keratinous debris lined by keratinising squamous epithelium with a distinct granular layer.

Complications: Infection, discharge of foul smelling, cheesy contents.

Malignant change has been reported (McDonald 1963) but is extremely rare

Multiple cysts occur in Gardener's syndrome.

Treatment: Complete surgical removal of entire cyst and its contents intact with an ellipse of overlying skin including the punctum. Recurrence occurs if even a small portion of the cyst lining is left behind. Can be done under local anaesthetic but large, multiple cysts may be removed under GA. Beware bleeding during excision of scalp lesions; have diathermy available, shave area for good access, use a local anaesthetic with adrenaline and close with mattress sutures to aid haemostasis. Mattress sutures are useful on the scalp but should be avoided on areas where cosmetic result is important.

2. Trichilemmal cysts

Clinically identical to epidermal cysts but not as common. 90% on scalp. 70% multiple. Genetic predisposition (autosomal dominant)

Pathology: derived from hair follicle epithelium. Lined by epithelial cells and do not have the granular layer from the epidermis which characterises the epidermal cysts.

Treatment: as for epidermal cyst.

Complications: calcification (not seen in epidermal cysts).

Pilar tumour: proliferation of epithelium lining cyst.

Ulceration and proliferation: may resemble a squamous cell carcinoma (Cock's peculiar tumour see fig opposite).

Malignant transformation: reported but rare

Treatment: as for epidermal cyst.

[78] Tenderness is a sign of infection.

[79] Most sebaceous cysts are found in the hair bearing parts of the body, especially the scalp, scrotum, neck, shoulders and back. They can occur wherever there are sebaceous glands (i.e. not the palms of the hands or soles of the feet.

[80] They can vary from a few millimetres to upward of 4 cm in diameter.

SEBACEOUS CYST/EPIDERMAL CYST[77]

Examination of lump, (see pg 29).

'There is a large non-tender[78] lump on the right side of the scalp[79]. It is 3 cm in diameter[80], spherical with a smooth surface and a well-defined edge. It is hard in consistency, not compressible or pulsatile. It moves with the skin freely over the underlying deep structures and although the surrounding skin is normal, the overlying skin shows signs of hair loss, excoriation, and inflammation. There is/is no evidence of a punctum/scar from previous excision/current infection and discharge. This is a sebaceous cyst.'

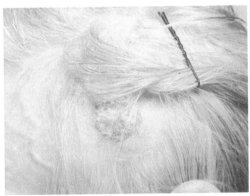

Cock's peculiar tumour

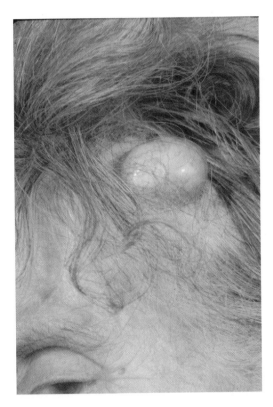

Sebaceous cyst

Neurofibroma
Very common case: seen by over 1 in 10 of the candidates surveyed.

[81] **Definition**: benign tumour containing a mixture of neural (ectodermal) and fibrous (mesodermal) elements. They are hamartomas (overgrowth of cell types normally found in that organ). They are often multiple.

Symptoms: most neurofibromas cause no discomfort. Subcutaneous neurofibromas related to a nerve trunk may be tender and may lead to paraesthesia or dysaesthesia in the distribution of the affected nerve.

Complications: nerve damage (including spinal cord and cranial nerves, typically the acoustic nerve). Malignant transformation in von Recklinghausen's disease (see below).

Treatment: excision is tricky due to the non-encapsulated diffuse nature of the lesions, the risk of bleeding and problems with nerve involvement. Regrowth is common.

von Recklinghausen's disease: autosomal dominant condition defined as multiple congenital familial neurofibromatosis associated with:

1. Fibroepithelial skin tags

2. Café au lait patches (light brown skin discoloration) 6 or more >1.5 cm in diameter is pathognomonic but 30% of von Recklinghausen's disease will have no cafe au lait spots.

3. Neuromas on major nerves especially acoustic neuromas and dumb-bell neuromas on the sensory roots of the spinal nerves.

4. Malignant change (neurofibrosarcoma) in 5–13% of von Recklinghausen patients but not generally seen in spontaneous neurofibromas. Usually arises from large nerve trunks. Carries a poor prognosis.

5. Phaeochromocytoma

Also associated with scoliosis, intracranial anomalies and mental retardation. Most of the neurofibromas are present at birth but they increase in size and number during life.

Plexiform neurofibroma: extremely rare condition involving excessive overgrowth of neural tissue in the subcutaneous fat. Looks like oedema but the lymphatics are normal. Called elephantitis neurofibromatosis due to the gross deformity, often of the hand or foot.

[82] To exclude nerve damage by neuromas.

[83] Because the acoustic nerve is the most commonly involved.

[84] Because phaeochromocytoma may cause hypertension.

[85] Because of the risk of malignant change (5–13%).

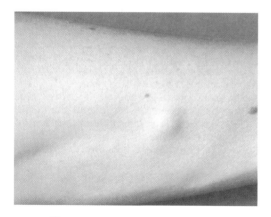

Neurofibroma

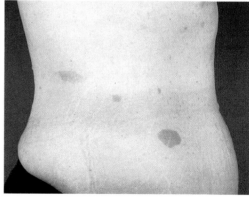

Café au lait spots

NEUROFIBROMA[81]

Spot diagnosis.

'This patient (of any age) is covered with non-tender nodules of varying sizes from minute lumps to large subcutaneous nodules. Some are in the skin, some are in the subcutaneous tissues and some are pedunculated. They vary in consistency from soft to hard but each one is discrete with well-defined edges. There are three well-demarcated areas of light brown skin discoloration – café au lait patches visible. The diagnosis is von Recklinghausen's disease or multiple neurofibromatosis.

A full examination of this patient should include a neurological examination concentrating on the cranial and spinal nerves[82], a hearing test[83] and a check of his blood pressure[84]. It is also important to ask if any of the lumps has suddenly increased in size or become more painful[85].'

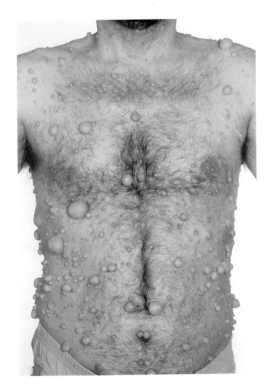
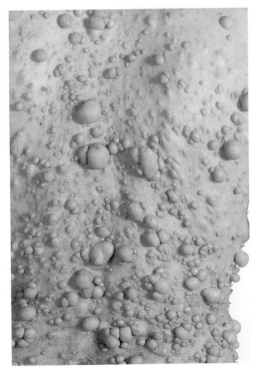

Multiple neurofibromatosis

PYOGENIC GRANULOMA[86]

Examination of a lump (see pg 29).

'There is a non-tender[87] lump on the back of the right hand[88]. It is a hemispherical nodule about 0.5 cm in diameter. The surface is friable and bleeds on contact and it stands proud of the skin with well-defined edges. It is soft, slightly compressible but not reducible or pulsatile. It arises from the skin to which its base is attached and is not fixed to any deeper structures. The surrounding skin is normal and the regional lymph nodes are not enlarged. This is a pyogenic granuloma. I would like to ask the patient about any previous injury to this area. It is important to exclude more serious differential diagnoses[89].'

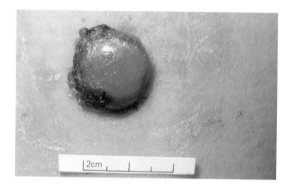

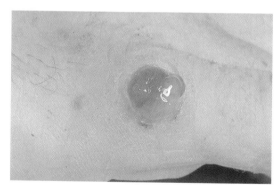

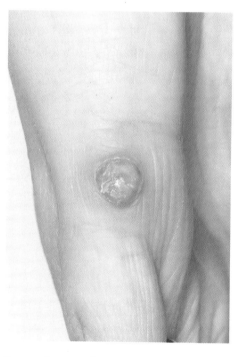

Pyogenic granuloma

Pyogenic granuloma

[86] This is neither pyogenic nor a granuloma. An overgrowth of granulation tissue, it is technically a rapidly growing capillary haemangioma. They may not always be secondary to trauma. They are treated by excision with diathermy of the base.

[87] Or slightly tender.

[88] Most common on those parts of the body likely to be injured such as the hands and face. They are also seen on the lips and gums of pregnant women.

[89] These include squamous cell carcinoma, non-pigmented melanoma and Kaposi's sarcoma. These can be excluded by excisional biopsy.

HISTIOCYTOMA/DERMATOFIBROMA[90]

Examination of a lump (see pg 29).

'There is (in this young/middle-aged woman[91]) a non-tender lump on the medial aspect of the lower leg[92]. It is 2 cm in diameter, hemispherical with a smooth surface and distinct edges. It feels firm and woody, and is not fluctuant, pulsatile, compressible or reducible. It is arising from the skin and moves with the skin, separate from and freely mobile over the deep structures. The overlying skin is loose, slightly crinkled and inseparable from the lump. It is brown in colour[93]. The surrounding skin is normal and the local lymph nodes are not enlarged. This is a histiocytoma also known as a dermatofibroma.'

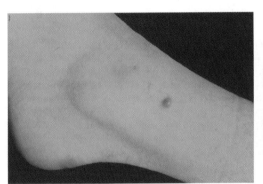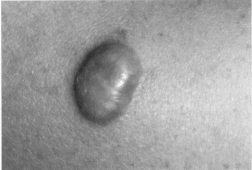

Histiocytoma

Histiocytoma/Dermatofibroma
Common case: seen by over 1 in 20 of the candidates surveyed.
[90] **Synonyms**: fibrous histiocytoma, sclerosing haemangioma, fibroma durum, sclerosing angioma
Definition: benign neoplasm of the fibroblasts of the dermis. The overlying epidermis is normal. Histologically some are cellular (histiocytes), some are fibrous (fibroblasts and collagen), some are angiomatous. Likely to come from dermal fibroblasts.
Treatment: do not resolve spontaneously. Treated by excision.
[91] Can occur in any adult but is more common in young and middle-aged women.
[92] They can occur anywhere but are more common on the limbs.
[93] Histiocytomas are covered in normal epidermis but can become pigmented to a brown colour due to haemosiderin deposition. May also be pink.

Dermoid congenital and implantation cysts

[94] A dermoid cyst is a cyst, deep to the skin, which is lined by skin. Skin can become trapped in the subcutaneous tissues either during fetal development (**congenital dermoid cyst**) or following an injury which forces skin into the deeper tissues (**acquired/implantation dermoid cyst**).

Congenital dermoid cyst

Definition: congenital subcutaneous cysts caused by developmental inclusion of epidermis along lines of fusion.

Histology: cysts lined by stratified squamous epithelium but unlike the epidermal (sebaceous) cyst the wall also contains functioning epidermal appendages such as hair follicles, sweat and sebaceous glands.

Sites: occur at sites of fusion of skin dermatomes, typically the lateral and medial ends of the eyebrow (external and internal angular dermoid) the midline of the nose (nasal dermoid), sublingually, the midline of the neck and at any point in the midline of the trunk, typically the perineum and sacrum.

Complications: may create a bony depression and penetrate down to the dura. Meningeal penetration is only a problem with midline dermoids along the cranio spinal axis but does not occur with internal/external angular dermoids. A nasal dermoid may look like a small superficial pit but may be an extensive cyst that passes between the nasal bones towards the sphenoid sinus.

Treatment: rarely troublesome and rarely get infected so can be left alone. Not to be excised by an SHO on the locals list! Needs experienced surgeon in case of deep extension. May need CT scan and skull X-ray preoperatively.

Acquired/implantation dermoid cyst: a cyst formed after the survival of a piece of skin forcibly implanted into the subcutaneous tissues by an injury such as a small deep cut or stab injury. The patient may not remember the injury. The histology is similar to the congenital dermoid.

Sites: occur in areas subject to repeated trauma (such as fingers) so tend to be troublesome, interfere with function, and can become painful and tender.

Management: excision. It is commonly confused with a sebaceous cyst, but the presence of a scar and history of an old injury is helpful in differentiating them. Dermoid cysts, unlike sebaceous cysts, rarely become infected.

[95] May transilluminate but more commonly will not as it is filled with thick, opaque mixture of sebum, sweat and desquamated epithelial cells.

[96] Unlike sebaceous cysts (arising from the skin) and implantation dermoid cysts (tethered to skin).

CONGENITAL DERMOID CYSTS[94]

Examination of a lump (see pg 29).

'There is a non-tender lump at the outer aspect of the left eyebrow. It is about 2 cm in diameter, ovoid in shape with a smooth surface and well-defined edges. It is soft and fluctuant but does not transilluminate[95]. It is dull to percussion, is not pulsatile, compressible or reducible. It arises in the subcutaneous tissues and is not attached to the skin[96] but appears to be fixed to the deeper structures. The overlying and surrounding skin and regional lymph nodes are normal. This is a congenital dermoid cyst.'

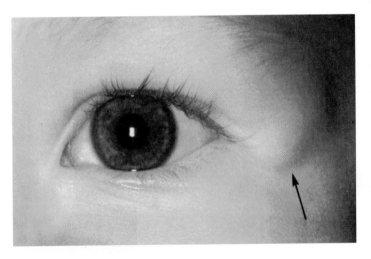

Congenital dermoid cyst at the angle of the eye

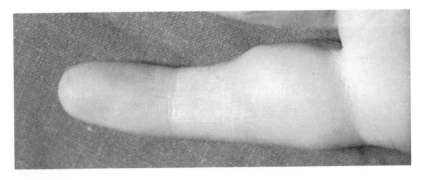

Implantation dermoid cyst which appeared two years after a small stab wound at the base of the finger

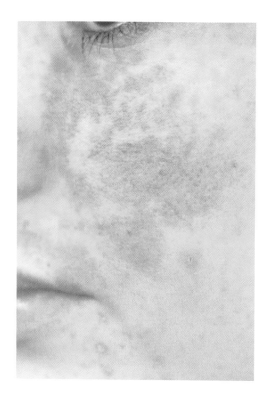 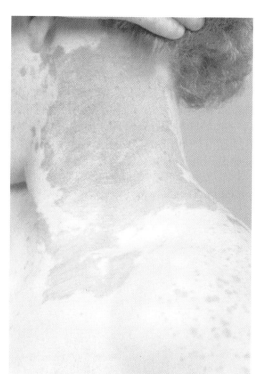

Port wine stain

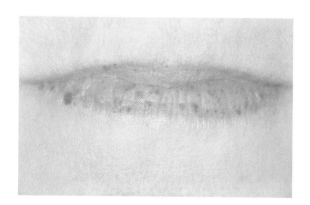

Telangiectasia

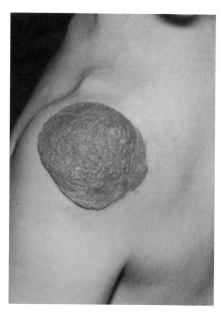

Large strawberry naevus on shoulder

HAEMANGIOMA[97]

Examination of a lump (see pg 29).

'There is (in this young child) a non-tender lump on the right side of the forehead. It dark red in colour, 2 cm in diameter, hemispherical and protuberant with well-defined edges and a smooth, pitted surface giving it a strawberry-like appearance. It is soft and compressible; gentle pressure empties the lump leaving it colourless and collapsed. It is not pulsatile. It arises from the skin and moves with it freely over the underlying structures. The surrounding skin is normal and the regional lymph nodes are not enlarged. This is a congenital intradermal haemangioma, or strawberry naevus.'

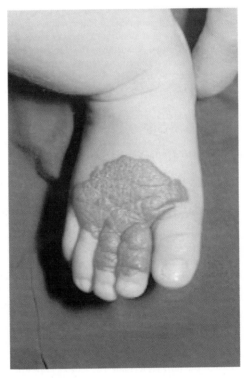

Strawberry naevus

Haemangioma

[97] **Definition**: haemangiomata are hamartomas – an overgrowth of a cell type normally found in that organ. A haemangioma (or vascular naevus) is an abnormal proliferation of the embryonic vascular network. Most display arterial, venous and lymphatic elements. Angiogenic and hormonal factors may be responsible. They are more common in females. They occur in 1–2.6% of new-borns 20% of whom have more than one lesion. All types may ulcerate and induce hyperkeratosis in the overlying stratum corneum. They hardly ever undergo malignant change.

Types of haemangioma

1. Strawberry naevus (congenital intradermal haemangioma or cavernous haemangioma): A bright red, lobulated lesion that stands proud of the skin and does, indeed, look like a strawberry. Formed by a network of capillaries radiating from an artery. Present at a few weeks of age, they often regress spontaneously within months or years. It is not associated with any other congenital vascular malformation apart from other haemangiomata.

2. Port wine stain (*also known as* naevus vingus, intradermal haemangioma): A congenital extensive collection of dilated venules and capillaries just below the epidermis, it is similar in histology to the strawberry naevus but does not stick out from the surface of the skin. It also does not tend to regress as the baby grows, but may fade in colour. They are common on the face and the junction between the limbs and the trunk and are very noticeable and disfiguring due to their deep purple-red colour. Occasionally, small vessels within the stain become prominent and bleed. It may present as part of a more extensive vascular abnormality. Sturge-Weber syndrome is a port wine stain in the distribution of the first and/or second division of the trigeminal nerve associated with ipsilateral intracranial haemangiomata and a history of epilepsy and/or mental retardation. In general, however, there are never any associated neurological abnormalities and the main symptom is deformity.

3. Vin rose patch (salmon patch, naevus flammeus neonatarum): another congenital intradermal haemangioma in which mild dilatation of the subpapillary dermal plexus gives the skin a pale pink colour. It is often associated with other vascular abnormalities such as extensive haemangiomata, giant limbs due to arteriovenous fistulae and lymphoedema. The vin rose patch can occur anywhere and causes no symptoms. Unlike the port wine stain it is not dark enough to be disfiguring and has often been accepted by the patient as a birthmark and forgotten about.

4. Spider naevus: a solitary dilated skin arteriole feeding a number of small branches that leave it in a radial manner. It is an acquired condition and is often associated with liver disease. In general > 5 are pathological.

5. Telangiectasis: a dilation of normal capillaries. Tend to arise after irradiation. Occurs on internal mucosal surfaces as well as the skin, and can lead to gastrointestinal haemorrhage, epistaxis, haematuria and intracerebral bleed.

6. Hereditary haemorrhagic telangiectasia (Osler-Weber-Rendu syndrome): a Mendelian dominant genetic condition with incomplete penetrance affecting 1–2/100,000. Tiny capillary haemangiomas scattered over mucus membranes and skin gives rise to bleeding (haematemesis, melaena, haematuria) and iron deficiency anaemia. The patient has telangiectasia on the face, around the mouth, on the lips and on the tongue, the fingers and the buccal and nasal mucosa. In some variants pulmonary arteriovenous aneurysms are common and increase in frequency with age (as do the telangiectases). Telangiectasia of the face also occurs in the **CREST** syndrome of **C**alcinosis, **R**aynaud's **S**yndrome, o**E**sophagitis, **S**clerodactyly and **T**elangiectasia.

7. Campbell De Morgan spot: very common, well-defined, uniformly brilliantly red capillary naevus 2–3 mm in diameter. Develops on the trunk in middle age. No clinical significance

Treatment of haemangiomata Apart from the strawberry naevus and the port wine stain, patients with the haemangiomata described above do not often seek treatment. Reassurance and waiting natural regression is the best line of management initially for the **strawberry naevus**, as premature treatment may lead to scarring which natural regression will not. Large, ulcerating or persistent lesions may need treatment that is difficult and controversial. Cryotherapy, laser photocoagulation, radiotherapy, sclerosants, electrolysis, steroids and excision with reconstruction have all been used. The **port wine stain** may fade but does not tend to regress, and many of the above methods have been used, with laser therapy currently the treatment of choice for most specialists. It is usually combined with conservative methods such as camouflage creams.

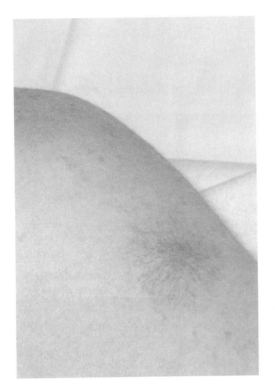

Spider naevus

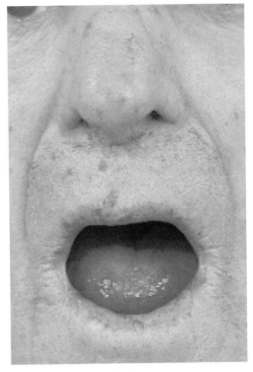

Osler-Weber-Rendu syndrome

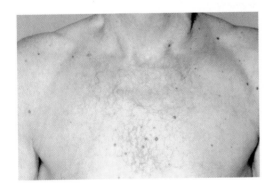

Campbell de Morgan spots

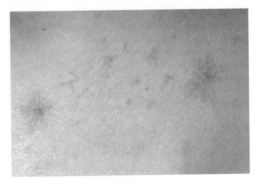

Spider naevi

Benign papilloma/skin tag

[98] **Definition**: simple overgrowth of all layers of the skin. It is not a benign neoplasm (it is a skin tag). Can occur at any age but is more frequent with advancing age. Also known as fibroepithelial papilloma, soft fibroma.

Complications: can catch on clothes. May become injured, red, swollen, ulcerated or infarct. Spontaneous ulceration is rare. The skin that forms a papilloma contains sweat glands, hair follicles and sebaceous glands all of which can become infected and make papillomata swollen and tender. If the granulation tissue that forms in response to the infection becomes exuberant, the swelling can look like a carcinoma.

Treatment is simple excision with a pair of sharp scissors under a local anaesthetic. Occasionally a single suture is needed to control bleeding from the feeding vessel.

[99] Can be single.

[100] Can be pigmented.

[101] They can be sessile.

Other benign skin lesions

<u>Seborrhoeic keratosis</u> (*also known as* senile wart, seborrhoeic wart, verruca senilis, basal cell papilloma) is a benign overgrowth of the basal layer of the epidermis containing an excess of small, dark staining basal cells. They occur in both sexes and are more common in the elderly (almost ubiquitous in over-70's). They become more prominent and are often multiple if the skin is not regularly and firmly washed (hence they are common in inaccessible areas such as the back of elderly patients). Colour varies from normal skin colour to grey or brown. Appear as raised plates of hypertrophic greasy skin with a distinct edge and a rough, papilliferous surface. Distinguishing feature is that it can be picked or scraped off leaving a pale pink patch of skin that may bleed slightly. No other skin lesion behaves like this. Generally do not need treatment but if they catch on clothes or become a nuisance they are easily scraped off. If infected they can look like a pyogenic granuloma, epithelioma or malignant melanoma.

<u>Warts</u> are patches of hyperkeratotic overgrown skin whose growth has been stimulated by the presence of a papilloma virus. They are commonest in children and young adults and may be present for months, most typically on the hands or feet (verrucas), but also on the knees, face and arms. They are greyish brown, hemispherical, only a few millimetres in diameter and frequently multiple. They have a rough, hyperkeratotic surface, are hard and non-compressible. Verrucas (plantar warts) look slightly different because they are pushed into the skin, causing a 'punched out' appearance of a pit containing a wart, surrounded by hardened, thickened, tender skin.

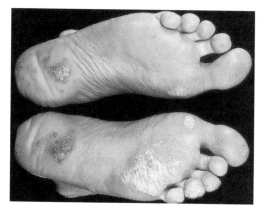

Verrucae (plantar warts)

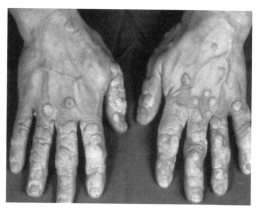

Warts on hand

BENIGN PAPILLOMA/SKIN TAG[98]

Spot diagnosis, or examination of lump (see pg 29).

'There are multiple[99] non-tender discrete skin-coloured[100] tags around the neck and axilla. They are less than 5 mm across, pedunculated[101], papilliferous polyps. They arise from the skin and move with it not invading deeper structures. They are soft, solid, and non-compressible. The surrounding skin and lymph nodes are normal. These are benign papillomata.'

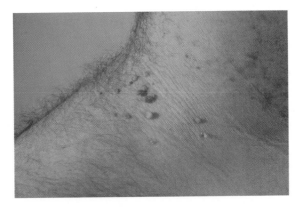

Benign papilloma/skin tags on the neck

Seborrhoeic keratoses on the back

69

Keloid or hypertrophic scars

[102] Keloid and hypertrophic scars are a result of an excessive tissue response during healing.

Hypertrophic scar - excessive fibrous tissue but it is:

<u>Confined to the scar</u> (between the skin edges)

<u>Not progressive</u> (tends not to advance after 6 months and may even regress)

<u>Frequent in children</u> (almost normal up to puberty, most common at the age of 8 and rare after 60 years)

<u>Burns commonly cause hypertrophy</u> (especially on posterior aspects)

Do not recur if excised properly.

Keloid scars - are also an excessive amount of fibrous tissue but:

<u>Extend beyond the original wound</u> into normal tissues

Has characteristics of a <u>local neoplasm</u>

<u>Continue to grow</u> for months, sometimes years after injury

<u>Rare before puberty</u>

May be <u>tender or itchy</u>

<u>Will usually recur</u> despite excision

Risk factors for keloid and hypertrophic scars

<u>Especially keloid</u>: pigmented skin (i.e. black and Asian patients), family history, previous history of keloid scarring.

<u>Especially hypertrophic</u>: burns, infected wounds, wounds under tension or scars in certain sites: e.g. across Langer's lines or over the sternum (high incidence in median sternotomy wounds).

Presentation: cosmetic disfigurement, itching (worse in the early stages) and contractures (if across a joint)

Management

1. <u>Prevention</u>:

Avoid scars across Langer's lines.

Warn of possibility pre-operatively in pigmented skin in high risk areas such as sternum.

Avoid tension.

Avoid infection.

2. <u>Wait</u>: never revise a scar in the first 6 months and advise waiting for two years postoperative in case regression occurs.

3. <u>Conservative</u>:

Pressure dressing immediately (e.g. burns).

Silicone gel sheeting (not proved).

Radiation (beware long-term effects).

Triamcinolone injections (subcutaneous steroid). Re-inspect for telangiectasia and skin thinning. If effective and no side effects, may be repeated 2 weeks after initial treatment. Thought to work by decreasing fibroblast proliferation and increasing collagen lysis.

4. <u>Surgical</u>: excise scar trying to avoid initial risk factors such as infection and tension. Realignment of the scar by 'Z' plasty to lie along tension lines. Can only be carried out if there is sufficient skin laterally to allow a tension free closure. Other techniques include shaving scar, skin grafting and pressure. Surgery should be combined with immediate conservative measures (see above) to prevent recurrence. Keloid scars are far more likely to reform.

Questions to ask patient

When and what was the original operation or injury?

Was there any infection or problems while it was healing?

Have you any other scars like this?

Is it itchy and painful?

Have you had any treatment for the scarring?

[103] If hypertrophic.

[104] If keloid.

KELOID OR HYPERTROPHIC SCARS[102]

Spot diagnosis.

'There is (in this often black or Asian patient) a scar which has had an excessive fibrous tissue response during healing which is confined to within the scar[103]/extending beyond the original margins of the scar[104]. This is a hypertrophic/keloid scar.'

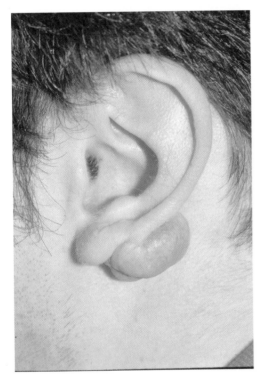

Keloid scar after ear piercing

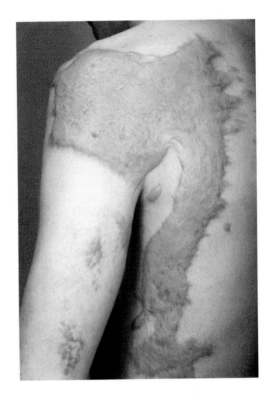

Hypertrophic scar after a burn

Keratoacanthoma

[105] Also known as adenoma sebaceum, molluscum pseudocarcinomatous, molluscum sebaceum.

Definition: a self-limiting overgrowth of hair follicle cells producing a central plug of keratin with subsequent spontaneous regression. Cause unknown – may be self-limiting benign neoplasm or an unusual response to infection.

Epidemiology: occurs in adults. 2–4 weeks to grow, 2–3 months to regress. Normally single lesions. More common in males.

Presentation: usually occurs on the face. The central core is hard and eventually separates. The lump collapses leaving a deep indrawn scar. Often mistaken for squamous cell carcinoma. Unlike a keratoacanthoma, a squamous cell carcinoma grows slower, does not have a dead central core, and gradually becomes an ulcer.

Treatment: should be excised to confirm diagnosis and to prevent depressed scar.

Differential Diagnosis – solar keratosis. A premalignant condition predisposing to squamous cell carcinoma. Usually found on sun-exposed areas especially on the back of hands, face and helix of ears.

[106] Usually found on the face but can occur anywhere where there are sebaceous glands

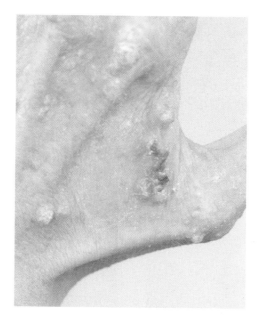

Solar keratosis

KERATOACANTHOMA[105]

Examination of a lump (see pg 29).

'There is a non-tender lump on the right cheek[106]. It is a skin coloured hemispherical nodule, about 2 cm in diameter, with a black sloughy centre. It has well-defined edges, is firm and rubbery but the central core is hard. It is not fluctuant, pulsatile or compressible. The lump arises from the skin and moves freely with it over the underlying structures. The surrounding skin and regional lymph nodes are normal. Clinically this is a keratoacanthoma rather than a squamous cell carcinoma but this should be confirmed by an excision biopsy.'

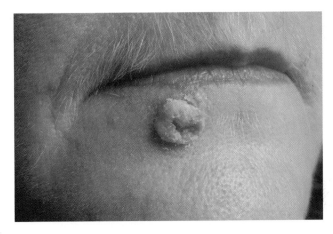

Keratocanthoma

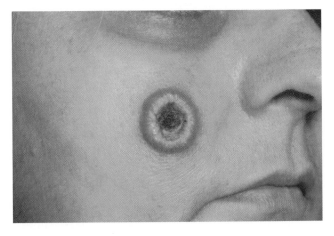

Keratocanthoma on the cheek with necrotic centre mimicking a basal or squamous cell carcinoma

Rhinophyma

[107] **Definition**: thickening of the skin over the tip of the nose caused by hypertrophy and adenomatous changes in its sebaceous glands. Probably a severe degree of acne rosacea. The nasal cartilages and bones are spared.

Aetiology: not associated with alcohol abuse, mostly occurs in old age. Twelve times more common in men than women.

Complications: malignant transformation (into basal or squamous cell carcinomas) has been reported but is extremely rare.

Treatment: surgical planing of the nose as far as the base of the sebaceous glands, trying to avoid full thickness débridement. Methods include scalpel, skin graft knife, laser, electrocautery, cryotherapy.

RHINOPHYMA[107]

Spot diagnosis.

'There is (in this elderly man) a marked overgrowth of the skin and subcutaneous tissues of the nose. This is rhinophyma.'

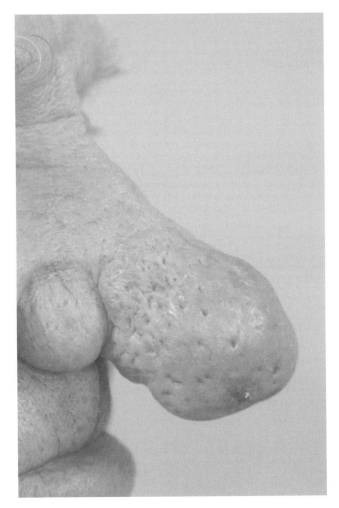

Rhinophyma

Hidradenitis suppurativa

[108] **Hidradenitis suppurativa** is an infection of the apocrine sweat glands seen most often in the axillae and groins of Caucasians living in tropical countries.

Can be associated with an underlying systemic disease such as diabetes. The condition is chronic and recurring. Many are sterile on culture. The severity of the disease varies from a single abscess that responds to incision and drainage to widespread 'watering can' sinuses that necessitate radical excision and skin grafting. Despite often having a negative culture, long-term oral metronidazole is commonly used to control flare-ups, as are vitamin E analogues (retinoids).

Related conditions include:

Acne conglobata: affects back, buttocks and chest

Perifolliculitis capitis: affects the scalp

Hyperhydrosis: (see pg 329 Circulatory System, chapter 4) not an infection but an increase in sweat production from sweat glands usually of the hands, axilla or feet. The majority are idiopathic, but secondary hyperhidrosis includes:

Hyperhydrosis erythematosus traumatica: a rare occupational form of the condition in which sweating occurs in skin in contact with a vibrating tool

Syringomyelia: can cause facial hyperhidrosis

Frey's syndrome: post parotidectomy (see pg 120) where 'gustatory sweating' is caused by disturbance of sympathetic and parasympathetic nerve fibres

Avoid total sympathectomy → postural hypertension

Hidradenoma is a benign tumour of a sweat gland and is rare. They occur from middle age onwards and are frequently multiple and disfiguring (known as a turban tumour). They are soft, non-tender and feel like cysts but do not fluctuate, as they are solid. Malignant change is rare.

[109] Although there may be due to infection.

[110] Especially if there are enlarged lymph nodes, as no abnormal lumps in the female axilla should be noted without checking for a primary breast cancer. It is best to mention that you would do the examination, but do not proceed with it unless instructed as it might be thought inappropriate in the examination setting (similarly with the groins).

[111] Commonly also affected.

[112] Such as steroids.

HIDRADENITIS SUPPURATIVA[108]

Examination of a lump (see pg 29). Don't forget to examine the other axilla.

'There are (in this young, obese, female patient) multiple tender swellings in both axillae which show evidence of purulent discharge. The worst of these is on the right and is 2 cm in diameter, red, hot, tender and inflamed. The swellings arise from the skin and move with it over the underlying structures. There is no associated lymphadenopathy[109]. There is evidence of previous surgery in the right axilla where there are two scars. This looks like recurrent hidradenitis suppurativa.

In a full examination I would like to examine the lady's breasts[110] and groins[111]. I would also ask her if she is diabetic or on immunosuppressant medication[112].'

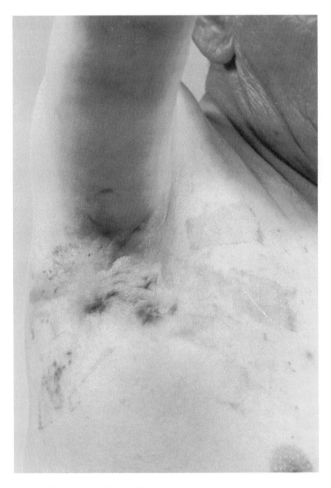

Hidradenitis of the axilla

Diffuse Goitre

Thyroid is a Top Five Case: seen by nearly a third of candidates surveyed. Accounted for 12.9% of the cases in the bay. A Goitre was seen by nearly a fifth of candidates surveyed.

[113] **Definition**: a non-toxic simple goitre diffusely involves the whole gland without producing nodularity and is not associated with hypo or hyperthyroidism. It is a compensatory hypertrophy and hyperplasia secondary to a reduction in T_3 and T_4 output which causes an increase in thyroid releasing hormone and thyroid stimulating hormone which in turn cause thyroid enlargement. It may revert to normal, may stay as a simple goitre or may progress to a multinodular goitre (see Case 2 pg 81) which may be toxic or euthyroid.

Causes of diffuse non-toxic simple goitre

1. Physiological goitre: due to increased demands for thyroid hormone e.g. in pregnancy and puberty.

2. Dietary iodine deficiency: now uncommon but traditionally the cause of goitres in areas far from the sea such as the Alps, Himalayas and Andes, or even closer to home (Derbyshire neck).

3. Dietary goitrous agents: such as uncooked Brassicas (cabbage, turnips), calcium or flouride in drinking water, para-aminosalicylic acid (PAS), lithium, phenylbutazone, thiouracil, carbimazole.

4. Hereditary congenital defects (in thyroid metabolism): very uncommon and do not usually require treatment but may account for familial goitre. Include iodine transport defects, de-iodinase deficiency, iodotyrosine coupling defects and thyroglobulin synthesis defects.

5. Treated Graves' disease: associated with a smooth, mild or moderate sized symmetrical goitre, hypervascularity, a bruit and typical facial signs (see pg 89). If untreated it is associated with hyperthyroidism.

6. Other rare causes of diffuse goitre: lymphoma, anaplastic carcinoma, autoimmune (Hashimoto's) thyroiditis, de Quervain's thyroiditis, thyroid amyloidosis.

Treatment of diffuse non-toxic simple goitre: if small, no treatment needed apart from reassurance and possibly iodine supplements. For cosmetic reasons subtotal thyroidectomy may be required.

GOITRE

Examination of a thyroid lump (see pg 33) and if appropriate, proceed to examination of thyroid status (see pg 35).

Bear in mind the patient could have:
- a diffuse goitre
- a multinodular goitre
- an apparently solitary nodule

Case 1 Diffuse goitre

'There is a smooth, firm, diffusely and symmetrically enlarged thyroid gland. It is non-tender, moves on swallowing and there is no evidence of retrosternal extension or bruit. The patient is clinically euthyroid and there is no evidence of Graves' disease or enlarged regional lymph nodes. This is a diffuse goitre[113].'

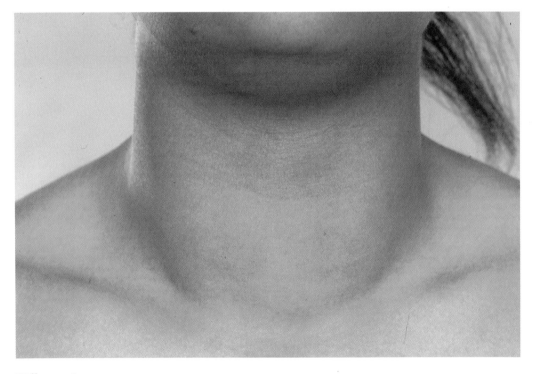

Diffuse goitre

Multinodular Goitre

[114] **Definition: a non-toxic multinodular goitre** occurs when a diffuse simple goitre progresses to a larger (up to 2kg) goitre with multinodular focal hyperplasia. The majority are euthyroid but some are hyper- or hypothyroid.

Causes of non-toxic multinodular goitre

1. Progressive enlargement of diffuse goitre caused by any of the factors listed above.
2. Sporadic multinodular goitre predominantly affecting middle-aged women.

Complications:

Local symptoms: stridor, SVC obstruction, dysphagia, cosmesis, retrosternal enlargement.

Toxicity (<50%): mild hyperthyroidism in the absence of Graves' disease: Plummer's syndrome.

Malignant change: 5% of untreated multinodular goitres.

Haemorrhage into cyst: can lead to sudden, painful enlargement.

Treatment: thyroxine will often prevent progression (should reduce TSH levels to 0).

Indications for surgery of a multinodular goitre:

- Local symptoms, e.g.: significant or symptomatic retrosternal extension, dysphagia, tracheal deviation or stenosis
- Enlarging dominant nodule (unless unequivocally benign)
- Recurrent laryngeal nerve palsy
- Cosmesis
- Hyperthyroidism

Surgery should be total thyroidectomy although some surgeons do a subtotal. Subtotal leads to the risk of recurrence and technically difficult further surgery.

Case 2 Multinodular goitre

'The thyroid gland is nodular and asymmetrically enlarged, the right lobe more so than the left. It is non-tender, moves on swallowing and there is no evidence of retrosternal extension or bruit. The patient is clinically euthyroid and there is no evidence of Graves' disease or enlarged regional lymph nodes. This is a multinodular goitre[114].'

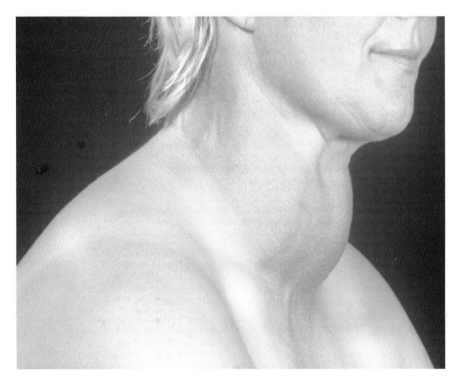

Multinodular goitre

Thyroid Nodule

[115] Only tracheal sarcomas and abnormal lymph nodes adherent to the thyroid can be mistaken for thyroid lumps, and these are both uncommon. Parathyroid adenomas are almost invariably impalpable.

[116] **Differential diagnosis of a thyroid nodule**:

5% of the adult population can be found to have a thyroid nodule.

In 50% this is a LARGE NODULE IN A MULTINODULAR GOITRE

In 50% this is a TRUE SOLITARY NODULE

Of the true solitary nodules 80% are ADENOMAS

10% are cancer (mostly papillary)

10% are cysts, fibrosis or thyroiditis.

Investigations: the two most sensible and universal investigations to say in an examination situation are **thyroid function tests (including autoantibodies)** and an **ultrasound scan** (to see if the lump is a prominent nodule in a multinodular goitre, a solitary nodule or a cyst). **FNA** is controversial, as it can miss follicular carcinoma, but should be requested if malignancy is suspected in a lump that would not otherwise need surgery. All true solitary nodules must either be excised or definitively shown to be benign by FNA aspiration. **Core biopsies** should be taken only from large or inoperable thyroid masses because they risk haemorrhage and damage to surrounding structures, even when performed under ultrasound control. A **Technetium isotope scan** is indicated if TSH is decreased to assess if there is a solitary hot nodule. **CT or MRI** are indicated if potential technical difficulty is suspected in surgery (e.g. large retrosternal element).

Management of a true solitary thyroid nodule: ask the following 2 questions:

1. **Hot** (i.e. functioning) **or cold** (i.e. solid or partly cystic non-functioning nodule)?

Hot: almost invariably benign – can be observed. Treat if patient becomes hyperthyroid.

Cold: may be neoplastic. Tissue diagnosis essential either by excision or FNA (see below).

2. **Needs removal clinically**? (e.g. pressure symptoms, cosmesis, patient wishes, suspicious of malignancy)

Yes: total lobectomy or subtotal thyroidectomy (if centrally placed or isthmic nodule). Never subtotal lobectomy for a true solitary nodule.

If frozen section histology during surgery confirms malignancy the surgeon should proceed to total thyroidectomy and adjuvant treatment. The exception is papillary carcinoma confined to the thyroid in which case total hemithyroidectomy plus isthmectomy is an acceptable minimum if the other lobe is palpably normal.

No: FNA needed (if definitely benign no further treatment needed). If definitely malignant proceed with surgery as above. If follicular (?benign ?malignant) total hemithyroidectomy and await result of paraffin section histology.

Thyroid cancers

70% papillary adenocarcinoma - seen in younger patients often with a history of irradiation to the neck. Most are TSH dependent, some are multifocal. Treatment is total thyroidectomy with thyroxine or unilateral lobectomy with thyroxine. 10 year survival 90%.

20% follicular carcinoma – unifocal treated by total thyroidectomy. FNA results unreliable. 10 year survival 85%.

5% medullary carcinoma – tumour of calcitonin secreting 'C' cells. Familial tendency can be part of the MEN (Multiple Endocrine Neoplasia) syndrome. Can be multifocal. Treatment total thyroidectomy.

<5% anaplastic carcinoma – seen in older patients. Worst prognosis. Treatment debulking surgery and external beam radiotherapy. Poor five year survival.

Case 3 Thyroid Nodule

Examination of a thyroid (see pg 33) followed by examination of thyroid status (see pg 35) if appropriate.

'There is a non-tender lump in the anterior triangle of the neck. It is about 2 cm in diameter, hemispherical, smooth with diffuse edges. It is firm, not fluctuant, pulsatile or compressible or reducible. It arises deep to the skin that moves over it, but moves on swallowing with the thyroid gland from which it is most likely to arise[115]. The overlying and surrounding skin and draining lymph nodes are normal. The patient is euthyroid. My diagnosis is a solitary thyroid nodule, or a prominent single nodule in a multinodular goitre[116].'

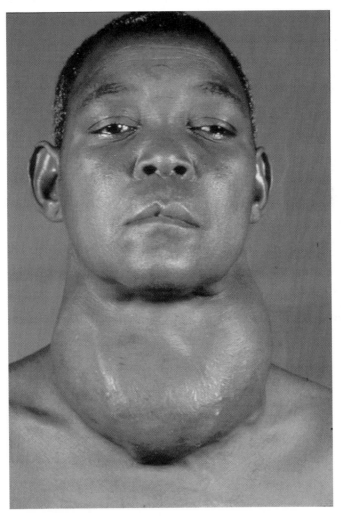

Malignant goitre

Thyroid Surgery

Preoperative assessment and preparation

<u>Thyroid status</u>: TFTs (T3,T4,TSH), thyroid auto-antibodies. Must treat/reduce thyroid activity pre-op. with carbimazole and beta blockers because operating on thyrotoxic patients can precipitate a thyroid crisis.

<u>Vocal cord check</u>: by ENT surgeon to ensure no pre-existing damage is present.

<u>For anaesthetist</u>: ECG, c/spine X-ray (due to neck extension needed on table), thoracic inlet X-ray, chest X-ray (to check for tracheal deviation).

<u>Frozen section</u>: if histology alters operation e.g. follicular carcinoma.

Consent should include

<u>Nerve damage</u>: recurrent laryngeal -> hoarseness. May need Teflon injections.

external laryngeal -> weak voice, only a problem for singers.

<u>Postoperative oral thyroxine</u> for life if total thyroidectomy (and a risk in subtotal).

<u>Others</u>: bleeding, thyroid crisis, recurrent thyrotoxicosis, hypocalcaemia, scar, abandoning tumour if inoperable

Positioning: supine, head up, head-ring, prep. from lower lip to nipples.

Incision: transverse 2 cm above suprasternal notch in existing skin crease beyond medial border of sternocleidomastoid.

Procedure

1. Elevate upper flap (with platysma) as far as upper thyroid cartilage and lower flap as far as the sternal notch.

2. Vertical midline incision between strap muscles through pretracheal fascia. Mobilise thyroid identifying important structures:

3. Superior thyroid artery and vein (transfix and ligate as the upper pedicle NEAR TO THE GLAND avoiding external laryngeal nerve).

4. Recurrent laryngeal nerve must be identified in the tracheo-oesophageal groove (more laterally on the right).

5. Middle thyroid vein ligated and divided entering internal jugular.

6. Inferior thyroid artery – beware as it crosses the recurrent laryngeal nerve just over the parathyroids – ligate the artery in continuity laterally FAR FROM THE GLAND to avoid nerve damage.

7. Ligate lower thyroid vein to free lower pedicle.

For subtotal thyroidectomy: mobilise other lobe and isthmus, cut through thyroid leaving lateral sliver in front of parathyroids and recurrent laryngeal nerve. Suture thyroid remnants to trachea.

For total lobectomy: identify and preserve recurrent laryngeal and parathyroids and dissect the thyroid free from these structures. Dissect isthmus from trachea and divide while oversewing and suturing cut end of isthmus to the trachea.

Closure: suction drains, approximate strap muscles, close skin with Michelle clips.

Postoperative: nurse semi-sitting for 24 hours to decrease venous pressure. Beware expanding haematoma. Check serum calcium daily for 2 days. Drains out after 24 hours. Alternate clips out day 3 final clips out day 4.

Complications of thyroid surgery:

Bleeding from	Torn middle thyroid vein
	Dissection in wrong plane
	Slipped tie on superior pedicle (always doubly ligate)
Nerve injury	Recurrent laryngeal ->hoarseness
	External laryngeal -> weak voice
Retrosternal goitre	Rarely needs sternotomy
Anaplastic tumour	Biopsy, decompress and close
Hypocalcaemia	+/- tetany / carpopedal spasm
Recurrent thyrotoxicosis	Radioactive iodine or medical treatment may be sufficient
Hypothyroidism	Needs thyroxine for life

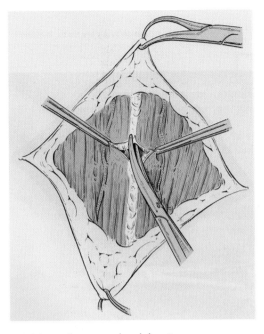

Division of pre-tracheal fascia

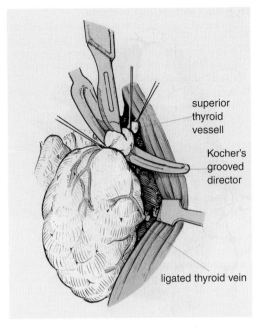

Transfix and ligate superior thyroid artery
and vein as upper pedicle

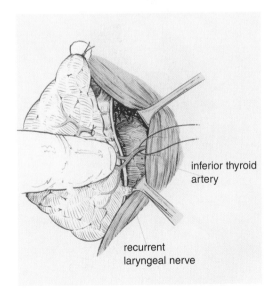

Ligating thyroid artery away from recurrent
laryngeal nerve

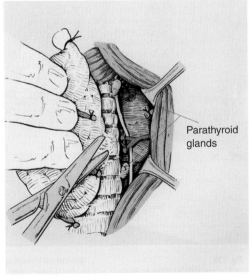

Total lobectomy

Hypothyroidism/myxoedema

[117] Thickened coarse facial features, periorbital puffiness and pallor.

[118] A Hashimoto's goitre is symmetrical, firm and finely micronodular.

[119] Evidence of previous Graves' disease suggests previous surgery (scar often difficult to see) or radioactive iodine treatment which has resulted in hypothyroidism.

[120] **Causes of hypothyroidism**

1. Iatrogenic (90%) due to previous total or subtotal thyroidectomy, radioactive iodine treatment for hyperthyroidism or exogenous irradiation for nearby neoplasm (e.g. lymphoma). No goitre but may have scar from surgery or signs of previous Graves' disease.

2. Primary idiopathic myxoedema usually autoimmune associated with other autoimmune diseases such as pernicious anaemia. TSH blocking autoantibodies so serum TSH is high but T4 is low. More common in women. No goitre.

3. Hashimoto's disease autoimmune disease – cytotoxic Tc cells and antibody action on follicular cells. Firm symmetrical enlarged goitre.

Associated autoimmune diseases:

Pernicious anaemia, Addison's disease, rheumatoid arthritis, Sjögren's syndrome, ulcerative colitis, lupoid hepatitis, systemic lupus erythematosus, haemolytic anaemia, diabetes mellitus, Graves' disease, hypoparathyroidism.

Treatment of hypothyroidism

Oral thyroxine for life.

[121] See pg 36 examination of thyroid status for list of questions.

[122] Should be slow relaxing (see pg 36 examination of thyroid status).

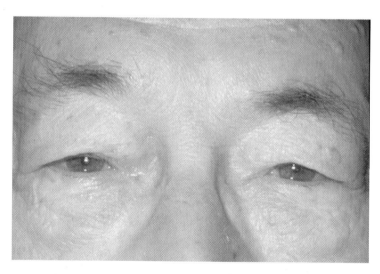

Myxoedematous eyes

HYPOTHYROIDISM/MYXOEDEMA

Examination of thyroid status (see pg 35).

'On initial inspection the patient (who is a middle-aged lady) is overweight with myxoedematous facies[117]. The hands are dry, cool and pale with rough, inelastic skin and non-pitting puffiness. She has/denies symptoms of carpal tunnel syndrome. She is/is not bradycardic. On inspection of the face there is thinning, dry brittle hair, loss of the outer third of the eyebrows and a yellowish complexion. There is/is no evidence of a goitre[118] or any evidence of previous Graves' disease such as exophthalmos[119]. The diagnosis is myxoedema[120]. I would like to ask her some questions[121] and check her reflexes[122].'

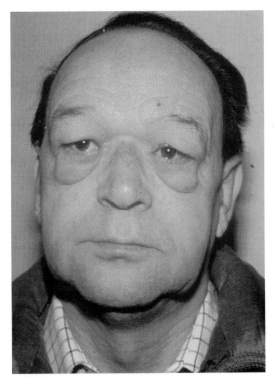

Myxoedemous facies

Thyrotoxicosis and Graves' disease

[123] **Causes of hyperthyroidism** (5% of all women).

1. Graves' disease (an autoimmune disease caused by stimulation of TSH receptors by autoantibodies which also cross-react with eye muscle and skin antigens. Commoner in women and associated with other autoimmune diseases such as diabetes and pernicious anaemia. The hyperthyroidism can be corrected in the usual way but the eye signs usually persist.)

2. Toxic multinodular goitre (multinodular focal hyperplasia. Less than half are thyrotoxic. Usually moderate thyrotoxicosis.

3. Toxic solitary adenomas (benign, solitary, discrete encapsulated nodules. Usually non-functioning but can cause mild hyperthyroidism.)

The above three disorders account for 99% of cases. Rarer causes of hyperthyroidism includes thyroiditis, carcinoma, choriocarcinoma, hydatidiform mole, teratomas, pituitary adenoma (TSH secreting), neonatal thyrotoxicosis (associated with maternal Grave's), iatrogenic (iodide or thyroxine induced).

Treatment of hyperthyroidism

Antithyroid drugs such as carbimazole

Surgery: for malignancy, pressure or cosmesis. 10% become hypothyroid, 5% have recurrent hyperthyroidism.

Radioactive iodine: almost always results in hypothyroidism.

[124] Thyroid acropachy resembles finger clubbing. New bone formation appears on X-ray as 'soap bubbles' on the bone surface with coarse spicules. Sometimes the new bone formation in acropachy is both visible and palpable along the phalanges.

[125] In the case of a toxic multinodular goitre.

[126] In the case of a toxic solitary adenoma/nodule (rarer).

[127] Graves' exophthalmos is due to cross reaction of autoimmune anti-thyroid antibodies with intra-orbital muscles. The proptosis (bulging eyes or exophthalmos) is due to increased retro-orbital fat and enlarged intra-orbital muscles infiltrated with lymphocytes and containing increased water and mucopolysaccharide. It may develop in the absence of hyperthyroidism and remit, persist or develop further despite successful treatment of hyperthyroidism. Complications of exophthalmos includes chemosis, ophthalmoplegia and diplopia.

[128] Pretibial myxoedema tends to develop after the hyperthyroidism has been treated especially with radioactive iodine.

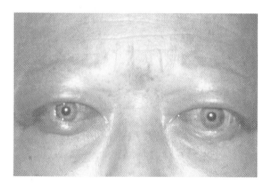

Periorbital swelling and chemosis in Graves' disease

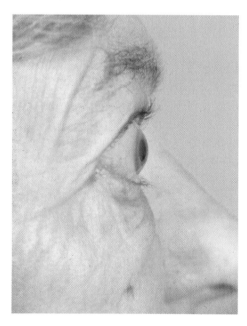

Exophthalmos and lid retraction in Graves' disease

THYROTOXICOSIS AND GRAVES' DISEASE[123]

Carry out examination of thyroid status (see pg 35).
Bear in mind the patient could be:

* thyrotoxic without Graves' disease
* thyrotoxic with Graves' disease
* euthyroid (due to surgery or treatment) with residual signs of Graves' disease
* hypothyroid (due to surgery or treatment) with residual signs of Graves' disease

Case 1

'On initial inspection this (middle-aged female) patient is thin, restless with a visible tremor. The hands are warm, sweaty with thyroid acropachy[124] and there is an irregular pulse. There is no exophthalmos, lid retraction or signs of corneal irritation. The lid lag test is positive. There is[125]/is no[126] sign of a goitre or a scar in the neck. This patient appears thyrotoxic but has no sign of Graves' disease. The presence of a goitre suggests toxic multinodular goitre/the absence of a goitre suggests a solitary toxic adenoma/the evidence of previous thyroid surgery suggests recurrent toxic multinodular goitre.'

Case 2

As for Case 1 but with the features of Graves' disease including exophthalmos[127], pretibial myxoedema[128], and a small diffuse goitre with a bruit. 'This patient is thyrotoxic with Graves' disease.'

Case 3

The features of Graves' disease (exophthalmos, pretibial myxoedema +/- goitre or scar of thyroid surgery) in a clinically euthyroid patient. 'This patient has Graves' disease and is clinically euthyroid/hypothyroid. It is likely that she has had hyperthyroidism treated in the past either by thyroidectomy or radioactive iodine (look for scar).'

Thyroglossal cyst

Very common case: seen by over 1 in 10 of candidates surveyed.

[129] **Definition**: a portion of the thyroglossal duct which remains patent

Embryology: the **thyroglossal duct/tract** is the (normally obliterated) remnant that marks the developmental descent of the thyroid gland. The thyroid appears as a midline diverticulum at the fourth week of gestation and descends ventrally from what will become the foramen caecum of the posterior third of the tongue down between the second branchial arches (see diagram showing descent of thyroid during development). The **thyroglossal cyst** is a dilatation along the thyroglossal duct, the rest of which may or may not be obliterated.

Histology: lined with stratified squamous epithelium or ciliated pseudostratified epithelium. May have thyroid or lymphoid tissue in the wall (site of ectopic thyroid which may develop a malignancy – usually papillary carcinoma).

History: they can appear at any age but generally between 15 and 30, more often in women. They are usually a painless lump, but can become painful, tender and enlarged if infected. They are removed for cosmetic reasons, discomfort or the risk of infection.

Differential diagnoses: congenital dermoid cyst, sebaceous cyst, enlarged lymph node, subhyoid bursa, pyramidal lobe of thyroid, thyroid nodule.

Complications: infection, thyroglossal sinus (see below), malignancy (papillary thyroid cancer)

Treatment: surgical excision. Preoperative assessment: ultrasound to confirm diagnosis and define a patent thyroglossal duct passing superiorly. Confirm normal thyroid function preoperatively.

Surgical procedure: transverse incision over cyst, dissect cyst out, look for downward tract (rare) and excise it, then follow main tract upwards to hyoid bone. Excise middle third of hyoid bone and excise rest of duct to its apex in continuity. Beware damage to thyrohyoid membrane and entering mouth via mucosa of foramen caecum (risk of infection, must close defect with absorbable sutures). Post-op. complications: haematoma, infection, recurrence.

[130] They can in fact lie anywhere from the chin (suprahyoid) and the second tracheal ring (pretracheal). The cyst can slip to one or other side of the midline, especially if it develops in front of the thyroid cartilage.

[131] Varies from 0.5 to 5 cm in diameter.

[132] Some cysts are too tense or too small to fluctuate but most do.

[133] The contents of the cyst are usually opaque because of desquamated epithelial cells, they may do if large.

[134] The thyroglossal duct is always closely related, and usually fixed, to the hyoid bone. When the hyoid bone moves the cyst also moves. The hyoid bone moves when the tongue is protruded. This is occasionally evident on observation (and is part of inspection of the neck examination pg xx which you should have performed on examining this lump) but more commonly can be felt as a tugging sensation during palpation. Ask the patient to open her mouth and keep her lower jaw still. Hold the cyst with your thumb and forefinger. Ask the patient to stick her tongue out. If the cyst is fixed to the hyoid bone you will feel it tugged upwards as the tongue goes out. This sign is absent from many thyroglossal cysts, however, especially those below the level of the thyroid cartilage.

[135] The overlying skin is normal most commonly.

[136] The overlying skin is inflamed if infected.

[137] A thyroglossal **sinus** is an acquired sinus which arises following rupture or surgery for a thyroglossal cyst. Unlike branchial fistulae these are never true fistulae, as they do not connect to the mouth. The physical signs include a sinus opening, usually in the midline, +/- a previous scar, often surrounded by a crescentic skin fold. The cyst may or may not be palpable.

[138] Whenever there is an abnormality of thyroid gland development, examine the base of the tongue for ectopic (lingual) thyroid tissue, which looks like a flattened strawberry sitting on the base of the tongue.

THYROGLOSSAL CYST[129]

Examination of neck lump (see pg 37).

'There is (in this young person) a non-tender lump in the midline of the neck at the level of the thyroid cartilage[130]. It is 2 cm in diameter[131], spherical and smooth with well-defined edges. It is firm but fluctuates[132] and does not transilluminate[133]. It is not pulsatile, compressible or reducible. It is tethered to deep structures, and can be moved sideways but not up and down. It moves on extending the tongue that suggests attachment to the hyoid bone[134].

The overlying skin is normal[135]/inflamed[136]/shows signs of a sinus[137] and the surrounding skin is normal. The regional lymph nodes are not enlarged. The base of the tongue shows no ectopic thyroid tissue[138]. This is a thyroglossal cyst.'

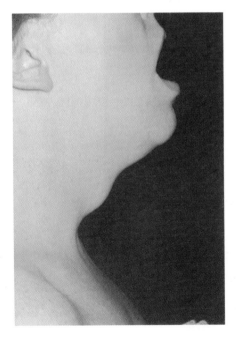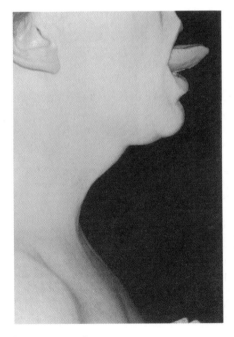

Thyroglossal cyst moving upwards on protruding tongue

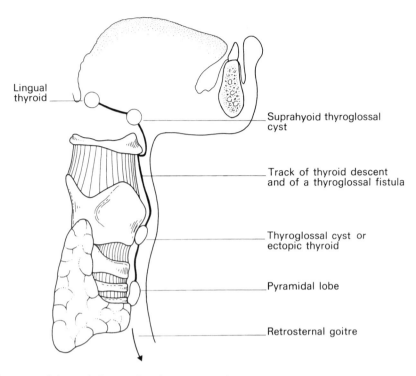

Lingual thyroid

Suprahyoid thyroglossal cyst

Track of thyroid descent and of a thyroglossal fistula

Thyroglossal cyst or ectopic thyroid

Pyramidal lobe

Retrosternal goitre

Path of descent of thyroid during development and sites of abnormalities of thyroglossal tract

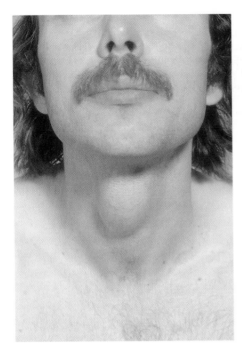
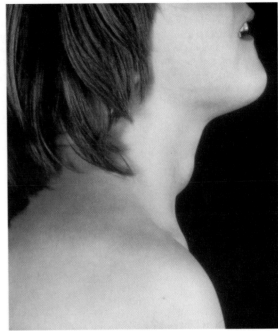

Thyroglossal cyst

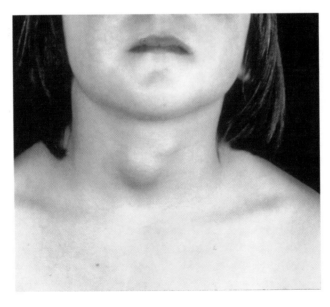

Infected thyroglossal cyst

Lymph node/s in the neck
Common case: seen by over 1 in 20 of the candidates surveyed.

[139] The commonest causes for cervical lymphadenopathy are **metastatic deposits** (in adults), **Hodgkin's and non-Hodgkin's lymphoma** in children and young adults and **tuberculous lymphadenitis** in young immigrant adults. Reactive lymphadenopathy secondary to **infection** (e.g. URTI, tonsillitis, glandular fever, toxoplasmosis) is also common, especially in babies, children and young adults. **Sarcoidosis** is another cause.

[140] **Metastatic deposits** of cancer cells in the cervical lymph nodes are the commonest cause of cervical lymphadenopathy in adults. The possible sites of primary cancer are legion (see below) but are most often in the buccal cavity (tongue, lips and mucus membranes) and larynx.

Sites of primary neoplasms that can metastasise to the cervical lymph nodes:

Head:	Glands:
Scalp	Parotid
Face	Submandibular
Ears	Thyroid gland
Neck	
Nose and nasopharynx	**Arms and trunk:**
Mouth:	Arms
Tongue	Chest wall
Gums	Breast
Mucosa	Lung
Tonsils	
Lips	**Abdomen**
Mandible	**Genitalia**

[141] Lesions above the hyoid tend to drain to the upper deep cervical nodes (see diagram of neck nodes, pg 38). The larynx and thyroid tend to drain to the middle and deep cervical nodes. An enlarged supraclavicular node commonly indicates intra-abdominal or thoracic disease (Virchow's node, Troisier's sign).

[142] In later stages tumour can invade the overlying structures and become tethered to the skin.

[143] Be careful how you say you think it is malignancy in front of the patient. It is insensitive even if you are right, and can be terrifyingly misleading for the patient if you are wrong. Methods of giving such a diagnosis in an examination include: discussing the case out of earshot of the patient (which the examiners may suggest or instigate); using the phrase 'related to a mitotic lesion' (although nowadays using jargon over the patient's head tends to be frowned upon) or saying it is 'important to exclude a malignancy' which has the advantage of sounding professional, not being scary and hedging your bets!

[144] **What you need to do before you can biopsy a lymph node in the neck**

History: most head and neck cancers occur in patients over 50 years. The symptoms depend on the primary e.g. sore ulcer on tongue, hoarse voice, weight loss, cough, dyspepsia, abdominal pain. Most commonly the patients are asymptomatic and present with a painless lump in the neck which has steadily enlarged. Ask if they are smokers.

Examination of the head, scalp, face, ears, neck. Look in the nose. Look in the mouth at the tongue, gums, mucosa and tonsils. Palpate the parotid, submandibular and thyroid glands. Examine the arms and chest wall, especially the breasts. Examine the abdomen and genitalia.

Investigations: full ENT examination under general anaesthetic including air sinuses, oropharynx, nasopharynx and buccal cavity. Chest X-ray (or CT if worrying signs or symptoms).

Principles of management of an enlarged neck node: full history, examination and investigations as above. If primary found, *en bloc* dissection or other appropriate treatment usually advised by relevant specialist. If no primary found, excision biopsy of the lymph node must be performed to confirm benign nature of node. If a biopsy of a lymph node is carried out without a full exclusion of a head and neck tumour, curative *en bloc* resection may be compromised if the node is found to be metastatic.

LYMPH NODE/S IN THE NECK[139]

Examination of a neck lump (see pg 37).

Case 1 Metastatic lymph node/s in the neck[140].

'There are (in this middle-aged/elderly man) a group of non-tender swellings at the anterior border of the sternocleidomastoid on the right side of the neck[141]. The lumps are matted together, and form an irregular shaped mass around five by two centimetres, with the long axis running down with the muscle. Some of the lumps are smooth and discrete, but the main mass is lobulated and craggy with indistinct edges. They are stony hard, not fluctuant, pulsatile, compressible, reducible or transilluminable. They are fixed to deep structures but not to the skin, which moves over the lumps[142]. They can be moved slightly in a transverse direction but not vertically.

This is a group of enlarged lymph nodes and I would want to exclude metastatic disease[143]. Other lymph nodes in the neck (say which) are also enlarged/not enlarged. If I saw this patient in clinic I would like to ask him some questions, examine him for a primary lesion and arrange some urgent investigations[144] which would include a full ENT examination.'

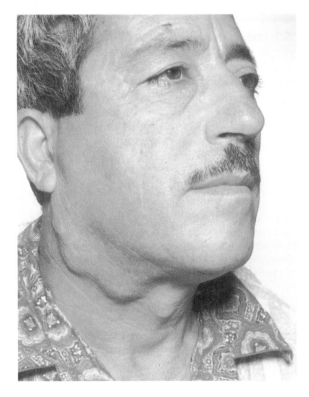

The patient presented with hard enlarged lymph glands in the neck. The primary lesion was the insignificant mole above his right eyebrow.

95

Lymphoma

[145] Lymphoma (Hodgkin's and non-Hodgkin's) is a huge topic worthy of a textbook in itself. If it appears in a surgical examination the main aims will be a thorough examination of the neck (see pg 37), identifying the features of a neck lump caused by a primary neoplasm of the lymph nodes (see this pg) and understanding of the principles of managing any suspected enlarged lymph node in the neck (see pg 95, metastatic lymph node).

[146] Any of the cervical lymph nodes can be affected. Lymphoma is one of the few conditions apart from infection that often causes lymphadenopathy in the posterior triangle.

[147] The nodes can be enlarged to any size.

[148] In Hodgkin's disease the lymph nodes remain separate and distinct even when enlarged unlike tuberculous nodes which quickly become matted together and indistinct.

[149] History: children and young adults, males more than females, will present most commonly with a painless lump in the neck. Associated symptoms include malaise, weight loss, pallor, night sweats, aching bones and pruritus.

[150] If asked 'would you biopsy this lesion?', remember the principles of managing any lump in the neck (see metastatic neck lump pg 95). A primary source of malignancy must be excluded before *en bloc* dissection is compromised by biopsy unless other evidence of lymphoma (e.g. on blood tests, chest X-ray or CT) is found.

Case 2 Lymphoma[145]

Examination of a neck lump (see pg 37).

'There is (in this young adult) a non-tender lump in the posterior triangle of the right side of the neck[146]. It is 3 cm in diameter[147] ovoid, smooth with discrete edges[148]. It is firm and rubbery, not fluctuant, pulsatile, compressible, reducible or transilluminable. It arises deep to the skin and the skin moves easily over it. Although not fixed, (the lump can be moved from side to side) it is tethered to nearby structures. The overlying and surrounding skin is normal. The surrounding lymph nodes are not/are (say which ones) also enlarged. This is an enlarged lymph node. In a patient of this age it would be important to exclude a primary lymphatic malignancy. In the clinical setting I would take a full history[149], perform a general examination looking especially at the liver, spleen, lymphadenopathy in the axillae or groins, and request a full blood count and chest X-ray in the first instance[150].'

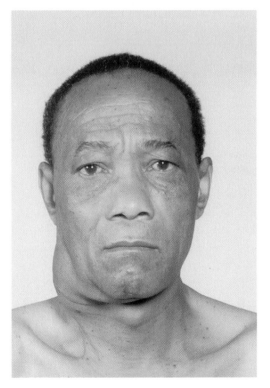 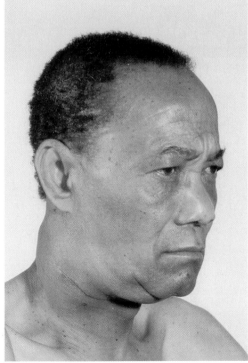

Cervical lymphadenopathy

Tuberculous lymphadenopathy

[151] The upper deep cervical nodes of the neck are the most commonly affected.

TB is less common in Great Britain because most people who have grown up here have been immunised. Immigrants from countries where TB is endemic and immunisation not widespread such as India and Pakistan commonly present in Britain with the disease. There is also a resurgence of TB, often drug resistant, in adults from deprived backgrounds (e.g. tramps, drug addicts) and in the immunocompromised (e.g. HIV patients). **History**: anorexia, weight loss (systemic symptoms unusual in the young), respiratory symptoms, previous history of TB, immunisation, family history, social history.

A typical mycobacterial lymphadenitis usually cervicofacial affecting children. The children it affects are not usually immunocompromised. Treatment is surgical as it responds very poorly to antibiotics.

[152] In the early stages the nodes are firm, discrete and between 1–2 cm in diameter. As caseation increases the nodes necrose, coalesce, become matted and grow larger. The deep cervical chain is usually involved (hence the lumps lie along the line of the sternocleidomastoid muscle) and the mass can become very large, distorting the neck.

[153] A mass of tuberculous lymph nodes may caseate, turn into pus and become a **tuberculous abscess** that, although not typically warm, may make the mass painful, tender and fluctuant, with the overlying skin becoming discoloured. If a tuberculous abscess develops, tachycardia, anorexia, weight loss and fever may be clinical features. A collar-stud abscess is one which has burst through the deep fascia and therefore consists of two collections of pus, one deep and one superficial, the contents of which can be compressed one into the other through a narrow connection.

[154] Once again, the principles of management of an enlarged lymph node in the neck (see pg 94) should be followed, with a biopsy only undertaken if TB is diagnosed by some other means or a primary malignancy which might have metastasised to the cervical glands is excluded. When it is performed, the biopsy or aspirated pus should be sent for a Ziehl-Neelsen stain to microbiology as well as for histology.

Case 3 Tuberculous lymphadenopathy[151]

Carry out examination of neck lump (see pg 37).

'There is (in this patient of any age, perhaps from India or Pakistan) a large lump along the upper half of the anterior border of the right sternocleidomastoid. The whole irregular shaped swelling measures about 7 × 3 cm, with the long axis extending along the line of the sternocleidomastoid muscle[152]. It is an indistinct, firm mass consisting of several discrete, smooth lumps that seem to be matted together in the centre. It is not fluctuant, pulsatile, compressible, reducible or transilluminable. It arises deep to the skin, which moves easily over it, and is tethered to the deep structures. It moves slightly from side to side but not vertically and appears to arise deep to the muscle. The overlying skin is normal[153] and there are no/are (say where) other enlarged lymph nodes nearby. These are enlarged lymph nodes, and I would be keen to exclude tuberculosis[154].'

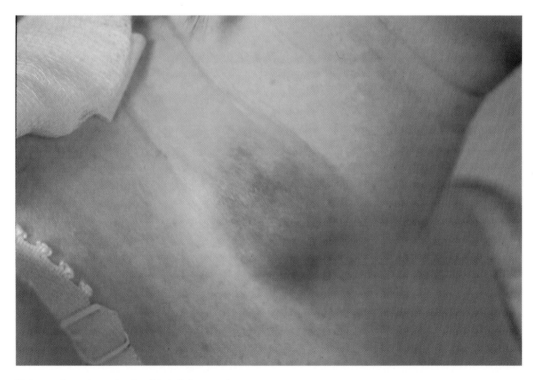

Tuberculous lymphadenitis of the neck

Branchial cyst

[155] **Definition**: a remnant of a branchial cleft – usually the second. Branchial cysts are rare, branchial sinuses are common.

Development: 2nd branchial arch grows down to cover the remaining arches. It leaves a temporary space lined with squamous epithelium. Usually disappears but may persist and distend with cholesterol containing fluid.

History: present at birth but do not distend and cause symptoms until adult life. The majority present between 15 and 25 years but may present in early middle age. It affects males and females equally. It is a painless swelling at the anterior border of the sternocleidomastoid muscle. It may become painful and swollen if it becomes infected.

Histology: lined with squamous epithelium but there are patches of lymphoid tissue in the wall which are connected with the other lymph tissue in the neck and which can become infected. May form an abscess or a sinus.

Complications: infection causes pain and swelling. A **branchial fistula** is a variation of the branchial cyst which occurs if fusion fails to occur distally leading to a persistent sinus which appears as a small dimple in the skin intermittently discharging clear mucus (or pus if infected). This external opening is situated at the junction of the middle and lower third of the sternocleidomastoid, or even lower at the suprasternal notch. If the upper end of the branchial tract is obliterated, this is a **branchial sinus**. If the whole branchial cleft has stayed patent, this is a true branchial fistula, connecting the skin with the oropharynx just behind the tonsil. Swallowing accentuates the openings on the skin.

Treatment: surgical excision. If not excised a branchial sinus or fistula will invariably become infected.

Preoperatively: exclude differential diagnoses (see below), treat an acutely inflamed or infected lesion with antibiotics and electively excise it when it has settled. Incision and drainage may be necessary, but subsequent surgery is made more difficult. Examine carefully for an external opening low in the neck suggesting a branchial sinus or fistula (see below).This may be tiny and is usually along the anterior border of the sternocleidomastoid muscle.

Operative technique and hazards: transverse incision over cyst (or elliptical incision around external opening if a sinus) expose cyst, free from carotid sheath and continue dissection cranially until the upper limit or oropharyngeal opening. Beware the mandibular branch of the facial nerve, hypoglossal nerve, accessory nerve, carotid sheath. Try not to rupture cyst. Complications include recurrence if inadequately excised, wound haematoma and infection, nerve palsies.

Preauricular sinus: Remnant of the first arch most commonly seen as a tiny pit in front of the ear.

[156] Most branchial cysts are between 5–10 cm in diameter.

[157] Most cysts are hard, but a lax cyst feels soft.

[158] This sign is difficult to elicit in the neck, especially if the cyst is small and the sternocleidomastoid muscle is thick.

[159] The contents of the cyst are usually opaque because of desquamated epithelial cells but if large and filled with fat globules and cholesterol crystals secreted by the lining sebaceous glands the cyst may transilluminate.

[160] Which differentiates it from a carotid body tumour (see pg 105) which is also situated slightly lower in the neck than a branchial cyst.

[161] From which it arises (not a sign of malignancy).

[162] Depending on if it was infected or not. If infected it is tender, with red inflamed overlying skin and difficult to differentiate from an abscess of any cause (e.g. infected sebaceous cyst).

[163] Examine carefully for evidence of an external communication which appears as a dimple along the anterior border of the sternocleidomastoid low down in the neck.

[164] If the surrounding lymph glands are enlarged you should reconsider your diagnosis in favour of a tuberculous abscess (see pg 99).

[165] **Differential diagnoses**: malignant cervical lymph node (pg 95 not fluctuant), pharyngeal pouch (pg 103, older patient, different history), carotid body tumour (pg 105 pulsatile, lower in neck), parotid lump (pg 119 branchial remnants can occur here and require parotidectomy for their removal).

Preoperative assessment: CT and/or full ENT assessment may be required.

BRANCHIAL CYST[155]

Examination of neck lump (see pg 37).

'There is (in this young or middle aged patient) a non-tender swelling arising from the anterior edge of the upper third of the right sternocleidomastoid muscle, bulging forward. It is ovoid, with its long axis running forwards and downwards, about 8 cm × 5 cm in size[156]. It has a smooth surface with distinct edges and is hard/soft[157] and fluctuant[158]. It does not transilluminate[159]. It is dull to percussion, is not pulsatile[160], compressible or reducible. The bulk of the mass is deep to the sternocleidomastoid muscle and it is fixed to the deep structures[161]. The overlying skin is normal/red and inflamed[162]. The surrounding skin is normal with no signs of external sinus openings lower in the neck[163] and the draining lymph nodes are not enlarged[164]. This is a branchial cyst, but I would like to order some investigations to exclude my differential diagnoses[165].'

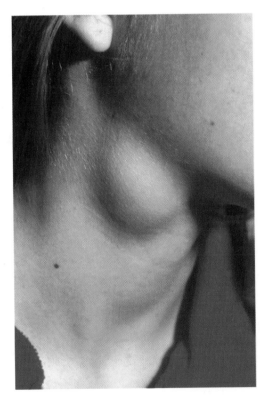

Branchial cyst

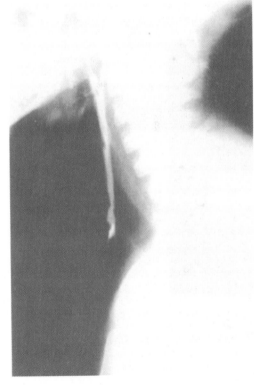

Sinogram showing contrast material that has been injected through an opening on the skin surface. The fact that the contrast fails to empty into the tonsillar fossa suggests that this is a sinus and not a fistula.

Pharyngeal pouch

[166] **Definition**: a pulsion diverticulum of the pharynx through the gap between the lowermost horizontal fibres and the higher oblique fibres of the inferior constrictor muscle.

Cause: unco-ordinated swallowing in which the lower sphincter-like fibres of the inferior constrictor do not relax, the weak unsupported area just above these fibres (Killian's dehiscence) bulges out. Eventually the bulge develops into a sac that hangs down (usually to the left side) and presses against the side of the oesophagus.

History: appears in middle to old age, more commonly in men. Long history of halitosis (bad breath) and recurrent sore throat. Common symptom is regurgitation of food that is undigested and comes up into the mouth at any time (no bile or acid taste). Regurgitation at night causes aspiration; nocturnal choking and coughing may lead to aspiration pneumonia and lung abscesses. It may also cause dysphagia and gurgling sounds and eventually malnutrition and weight loss.

Investigations: barium swallow. Careful endoscopy by experienced endoscopist.

Treatment: surgical excision. Starve for at least 24 hours. Beware inhalation during induction of GA (Mendelsohn's syndrome). NG tube (difficult but advised). Pouch packed with proflavine gauze to make identification easier. Pharynx approached via incision along inferior half of the sternocleidomastoid muscle. Dissect out pouch. Remove proflavine gauze via mouth. Clamp and excise neck of pouch. Concomitant cricopharyngeal myotomy is recommended but may lead to reflux. Send pouch for histology to exclude carcinoma.

Dohlman's procedure is another surgical option: endoscopic resection that consists of simple inversion and oversewing of pouch from inside the pharynx. Suitable in high-risk patients but may miss carcinoma, as pouch is not excised.

Endoscopic stapling is becoming the treatment of choice and is replacing surgical excision.

[167] Most pouches are not palpable below 5 cm and rarely enlarge to be bigger than 10 cm.

[168] A pouch can occasionally be emptied manually by compression (this may cause regurgitation) and the pouch will not recur until the patient eats again (hence compressible but not reducible).

[169] A pharyngeal pouch lies deep to the deep fascia, behind the sternocleidomastoid muscle. On palpation it can be appreciated that it originates from behind the trachea and is fixed deeply (in fact to the pharynx, but this attachment cannot be felt).

[170] Look for aspiration pneumonia, collapse of a lobe or a lung abscess.

[171] The diagnostic investigation of choice.

PHARYNGEAL POUCH[166]

Examination of neck lump (see pg 37).

'There is (in this middle-aged/elderly patient) a non-tender bulge behind the sternocleidomastoid muscle below the level of the thyroid cartilage. The lump is a deep structure with an indistinct shape and edges, but appears to be about 7 cm in diameter[167]. It has a smooth surface and is soft and compressible but not reducible[168]. It is dull to percussion, is not pulsatile and does not fluctuate or transilluminate. It arises from the deep structures in the neck, to which it is firmly attached and cannot be moved freely[169]. The overlying and surrounding skin is normal and the regional lymph nodes are not enlarged. This is a pharyngeal pouch. I would like to see the chest X-ray[170] and barium swallow[171].'

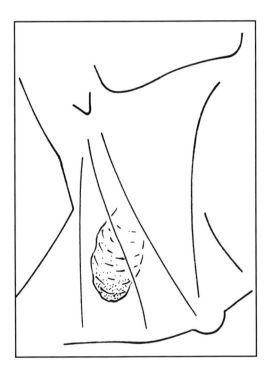

A pharyngeal pouch rarely causes a detectable swelling. If it does, the swelling is behind the sternomastoid muscle.

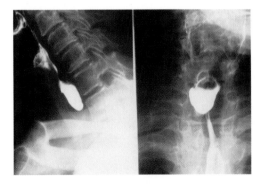

Barium swallow of pharyngeal pouch

Carotid body tumour

[172] A rare tumour of the chemoreceptors of the carotid body (a chemodectoma). It is usually benign but has malignant potential (5–10% of untreated tumours develop metastases within 10 years). It is more common in high altitude areas such as Peru and Mexico.

History: a painless slowly growing pulsatile lump in a patient aged 40–60 years. There may be associated transient ischaemic attacks due to pressure on the carotid artery.

Investigations: carotid arteriography by catheter, needle or intravenous digital subtraction arteriography shows a splayed carotid bifurcation containing a highly vascular tumour and gives information on cerebral circulation and potential collateral's (unlike USS and CT).

Treatment: surgical excision is strongly recommended due to risk of malignant transformation and progressive enlargement making surgery more risky. The procedure may require sacrifice of the external carotid artery and/or bypass, vein grafting or shunting of the internal carotid. Preoperative embolisation may be used in larger tumours. Older patients may decline surgery, as there is a risk of mortality (1–2%), hemiplegia and nerve injury. Radiotherapy may be an alternative for these.

[173] Vary from 2–10 cm diameter.

[174] Often called 'potato tumours.'

[175] Either transmitted pulsation by virtue of close association with the carotid bifurcation, or true expansile pulsatility due to vascularity of the tumour itself.

[176] It may indeed be compressible if it is very vascular but is more often solid.

[177] Due to attachment to the carotid sheath.

[178] In 20% of cases.

[179] A third of familial and 10% of non-familial carotid body tumours are bilateral.

[180] 30% are incorrectly diagnosed on clinical examination. If a tumour is found unexpectedly at operation, further dissection should be abandoned without a biopsy being taken.

[181] See pg 95. Only distinguishable from carotid body tumour by virtue of the relationship with the carotid arteries.

[182] See pg 101.

[183] See pg 314.

CAROTID BODY TUMOUR[172]

Perform examination of neck lump (see pg 37).

'There is (in this middle-aged patient) a non-tender lump in the upper part of the anterior triangle of the neck at the level of the hyoid bone on the right. It is irregular but basically round in shape, about 5 cm in diameter[173]. It is hard, solid[174], dull to percussion, non-fluctuant and non-transilluminable. It is pulsatile[175] but not compressible[176]. The skin moves over the lump freely, and the lump can be moved from side to side but not up and down[177]. The lump is deep to the cervical fascia and beneath the anterior edge of the sternocleidomastoid muscle. It does not move on swallowing or extending the tongue. The common carotid artery is palpable below the mass and the external carotid artery passes over its superficial surface. There is a bruit on auscultation[178]. There are no regional enlarged lymph nodes palpable, and there is no similar lump on the other side[179].

This is likely to be a carotid body tumour, but my differential diagnosis[180] is an enlarged lymph node[181], a branchial cyst[182] or a carotid artery aneurysm[183].'

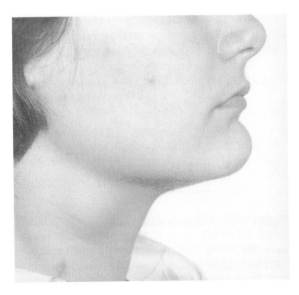

Carotid body tumour

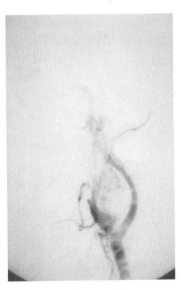

Digital subtraction angiogram of the carotid circulation showing splaying of the carotid bifurcation and contrast filling small vessels in the region of the bifurcation- typical signs of a carotid body tumour.

Cystic hygroma

[184] This is a type of **lymphangioma** – a congenital cluster of lymphatic channels that forms a lymph cyst. The majority are present at birth but some are aggravated by infection and present in adult life. The only symptom is disfigurement, which can be very distressing in a new-born. Regression by the age of 4 years is possible and therefore a watch and wait policy avoids surgical scarring or nerve damage. Persistence into adolescence may be treated by attempts at aspiration and injection of sclerosing agents. Surgical excision is technically demanding and often incomplete risking collateral damage and lymph leaks.

Other types of lymphangiomas

Solid or diffuse lymphangiomas and lymphohaemangiomas can involve any part of the body and are usually present at birth. Growth usually occurs at the same rate as the rest of the body, but they may be associated with local overgrowth of surrounding soft tissue and bone, especially in the face and neck. It is diffuse, difficult to excise and prone to recurrence.

Cutaneous lymphangioma presents as small multiple transparent or red vesicles of skin and mucosa that present at birth or in childhood. They can occur alone or with solid lymphangiomas and lymphohaemangiomas. They are disfiguring and can become infected and bleed. They are treated by local diathermy or extensive subcutaneous excision of the lymphatic cisterns in the dermis. It is difficult and recurrence is common.

[185] It can be very extensive and involve the whole of the subcutaneous tissue of one side of the neck. Lymph cysts typically occur near the junction of the arm and the leg with the head or the trunk.

[186] An examination of the oropharynx would exclude extension into the retropharyngeal space.

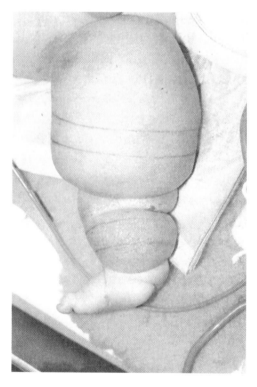

Solid or diffuse lymphangioma

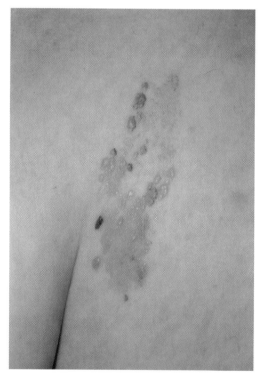

Cutaneous lymphangioma

CYSTIC HYGROMA[184]

Carry out examination of neck lump (see pg 37).

'There is (in this child/young person) a large non-tender mass at the base of the neck in the posterior triangle[185]. It is about 10 cm in diameter, lobulated and flattened with an indistinct surface and edges. It is soft, fluctuant and dull to percussion. Of note, it transilluminates brilliantly, emphasising its superficial nature and its clear, fluid content. It is not reducible. It arises from the subcutaneous tissues deep to the skin but is not fixed to skin, and is superficial to the underlying muscles[186]. There are no enlarged lymph nodes in the region or local lymphoedema. This is a cystic hygroma.'

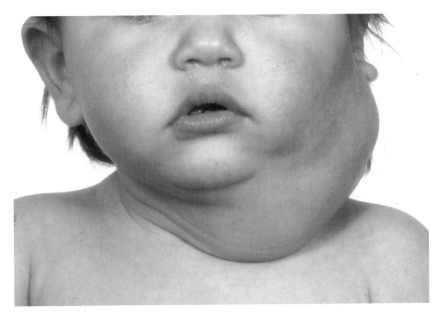

Cystic hygroma

Carcinoma of the breast

**Breast pathology was a Top Five Case: seen by over a quarter of the candidates surveyed. Accounted for 10.6%
of the cases in this bay.**

[187] **Carcinoma of the breast**

70% invasive ductal: firm hard scirrhous mass

10% lobular: bilateral in 20%, multicentric

10% tubular: picked up on screening, small stellate lesions

10% other: medullary (good prognosis, soft, fleshy)

mucoid (good prognosis, rare)

Paget's (poor prognosis, nipple excoriation and underlying intraductal tumour)

Staging of breast cancer (TNM):

T_{is} (Ca in situ); T_1 (<2 cm); T_2 (2–5 cm); T_3 (>5 cm)

T_{4a} (involves chest wall); T_{4b} (involves skin); T_{4c} (chest wall and skin); T_{4d} (inflammatory)

N_0 (no regional nodes); N_1 (mobile ipsilateral axillary); N_2 (fixed ipsilateral axillary); N_3 (internal thoracic
ipsilateral).

M_0 (no mets); M_1 (distant mets including any contralateral axillary nodes and ANY supraclavicular nodes)

[188] **Investigation of breast lump** (triple assessment is mandatory). The important rule to remember is that if any
one of the triple assessments suggests malignancy, a biopsy at the very least should be performed even if the
other two tests suggest benign disease.

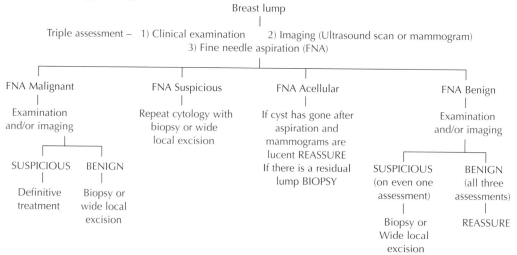

[189] It may be appropriate to say 'the diagnosis is carcinoma of the breast' if, for example, the examiners have said
'the lady is aware of her diagnosis' or 'tell us freely what you think this is' or ask you the diagnosis after you
have moved away from the patient. If you are not sure, however, tact counts for a lot, so be clear about
identifying the malignant features and then use a phrase such as 'concerned to exclude carcinoma'. Remember,
however, that by the rules of triple assessment, a benign FNA and mammogram does not exclude carcinoma if
clinical assessment is suspicious; that can only be excluded by an excision biopsy.

CARCINOMA OF THE BREAST[187]

Examination of the breast (see pg 39).

'On initial inspection this (middle-aged or elderly) lady looks well with no signs of systemic disease. On inspection of the breasts there is fullness in the upper outer quadrant of the left breast. There are no obvious nipple changes, and the skin initially appears normal, but on raising the arms there is evidence of tethering and peau d'orange in the area. There are no signs of previous surgery or radiotherapy. On examination of the breast, there is a non-tender lump in the upper outer quadrant of the left breast. It is about 4 cm in diameter, hemispherical in shape with an irregular surface and indistinct edges. It is stony hard and craggy, and does not fluctuate, transilluminate and is not pulsatile, compressible or reducible. It arises deep to the skin, but the skin is tethered to it and can be seen to dimple when moved over the lump. The lump is also fixed to the underlying pectoralis muscle. There are enlarged axillary glands on the left, but the supraclavicular nodes, contralateral breast and axilla are free of palpable lumps. There is no evidence of lymphoedema in the left arm, and the patient denies alteration of power and sensation.

If I saw this lady in clinic I would examine the chest and abdomen, and be concerned to investigate[188] the breast lump with urgent mammography and fine needle aspiration cytology[189] or Trucut histology.'

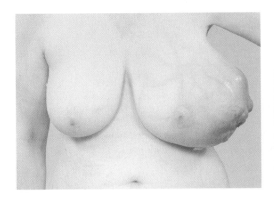

Advanced breast carcinoma

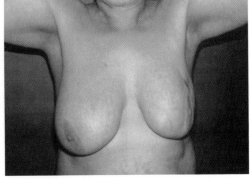

Breast carcinoma showing skin tethering asymmetry and nipple retraction

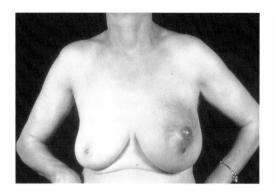

Carcinoma of the left breast showing erythema, asymmetry, enlargement of breast, ulceration and nipple retraction

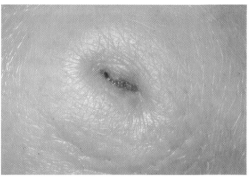

Carcinoma of the breast showing 'peau d'orange'

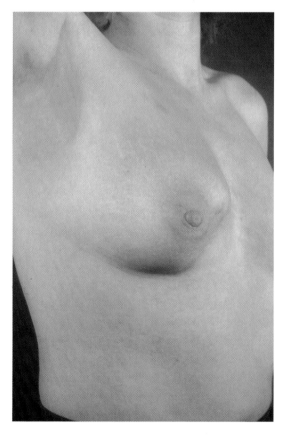

Carcinoma of the right breast showing skin tethering when arms are raised

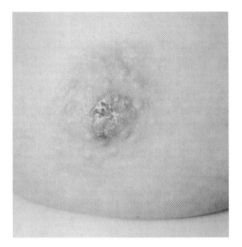

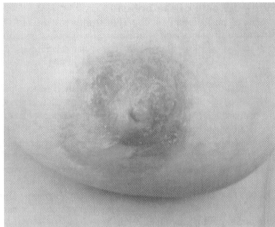

Paget's disease of the nipple   Eczema of the nipple

Differentiating this benign condition eczema from the malignant Paget's disease is difficult but benign disease is suggested by

a) Areolar area rather than nipple affected
b) No underlying lesion on mammography
c) Benign imprint or scrape cytology after pressing or scraping the lesion onto a slide

NB an incisional biopsy of the affected skin is the only definitive investigation

111

Fibroadenoma of the breast

[190] **Fibroadenosis/fibrocystic disease/benign breast disease**

Aberrations of normal development and involution. Common (90% of autopsies). Peaks in premenopausal years. Proliferation of epithelial cells. Often associated with cysts. Breasts often feel generally nodular. Cyclical changes typical. Surgery not needed if triple assessment negative.

Cysts

Part of the fibrocystic disease spectrum. Dilatation of acini and terminal ductules. Usually multiple. Can become very large. Typical appearance on imaging, especially ultrasound. Aspiration usually deflates cyst producing greenish acellular aspirate. No treatment needed if clinical and imaging assessment negative **and** aspirate not bloodstained **and** no residual lump felt after aspiration. Often recur.

Fibroadenoma

Most common benign tumour of the breast. New growth of fibrous and glandular tissue. Common in premenopausal women. May change with cycle. Well circumscribed. Clinically feels like a mobile, smooth 'breast mouse'. Histologically characteristic delicate cellular fibroblastic stroma enclosing glandular cystic spaces within an epithelial lining. Typical mammographic and ultrasonographic appearance. Does not require excision if definitively diagnosed on triple assessment but patient may be happier with lump excised.

Rare phylloides tumour are giant fibroadenomas 10–15 cm or more. Can cause pressure necrosis, gross deformity and may become malignant, so must be excised.

FIBROADENOMA OF THE BREAST[190]

Examination of the breast (see pg 39).

'On general inspection this (young) lady looks well with no signs of systemic disease. Inspection of the breasts reveals no asymmetry, skin changes or nipple changes and no evidence of previous surgery or radiotherapy. On examination of the breasts there is a small, non-tender lump in the upper outer quadrant of the left breast. It is 2 cm in diameter, round and smooth with well-defined edges. It is firm and rubbery, not fluctuant, pulsatile reducible or compressible. It arises from the subcutaneous tissue and is very mobile, tethered neither to skin nor underlying pectoralis major. There are no palpable lumps in either axilla, supraclavicular region or in the contralateral breast. My clinical diagnosis is a benign fibroadenoma.'

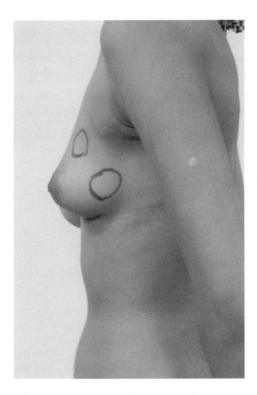

Fibroadenomas (outlined in pen)

Post mastectomy
[191] Treatment of breast cancer

Surgery
Excision biopsy: to diagnose not to treat e.g. in lesions suspicious on mammography but not palpable or borderline suspicious FNA but mammogram and clinical examination suggest benign disease. May need wire localisation under mammographic control preoperatively if impalpable screen-detected lesion. Should remove no more than 20 g of tissue (not aiming for complete clearance as it is for diagnosis, not treatment). Will need definitive treatment if histology is positive and clearance is not complete.

Wide local excision (breast conservation surgery): single, small (<4 cm diameter in small breast) node negative local disease. Aim is cure with good clearance. If margins not clear → mastectomy.

Mastectomy: large/central/multifocal disease or patient's preference. Also may be indicated in recurrence or inadequate clearance (affected margins) after wide local excision.

Axillary sampling: removing at least 4 nodes OR level 1 nodes OR level 1+2 nodes. If no positive nodes, no further treatment needed. If positive node, need level 3 dissection or radiotherapy to treat axilla.

Axillary clearance: removing level 1, 2 and 3 nodes (lateral, behind and medial to pectoralis minor). Even if nodes are positive, radiotherapy not needed after level 3 clearance unless recurrence detected later.

Complications of mastectomy: seroma, infection, flap necrosis.

Complications of axillary surgery: nerve damage, lymphoedema, wound infection, reduced range of movement

Radiotherapy
Breast: all patients after breast conservation surgery. High risk mastectomy patients (pectoralis major involvement or any two of the following: axillary lymph node involvement, lymphatic or vascular invasion, Grade 3 cancer, Tumour > 4 cm diameter).

Axilla: if axillary sampling shows positive nodes or in axillary recurrence if no previous radiotherapy (can only be given once).

Complications of radiotherapy: skin reactions, telangiectasia, cardiac damage, pneumonitis, osteoradionecrosis, lymphoedema in axillary radiotherapy (especially when combined with axillary surgery).

Adjuvant treatment
Chemotherapy: most effective in premenopausal patients: not widely used in patients over 50 years in UK. Cyclophosphamide, methotrexate and fluorouracil are the common agents used in UK. Side-effects include fatigue, alopecia and nausea.

Oophorectomy (or ovarian ablation by radiotherapy or gonadotrophin releasing hormone): only of benefit in premenopausal women.

Tamoxifen: all high risk or node positive postmenopausal women. Effective in all age groups. Greatest benefits in oestrogen positive tumours. Side-effects include vaginal dryness, loss of libido and hot flushes.

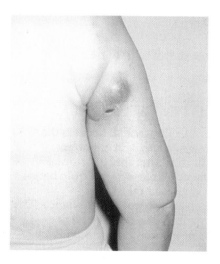 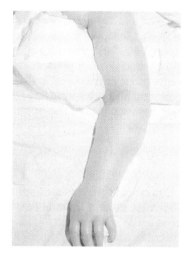

Lymphoedema due to recurrent axillary metastatic breast cancer

POST MASTECTOMY[191]

Carry out examination of the breast (see pg 39).

'On general inspection this (middle-aged or elderly) lady looks thin, pale and short of breath at rest. Immediately evident is her previous left mastectomy, and the oedematous left arm. She also shows signs of chemotherapy with hair loss and a cushingoid, flushed facial appearance. On inspection of the chest wall, there is a scar of previous mastectomy and axillary surgery on the left and ink markings and telangiectasia indicating radiotherapy. On examination there is no evidence of recurrence in the scar, but there are palpable nodes in the left axilla. The right axilla and breast and both supraclavicular areas are clear clinically. The left arm is markedly swollen with pitting oedema. The patient denies weakness and numbness. My diagnosis is previously surgically treated carcinoma of the breast with recurrent or residual disease being treated by adjuvant therapy. I would like to listen to the chest and examine the abdomen to complete my examination.'

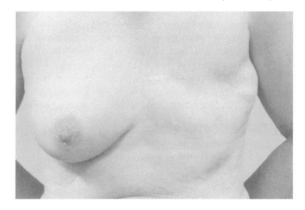

Mastectomy scar

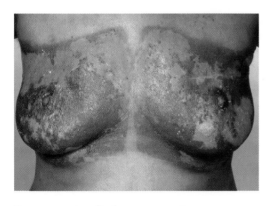

Severe post radiotherapy reaction

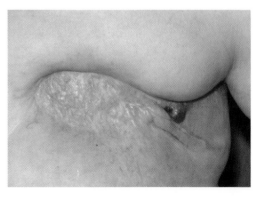

Recurrence carcinoma in mastectomy scar

Breast reconstruction

[192] **Options for breast reconstruction**

Immediate

Reduces the psychological trauma of the change in body image experienced after mastectomy

No evidence that it increases rate of local or systemic relapse

Radiotherapy can be carried out while prosthesis or expander is in situ

Should be more widely available to patients

Delayed

More widely available

Needs well healed scar and (except in the case of myocutaneous flaps) has poor results after radiotherapy

Prosthesis

Suitable in small breasts with adequate skin flaps

Mostly silicone or saline

Problems include: fibrous capsules and contracture (reduced by textured prostheses), infection (5% of cases need removal), implant rupture (1%) resulting in silicone leakage which, contrary to media stories has not been shown to increase the incidence of carcinogenesis, problems with other organs or connective tissue disorders.

Tissue expansion: suitable if there are adequate skin flaps and good skin closure in small to medium sized breasts. Silicone bag with filler port is initially inserted, and the expander has saline injected weekly. It should be overexpanded to produce ptosis. It is then replaced with a permanent prosthesis.

Myocutaneous flaps: Suitable in large skin incisions, doubtful skin closure and large breasts. Can be used in delayed reconstruction if there has been previous radiotherapy (see fig below). Complications include flap necrosis, infection and abdominal hernias (in TRAM flaps).

Nipple reconstruction: best done after 6 months. Areola is reproduced using upper inner thigh skin, contralateral areola or tattooing. The nipple can be reconstructed using local tissue, the contralateral nipple or artificial adhesive nipples worn for a month at a time.

Other techniques: reduction mammoplasty or mastopexy of remaining breast may be indicated.

[193] Or the right side of the back in the case of a latissimus dorsi myocutaneous flap.

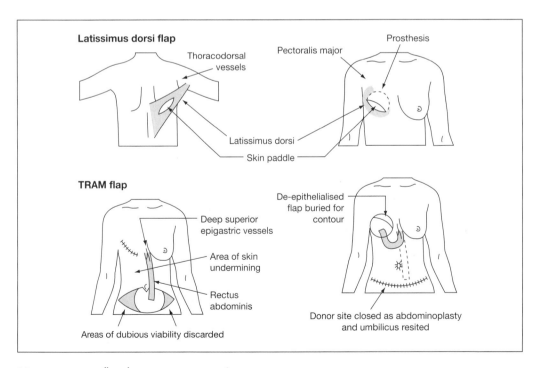

Myocutaneous flap breast reconstruction

BREAST RECONSTRUCTION[192]

Examination of the breast (see pg 39).

'On general inspection the patient looks well with no signs of systemic disease. On inspection of the chest there has been previous surgery on the right breast. There is an ovoid scar over the breast and there is no nipple on the right. There is a transverse scar across the lower abdomen[193] indicating the donor site of what I presume to be a myocutaneous flap reconstruction. On examination of the breasts there is no evidence of recurrence in either breast, axilla or supraclavicular fossa. A full examination would include listening to the chest and examining the abdomen. My diagnosis is previous mastectomy, probably for carcinoma of the breast with immediate or delayed reconstruction using a TRAM (transverse rectus abdominis myocutaneous) flap.'

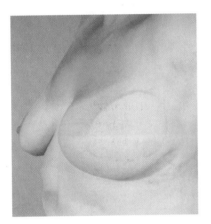 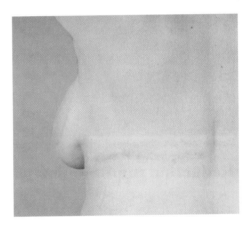

Latissimus dorsi myocutaneous flap

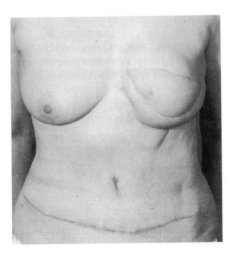

TRAM flap

117

Pleomorphic adenoma of the parotid

Salivary gland pathology was a Top Five Case: seen by nearly one fifth of candidates surveyed. Accounted for 7.6% of the cases in this bay. Parotid gland lumps were seen by over 1 in 10 of candidates surveyed.

[194] Although adenomas can arise anywhere in the gland, this is the most common site for **pleomorphic** adenomas.

[195] They can vary in size from just palpable to 20 cm in diameter but often will be noted between 1–3 cm.

[196] **Adenomas** account for 90% of salivary gland neoplasms, and of these 2/3 are pleomorphic (see opposite). Neoplasms in other salivary glands are rarer than in the parotid and are more frequently malignant. On the other hand, **calculi** and **sialadenitis** (infection) are less common in the parotid than in the other salivary glands, probably because it is chiefly a serous secreting gland (more watery), not mucus secreting.

Monomorphic adenomas account for the remaining 1/3 of salivary gland adenomas. The commonest of these is **Warthin's tumour** (adenolymphoma), which is similar to pleomorphic adenoma except for the following features:

Histologically there is no sign of stroma.

It tends to arise in the lower part of the parotid gland, lower than the common site of a pleomorphic adenoma. They are soft and often fluctuate.

They are more commonly bilateral.

Pleomorphic adenomas of the palate: the hard palate contains many small glands identical in structure and function to the salivary glands. Pleomorphic salivary adenomas can therefore arise on the palate. If it is not treated this non-tender lump can slowly enlarge and make speech and eating difficult.

PLEOMORPHIC ADENOMA OF THE PAROTID

Carry out examination of a parotid lump (see pg 42).

'There is (in this middle-aged man) a non-tender lump just anterior and superior to the angle of the jaw[194] on the right. It is 2 cm in diameter[195], hemispherical with a smooth surface and distinct edge. It is hard and rubbery, dull to percussion and not fluctuant, compressible, reducible or transilluminable. It arises from the subcutaneous tissues and the skin moves freely over it. It can be moved over the deep structures. The overlying and surrounding skin is normal, and the regional lymph nodes are not enlarged. The rest of the parotid gland and the contralateral gland are normal, and the facial nerve is not affected. There is no evidence of stones or inflammation of the gland. The most likely diagnosis is a pleomorphic adenoma of the parotid gland[196].'

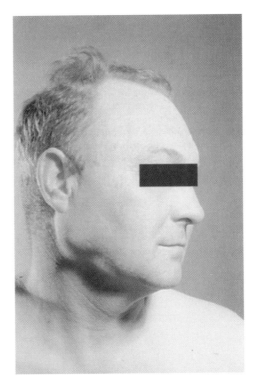

Pleomorphic adenoma of the parotid

Anatomy of the parotid gland

Largest of the salivary glands, mostly serous (not mucus). Situated below external auditory meatus behind the ramus of the mandible and in front of the sternocleidomastoid muscle. The facial nerve runs through the gland and divides it into superficial and deep lobes. The structures within the parotid gland are (lateral to medial). The facial nerve and its five terminal branches supplying the muscles of facial expression (the temporal, zygomatic, buccal, mandibular and cervical branches) the retromandibular vein, the external carotid artery (and its branches, the superficial temporal artery and the maxillary artery) and lymph nodes.

The parotid duct emerges from the facial process of the gland and runs forward over the lateral surface of the masseter muscle, piercing the buccinator muscle and opening in the mouth opposite the upper second molar tooth. It can be palpated 1 cm below the zygomatic arch if the teeth are clenched.

The nerve supply is via parasympathetic secretomotor fibres from the inferior salivary nucleus of the ninth cranial nerve, which 'hitchhike' on the tympanic branch of the ninth cranial nerve, the lesser petrosal nerve, the otic ganglion and the auriculotemporal nerve. Disruption of these fibres lead to postoperative gustatory sweating (see below).

Management of a parotid lump

Investigations are controversial. Ultrasound and FNA are advocated by some but may be difficult to distinguish between malignant and benign tumour. **Golden rule: do not cut into a parotid lump** (increases risk of implantation and recurrence). So no wedge biopsies, no Trucut.

If clinically benign: wide local excision or superficial parotidectomy. Low incidence of recurrence.

If clinically malignant: radical *en bloc* surgery plus radiotherapy. Very poor prognosis (<20% 5yr survival)

Parotidectomy

Definitions:

Conservative parotidectomy – all named branches of facial nerve preserved

Radical parotidectomy – facial nerve sacrificed

Superficial parotidectomy – removal of superficial part of parotid gland

Total parotidectomy – removal of whole gland (conservative or radical)

Incision: S shaped incision starting from tragus, curving under pinna to mastoid process then forward in the upper skin crease of the neck. Deepen incision, looking for facial nerve just below and in front of the auditory meatus deep to the stylomastoid artery.

Procedure: follow facial nerve forward following the superior branch each time. When the anterior border is reached, reflect the superficial lobe forward and dissect it from the skin flap. Divide the parotid duct as far forward as possible and ligate it with catgut skin closure over drain.

Beware: facial nerve, jugular vein, tumour in the deep lobe (requiring external carotid artery sacrifice).

Postoperative complications of parotidectomy:

- Haemorrhage
- Sloughing of skin flap
- Parotid duct fistula
- Facial nerve palsy (temporary or permanent)
- Frey's syndrome: sweating on the cheek during a meal (gustatory sweating) due to inappropriate cross-regeneration of sympathetic and parasympathetic nerve fibres divided during the operation.

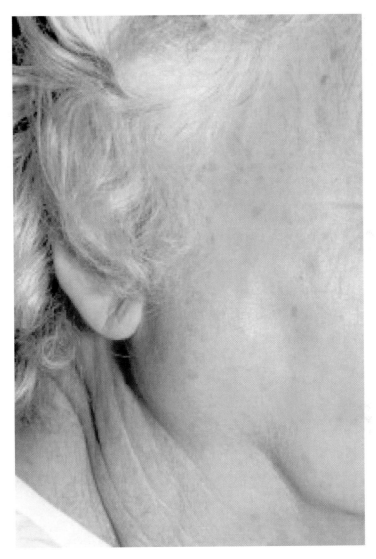

Adenolymphoma/Warthin's tumour

Carcinoma of the parotid gland

[197] The mass may infiltrate and become tethered to the skin.

[198] **Facial nerve palsy** (results in a Bell's palsy): absence of tone of the facial muscles on the affected side, asymmetry and less noticeable nasolabial fold, drooping of the corner of the mouth and drooping of the lower eyelid. On closing the eyes, the eyelids fail to close on the affected side (see fig opposite).

Testing the facial nerve (seventh cranial nerve): 'raise your eyebrows, screw your eyes up tight, puff your cheeks out, whistle, show me your teeth'. *NB* The facial nerve supplies the muscles of facial expression only and not facial sensation (supplied by the trigeminal nerve – the fifth cranial nerve). For the course of the facial nerve within the parotid (see pg 120).

[199] **Management of malignant parotid lump:** radical *en bloc* surgery plus radiotherapy. Very poor prognosis (<20% 5-year survival). If a lump thought to be benign is removed by superficial parotidectomy and then found to be malignant, the options are:

- Wait and See (if completely excised, acinic or mucoepidermoid tumour).
- Post-op radiotherapy (if adenoid cystic carcinoma or frank carcinoma), or
- Further more radical surgery (if completely excised).

If doubt exists clinically, wide excision biopsy is appropriate.

Golden rule: DO NOT cut into a parotid lump (see pg 120, Management of a parotid lump).

CARCINOMA OF THE PAROTID GLAND

Carry out examination of the parotid lump (see pg 42)

'There is (in this older patient) a painful, warm but non-tender swelling over the angle of the jaw on the right. It is hemispherical measuring 3 cm in diameter with an irregular surface and indistinct edges. It is firm/hard, dull to percussion, not pulsatile, reducible, compressible or transilluminable. It arises from the deep structures and is fixed to them, but the skin moves over the lump with no sign of tethering[197]. The overlying skin is hyperaemic and hot. The surrounding skin is normal but there are enlarged lymph nodes (say where). The facial nerve is intact[198]. This is a hard, warm, fixed parotid mass with associated lymph nodes and I would be concerned to exclude a malignant lesion[199].'

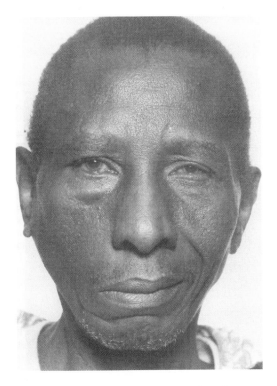 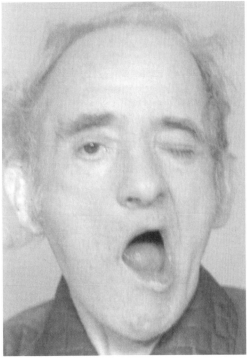

Facial nerve palsy from carcinoma of parotid gland on the right

Facial nerve palsy- note drooping of right side of mouth, loss of nasolabial fold on right and inability to close right eye

Chronic parotitis

[200] **Chronic inflammation of the parotid gland** is usually caused by a small calculus (rarer in the parotid – a serous secreting gland – than in the other salivary glands which secrete a more mucus solution) or a fibrous stenosis blocking the mouth of the parotid duct.

History: recurrent swelling and aching pain of the parotid gland, worse before eating. Occasionally bilateral. The gland can eventually become permanently swollen.

Investigations: plain film (65% of submandibular gland stones are radiopaque whereas 65% of parotid stones are radiolucent). Sialogram outlines the ducts demonstrating calculi, duct stenosis and sialectasis.

Treatment: stones can be removed trans-orally. Gland resection may be required.

Acute parotitis, in contrast to chronic parotitis, is acutely tender, with generalised swelling of the whole parotid gland to up to three or four times larger than normal. The gland is red and hot, firm but indentable, not mobile and often associated with enlarged lymph nodes. A purulent discharge may be expressed from the duct. **Mumps** is the commonest cause of parotitis, (typically occurring in children during viral epidemics), but **acute bacterial parotitis** (usually staphylococcal) can occur in the elderly or debilitated, usually due to poor oral hygiene, dehydration and obstruction of the parotid duct by a stone or scarring. The symptoms are of an acute onset of continuous throbbing pain and swelling over the parotid gland worse on speaking and eating. There are also systemic signs of infection such as fever, rigors and malaise.

Other causes of enlargement of the salivary glands (sialomegaly) include the following:

Mikulicz's syndrome: is an autoimmune disorder involving enlargement of one or all of the parotid and submandibular glands, combined with a visible enlargement of the lachrymal glands and a dry mouth.

Sjögren's syndrome: also an autoimmune disease, presents with the features of Mikulicz's syndrome plus dry eyes and generalised arthritis.

Drugs: the contraceptive pill, thiouracil, co-proximal, isoprenaline, phenylbutazone.

Sialectasis: a disease of unknown origin recognised by progressive destruction of the alveoli and parenchyma of the gland, with duct stenosis and cyst formation. Calculi may be found in the main ducts. The priority of management is excluding malignancy.

Sialadenosis

Chronic parotitis[200]

Examination of parotid gland (see pg 42).

'The right parotid gland is generally enlarged and firm with distinct edges. It is tender and rubbery hard. A stone can/cannot be felt in the duct. The other salivary glands are normal. This patient has the signs of chronic parotitis secondary to calculi.'

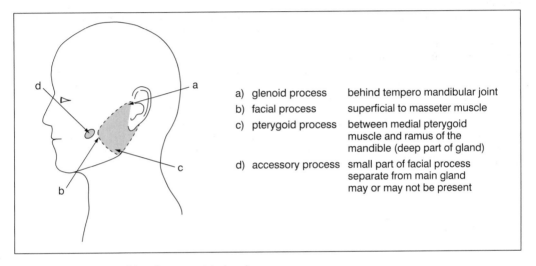

a) glenoid process — behind tempero mandibular joint
b) facial process — superficial to masseter muscle
c) pterygoid process — between medial pterygoid muscle and ramus of the mandible (deep part of gland)
d) accessory process — small part of facial process separate from main gland may or may not be present

Typical area covered by the parotid gland

Submandibular calculi

[201] Submandibular calculi are common because:

1. Gland lies below opening of duct (impedes drainage, encourages stasis)
2. Submandibular gland is a mucus-secreting rather than serous secreting gland

A salivary gland calculus is composed of similar mixture to the 'tartar' dentists scrape off your teeth: cellular debris, bacteria, mucus and calcium and magnesium phosphates.

History: young to middle-aged adults who complain of recurrent pain and swelling beneath the jaw worse before and during eating. Gland may become persistently enlarged.

Anatomy: the **submandibular gland** is divided into deep and superficial parts by the posterior border of the mylohyoid. It is a mixed salivary gland, secreting mucus and serous saliva as opposed to the parotid that is mainly a serous gland and the sublingual gland which is mainly mucous-secreting. The submandibular duct emerges from the superficial part of the gland, runs between mylohyoid and hyoglossus and enters the floor of the mouth next to the frenulum. Nerves at risk in excision of submandibular gland are the mandibular branch of the facial nerve, the hypoglossal and the lingual nerves.

The **sublingual gland** lies in front of the anterior border of the hyoglossus and medial to genioglossus. The glands form the sublingual fold of mucosa in the floor of the mouth and meet each other anteriorly.

Submandibular salivary gland tumours: pleomorphic adenomas, monomorphic adenomas and carcinomas of the submandibular gland are rare compared with the parotid gland but present in a similar way. Numbness of the anterior two-thirds of the tongue suggests infiltration of the lingual nerve.

Submandibular sialadenitis: infection of a submandibular gland is secondary to the presence of a stone in its duct or stenosis caused by previous stones passing through. The pain is more severe, throbbing and continuous than in the presence of stones without infection. The gland is more swollen and is red, hot and tender on examination.

[202] Unless infected.

[203] When the muscles of the floor of the mouth are tested, by asking the patient to push his tongue against the roof of the mouth, the gland becomes less mobile.

[204] Bimanual palpation: feel the lump between the gloved index finger of one hand inside the mouth and the fingers of the other hand on the outer surface of the lump.

[205] If the patient opens his mouth and lifts his tongue the orifices of the submandibular ducts are evident as small papillae on either side of the frenulum of the tongue. A stone may be visible impacted at the orifice of the duct. The presence of a stone in the duct may appear as a pink swelling along the floor of the mouth. The duct should be gently palpated to see if any swellings or stones can be appreciated, and if any discharge can be expressed.

[206] To exclude systemic disease such as Sjögren's syndrome (see pg 128).

SUBMANDIBULAR CALCULI[201]

Examination of a neck lump (see pg 37) as well as examination of the inside of the mouth and bimanual palpation of the gland as described below.

'There is (in this young or middle-aged adult) a non-tender[202] but apparently intermittently painful lump beneath the horizontal ramus of the mandible on the mylohyoid muscle about 3 cm in front of the anterior border of the sternocleidomastoid muscle. It is a 4 cm wide, flattened ovoid, smooth with distinct anterior, posterior and inferior edges. It is rubbery hard, does not fluctuate or transilluminate, and is non-compressible, non-reducible and non-pulsatile. It is dull to percussion. The skin is freely moveable over the lump, which is tethered to the deep structures[203]. On examining and palpating the floor of the mouth, there is no lump or ulcer evident from inside the mouth. Bimanual palpation of the lump shows it to lie beneath the floor of the mouth[204]. There is no visible or palpable stone in the submandibular duct, and I cannot express any pus from the orifice of the duct[205]. The overlying and surrounding skin is normal, and the regional lymph nodes are not enlarged. This is an enlarged submandibular gland. The history suggests a submandibular calculus. To complete my examination, I would like to examine the opposite submandibular gland and the parotid glands[206].'

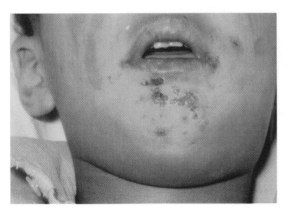

Enlarged submandibular gland (this case is due to adenoma, not calculi)

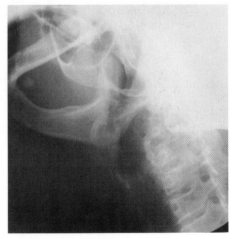

Radiograph of stone in submandibular duct

Other causes of a swelling on the floor of the mouth

Ranula: a large mucus containing cyst probably from acini of the sublingual gland secondary to obstruction. It is a tense, grey, translucent, spherical swelling just below the mucosa of the floor of the mouth and presents in children and young adults. A 'plunging' ranula is a rare variant that extends through the mylohyoid muscle into the neck.

Sublingual dermoid cyst: this is a non-tender swelling above or below the mylohyoid muscle in the midline which is caused by entrapment of a portion of epidermis during embryological fusion of the facial processes. It usually presents between the ages of 10 and 25 years as a swelling under the tongue or just below the point of the chin looking like a double chin. It is spherical, non-tender, smooth and well-defined, and although firm, it fluctuates. Bimanual palpation combined with asking the patient to contract the muscles of the floor of the mouth should make it clear whether the dermoid cyst is supra-mylohyoid or infra-mylohyoid.

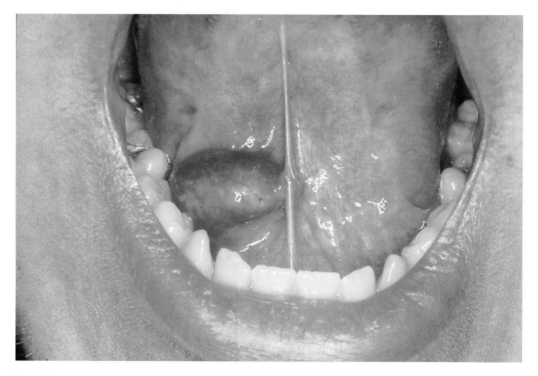

Ranula

D   Detailed Results of Questionnaire

SUPERFICIAL LESIONS BAY

Total 132 cases reported in the survey

TOP 5 CASES (Accounted for 64.4% of all Superficial Lesion cases)

Type of case	Number seen in survey	Breakdown and details of cases
Lipoma	22	17 Lipoma 5 Dercum's disease Four of these occurred in the Abdomen bay. Questions included differential diagnosis, management, incision lines, malignant potential.
Skin cancer	22	15 Basal cell carcinomas on face or scalp 1 Superficial spreading malignant melanoma 2 Same lady post malignant melanoma excision with skin graft behind knee and radiotherapy tattoo. 2 Squamous cell carcinoma 1 Bowen's disease 1 Marjolin's ulcer under nail Questions included describe, examine, differential diagnoses, treatment (surgery vs radiotherapy), complications, skin closure, where else would you examine in malignant melanoma?
Thyroid	17	10 Goitre 5 Lump 2 Graves Questions included 'describe full examination', differential diagnosis, effects of retrosternal extension, causes of thyroid lump.
Breast	14	8 postoperative 3 breast lump 3 post reconstruction Four cases seen in Abdomen and Thoracic bay. Questions included sentinel nodes, tram flap, radiation side effects, tamoxifen side effects.
Salivary glands	10	3 Parotid Lump ?cause 1 Pleomorphic adenoma, parotid 1 sebaceous cyst over parotid gland 1 post total parotidectomy 1 Warthin's with bilateral parotid swelling 2 swollen submandibular gland, one with calculus 1 pleomorphic adenoma of salivary gland in palate Questions included differential diagnoses, bimanual palpation, management of calculi, principles of parotid surgery, risks of surgery, course of facial nerve, follow-up.

OTHER CASES

Type of case	Number seen in survey	Breakdown and details of cases
Sebaceous cyst	8	All on head and neck.
Thyroglossal cyst	7	Questions included movement on swallowing/sticking out tongue.
Neck lumps	7	3 lymph node cases, two with tracheostomies 4 neck lumps? cause
Neurofibromata	6	All neurofibromatosis. One lower limb amputation due to neurofibromatosis (in orthopaedics bay). Questions included von Recklinghausen's syndrome, acoustic neuroma, MEN II, café au lait spots, genetics, associated disorders.
Tracheostomy	4	Also a feature in two 'lymph nodes in the neck' cases. Questions included long term requirements, indications, types, complications, side vs end tracheostomies and sudden airway obstruction.
Histiocytoma	2	
Dermoid cyst	2	1 congenital 1 implantation
Haemangioma	2	both periorbital
Benign papilloma	1	
Cervical rib	1	
Hypertrophic scar	1	
Keratoacanthoma	1	
Branchial cyst	1	
Seborrhoic keratosis	1	
Pharyngeal pouch	1	
Laryngectomy	1	With oesophageal speech
Seroma of vein harvest Scar on leg	1	

CHAPTER THREE

CLINICAL BAY 2
ORTHOPAEDICS AND NEUROLOGY

CONTENTS

E   Detailed results of questionnaire   **254**

ORTHOPAEDICS AND NEUROLOGY

A   The Bay

In the MRCS (Eng) examination the Orthopaedic and Neurology bay lasts ten minutes. This will be extended to 15 minutes after December 2002 (see pg 5 for details of the changes). There are two examiners, one asking the questions and the other taking down the marks. During this bay you are expected to see 3–4 patients. The bay is worth 5 marks, of which 3 are awarded for clinical approach and 2 for discussion and investigations. The MRCS(Eng) Regulations describe this bay as follows:

'The aim of this bay is to ensure that the candidate has a system for taking a history in the musculoskeletal system and is able to undertake an examination of any part of the musculoskeletal system. The findings should be interpreted to reach a possible diagnosis. Investigation results may be shown to corroborate the diagnosis.

The candidate may be asked to carry out simple procedures such as simulation of fracture reduction for Colles' fracture. Surgical shoes, walking sticks and splints may also be used as points for discussion. Real life implications in terms of function for the patient are important.

One examiner will be an orthopaedic surgeon; one will be a non-orthopaedic surgeon.'

B   The Examinations

EXAMINATION OF THE HIP

'Hello, I'm Dr Parchment Smith. Would you mind if I examine your hips? Can you stand in front of me? Do you mind if I talk about you as I go along?'
Stand back, hands behind the back and LOOK.
'On inspection from the front I am looking for pelvic tilting[1], muscle wasting[2] or rotational deformity[3]. From the side I am looking for scars[4] and an increase in lumbar lordosis[5]. From behind I am looking for scoliosis[6], gluteal muscle wasting and sinus scars. Now will you lie on the bed? Let me get your hips straight.'
Assess for SHORTENING.
'There is/is no obvious shortening[7]. Ideally I would like to measure the true length and the apparent length[8]. If there is any discrepancy I would like to flex the knees and see if the shortening is of the femur or the tibia[9]. I can further assess femoral shortening by palpating the greater trochanters[10]. Now I would like to palpate the joint.'

---

[1] For example from adduction or abduction deformity of the hip, short leg, scoliosis.
[2] Due to infection, disuse or polio.
[3] Common in osteoarthritis.
[4] Previous surgery, old TB sinuses.
[5] Suggests fixed flexion deformity of the hip.
[6] May be secondary to pelvic tilting, adduction deformity and/or shortening of a leg.
[7] **Causes of shortening of the leg**
1.True shortening: affected limb physically shorter than the other
   a) Causes distal to the trochanters: old femoral or tibial fractures, growth disturbance (polio, bone or joint infection, epiphysial trauma).
   b) Causes above the trochanters: coxa vara (from neck fractures, slipped epiphysis, Perthes' disease, congenital coxa vara), loss of articular cartilage (infection, arthritis), or dislocation.
   c) Lengthening of other limb (rare): stimulation of bone growth by increased vascularity (after tumour or fracture in children), coxa valga (following polio).
2. Apparent shortening: limb not altered in length but appears short as a result of an adduction contracture of the hip which has to be compensated for by tilting of the pelvis.
[8] Lie patient square on couch. Adjust anterior superior iliac spines (ASIS) to be parallel. Heels should now be level. Measure ASIS to medial malleolus for true length, xiphisternum to medial malleolus for apparent length.
[9] Put heels together and flex knees to 90°. If the knee of the short leg is sitting proximal to the normal knee, the femur is short. If it sits distally, the tibia is shortened. This can be confirmed by measuring from the tibial tubercle to the medial malleolus.
[10] Put thumbs on ASIS and feel for greater trochanters with the fingers. If the distance is shorter on one side this suggests the pathology lies above the trochanters. It is not very reliable to measure the femoral shaft but in thin people the tip of the trochanter to the lateral joint line are the landmarks. NELATON'S LINE runs from the ASIS to the greater tuberosity and should pass the tip of the trochanter.

FEEL for the greater trochanter.
'I have just palpated the greater trochanter.'
'Now the head of the femur which should lie below the inguinal ligament just lateral to the femoral artery. Does it hurt when I rotate it like this? I'm listening for crepitations.'
Abduct the bent leg.
'I'm now palpating adductor longus which can be tender[11], and just below it, the lesser trochanter. In a young patient with hip pain I would palpate the ischial tuberosity if I suspected hamstring strain was the source of the hip pain. I would now like to examine the MOVEMENTS at the hip[12].'
Place your hand behind the lumbar spine to assess its position. Now flex the <u>good</u> hip fully, observing with the hand that the lumbar curvature is fully flattened.
'I felt the lumbar spine flatten and the opposite hip has remained on the bed. This is Thomas' test for a fixed flexion deformity[13], and it is negative in this case indicating no gross loss of EXTENSION.'

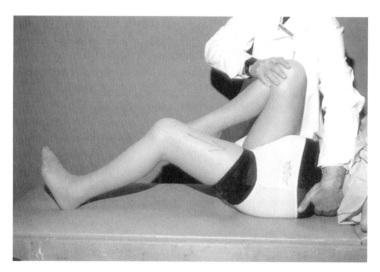

Thomas' test demonstrating a fixed flexion deformity of the left hip

---

[11] Especially in sports injuries (strain of adductor longus).

[12] For timesaving purposes most examiners would only expect you to examine the bad hip. 'Examine this patient's left hip', although technically you should examine both sides and compare the range of movements. Be prepared to do either as required.

[13] **Thomas' test** is a test of hip extension. If the hip being examined (the 'bad' hip) rises from the couch when the <u>other</u> hip is being flexed in the presence of a normal lumbar spine there is a fixed flexion deformity/loss of extension of the 'bad' hip.

Ask the patient to hold the good hip in the position which obliterates lumbar

lordosis.

'Just hold your good leg there while I assess the FLEXION of your bad hip – how far can you bend your bad leg[14]?'

To the examiners:

'I would like to test ABDUCTION and ADDUCTION now. Both legs out straight, please. I need to make sure the pelvis does not contribute.'

Place your hand over the ASIS, fingers on one, thumb on the other.

'How far can you bring your leg out[15] and how far can it swing in over the other leg[16]?

Adduction and abduction are normal. Now I am going to test INTERNAL AND EXTERNAL ROTATION[17]. Can you bend your knee up for me?'

With the knee and hip flexed to 90°, steady the knee over the hip and pull the foot out laterally.

'This is internal rotation of the hip[18].'

Now move the foot medially.

'This is external rotation of the hip[19]. Thomas' test earlier showed me that there was no gross loss of extension, but a more subtle test if I were concerned would be to turn the patient prone and check for extension in that way[20].

---

[14] Flexion is tested using one hand under the pelvis to check no further movement occurs, and with the opposite hip held by the patient in enough flexion to obliterate the lumbar lordosis. Normal range 120°. The thigh should touch the abdomen.

[15] Normal range of abduction is 40°.

[16] Normal range of adduction is 25°. The legs should cross around mid-thigh.

[17] These tests are for hip rotation **in 90° of flexion**, the commonest way of testing rotation. Internal and external rotation of the hip **in extension** can be assessed by making the patient lie with legs extended and simply rolling the straight leg laterally and medially, observing any play at the knee. Alternatively, the patient can lie prone with his knees bent, feet in the air. (The hips will be extended although the knees are flexed.) The normal range of external and internal rotation in extension is 45° and 35° respectively.

[18] Normal range is 45° from the midline. Loss of internal rotation is common in most hip pathology.

[19] Normal range is 45° from the midline. Loss of external rotation is common in most hip pathology.

[20] To test for extension, turn the patient face down, put your hand on the small of his back to steady his pelvis and lift each straight leg up out behind him. This test is not usually necessary if you have done Thomas' test and is awkward in older, obese or immobile patients.

I would now like to perform TRENDELENBURG'S TEST. Could you stand up

please? The Anterior Superior Iliac Spines are level. Now turn your back to me with your feet together. Now, keeping your knees together, just lift the foot of your good leg back off the floor and hold it there, standing on your bad leg. The pelvis on the opposite side to the supporting leg should rise. If it falls, the Trendelenburg's test is positive[21].'

'Finally, to complete my examination I would like to see the patient WALK[22], do a NEUROLOGICAL examination and see the X-RAYS.'

---

[21] **Trendelenburg's test**: standing on one leg tests the abductors of the supporting leg (gluteus medius and minimus) which would normally pull on the pelvis causing it to tilt (and the opposite side of the pelvis to rise) to bring the centre of gravity over the supporting foot (see Osteoarthritis of hip pg 181).

Reasons for a positive Trendelenburg's test include:
   1) Gluteal paralysis or weakness (e.g from polio or a muscle wasting disease)
   2) Gluteal inhibition from pain arising in the hip joint (most common cause in exam)
   3) Coxa vara which shortens the distance between the origin and insertion of the gluteal muscles causing gluteal insufficiency
   4) Congenital dislocation of the hip (see Osteoarthritis of hip pg 181)

[22] Assess stride, dwell time on each side, pain, stiffness, shortening, Trendelenburg's gait. In cases of unilateral Trendelenburg's, there is a dipping movement on the affected side. In bilateral cases there is a waddling gait.

EXAMINATION OF THE KNEE

'Hello, I'm Dr Parchment Smith. Would you mind if I examined your knee? Could you lie flat? Do you mind me talking about you to these doctors as I go along?'

Stand back, hands behind the back, and LOOK.

'On inspection the knees look symmetrical. I am looking for generalised[23] or localised[24] swelling, bruising[25], scars[26], signs of inflammation or a rash[27]. I am also looking for obvious deformity and quadriceps wasting[28].'

To the patient:

'Which is the bad knee? Is it tender?'

Begin to FEEL starting with the back of the hand comparing both sides and the feet for temperature.

'The knee is not hot[29]. I would like to start by examining the EXTENSOR APPARATUS.'

Place a hand behind the knee and feel the quadriceps with the other hand.

To the patient:

'Can you press your leg down against my hand? Now do it again with your foot turned in, toes pointing up to the ceiling[30].'

To the examiners:

'Quadriceps function appears normal. If I had any doubt, I would compare the circumference of the legs 18 cm above the joint line. I am now feeling for the position of the patella.

The upper borders of the patella are equal[31] and there is no tenderness or loss of soft tissue above the upper border[32], across the patella[33], across the lower border[34] or over the tibial tubercle[35]. The extensor apparatus appears intact but ideally I should assess the straight leg raise[36].'

---

[23] Swelling confined to the limits of the synovial cavity and suprapatellar pouch suggest effusion, haemarthrosis, pyarthrosis or a space occupying lesion within the joint. Swelling beyond the limits of the joint suggests infection, tumour or major injury.

[24] Bursitis presents as localised swelling most commonly in the prepatellar or infrapatellar bursa. Meniscal cysts are localised swellings in the joint line. Exostoses occur on the bone.

[25] Suggests trauma to superficial tissues or ligaments (not usually seen in meniscal injuries).

[26] Of previous injury, arthroscopy or surgery.

[27] Psoriasis is associated with arthritis.

[28] Wasting of the quadriceps occurs because of disuse, generally from a painful or unstable lesion of the knee, or from infection or RA.

[29] A hot joint suggests active rheumatoid arthritis or infection.

[30] Extending the hip with the foot dorsiflexed and inverted emphasises the vastus medialis which is involved in recurrent dislocation of the patella.

[31] If not, suspect patellar fracture, rupture of the patellar ligament, avulsion of the tibial tubercle.

[32] This suggests rupture of quadriceps tendon.

[33] This suggests fracture of patella.

[34] This suggests rupture of patellar ligament.

[35] This suggests avulsion of tibial tubercle.

[36] Give them the opportunity to move you on if they are getting impatient.

If they say you should do this, ask the patient to sit with legs dangling off the couch, support the ankle with your hand and ask them to straighten the knee while feeling the muscle.

'The extensor apparatus is functionally intact. I will now examine for an EFFUSION.'

Slide your hand firmly from 15 cm above the knee to the level of the upper border of the patella. Tap the patella firmly with three fingers and the thumb. Listen and feel for a click.

'The patellar tap test is negative[37].'

Stroke the medial side of the joint to empty it. Then watch the medial side as you stroke the lateral side. Excess fluid will distend it.

'The fluid displacement test is negative[38]. If I suspected a haemarthrosis[39] or pyarthrosis[40] at this point I would aspirate the joint before proceeding with the examination.'

Pick up the skin and the relaxed quadriceps tendon above the patella[41].

'The synovium does not feel grossly thickened[42]. I will now assess for TENDERNESS.'

To the patient:

'Can you bend your knee please? Let me know if this feels sore.'

---

[37] If the effusion is too slight or too tense the test will be negative.

[38] If the effusion is too tense the test will be negative.

[39] A haemarthrosis usually occurs within half an hour of injury and gives a doughy feel to the suprapatellar region. It should always be aspirated before examination of the joint because of pain and ability to examine structures.

[40] The tenderness in pyoarthrosis usually impedes examination. It is also vital to get early exclusion of the diagnosis by microscopy.

[41] To assess the thickness of the synovial membrane in the suprapatellar pouch.

[42] It is thickened in rheumatoid arthritis and other inflammatory conditions such as villo-nodular synovitis.

To the examiners:

'I am PALPATING the joint line for meniscus and fat pad injury[43]**, the collateral ligaments and their attachments**[44]**, the tibial tubercle for avulsion injuries or Osgood-Schlatter's disease**[45]**, and the femoral condyles, especially medially, for osteochondritis dissecans**[46]**. I would now like to assess MOVEMENT of the joint.'**

To the patient:

'Can I just lift your foot? You relax with the leg straight.'

Lift leg by ankle and check for full EXTENSION[47]*. Then try active extension*[48]*.*

'I'm just going to press on the knee to try to straighten your leg.'

Compare with the other side.

To the examiners:

'The knee lacks X° of extension. There is no hyperextension[49]**.'**

To the patient:

'Can you bend the knee? Pull your heel into your bum as far as it will go. Now the other side.'

To the examiners:

'There appears to be full FLEXION of 135°, but ideally I would measure the angle or do serial heel to buttock distance (1cm=1.5° approximately).

---

[43] The fat pad may become tender and swollen and give pain on extension of the knee especially when nipped between femur and tibia. Seen in osteoarthritis or young women with pre-menstrual fluid retention. Cured by excision of fat pad.

[44] Lateral ligament from lateral femoral epicondyle to head of fibula. Medial ligament consists of superficial and deep parts attached above to medial epicondyle and below to medial tibia either side of the semimembranosus groove.

[45] Occurring in the 10–16 age group. Recurrent pain over tibial tuberosity that becomes tender and prominent. May be caused by partial avulsion of the tuberosity by the patellar ligament. Pain usually ceases with closure of the epiphysis. Management conservative so long as not completely avulsed.

[46] In teenage males as a result of the impingement of the femoral condyle against the tibial spines or cruciate ligaments. A segment of bone undergoes avascular necrosis. May separate and cause a loose body. Aching pain and recurrent effusion +/- locking. Conservative treatment includes quadriceps exercises. Fragment may be pinned or excised. Cavity may be drilled to encourage vascularisation.

[47] Full extension is 0°.

[48] A springy block to full extension is suggestive of bucket handle meniscus tear. A rigid block to full extension is common in arthritic conditions (fixed flexion deformity).

[49] If hyper-extended (X° of hyperextension) check the other leg and the elbow ?rare Ehlers-Danlos syndrome. Hyperextension (genu recurvatum) is seen in girls and is associated with a high patella, chondromalacia patellae, recurrent patellar dislocation and sometimes tears of the anterior cruciate, medial meniscus or medial ligament. It may be associated with ballet or high heels that retard upper tibial epiphysial growth. Polio and Charcot's disease are rare causes.

I will now examine the stability of the knee[50] **starting with the COLLATERAL LIGAMENTS.'**

Extend the knee fully. Grasp knee with one hand, heel of hand against the lateral knee, fingers under knee. Grasp the lower tibia with the other hand and push them in opposite directions stressing the knee in valgus. Look for the knee opening up[51]. *Compare the two sides. Repeat with knee flexed 30° and foot internally rotated*[52].

'Valgus stress instability test shows there is no gross instability of the medial ligaments.'

Repeat, heel of hand medially, stressing the lateral side looking for varus stress instability[53].

'Varus stress instability test shows there is no gross instability of the lateral ligaments. If there were, I should check the distribution of the common peroneal nerve[54] **to ensure it has escaped injury. Now I would like to examine the stability of the CRUCIATES.'**

Flex both knees to 90°; look from the side.

'I'm looking for tibial subluxation.'

Sit on the foot. Grasping the tibia with both hands, pull tibia forward (see fig on pg 146).

---

[50] **Summary of instability in knee**
1. Valgus stress test +ve if medial ligament torn
2. Varus stress test +ve if lateral ligament torn
3. Anterior drawer test +ve if anterior cruciate torn
4. Posterior drawer test +ve if posterior cruciate torn
Rotatory instabilities:
5. Anteromedial instability with 1+3
    medial tibial condyle subluxates anteriorly on anterior drawer test
6. Anterolateral instability with 2+3
    lateral tibial condyle subluxates anteriorly on anterior drawer test
    test with MacIntosh test, Losee test or pivot shift test
7. Posterolateral instability with 2+4
    lateral tibial condyle subluxates posteriorly on post-drawer test

[51] Moderate valgus is a sign of major medial and posterior ligament rupture. Severe valgus indicates additional cruciate (esp. posterior cruciate) rupture. The medial ligament may be slightly torn (sprain), calcified after haematoma (Pellegrini Stieda disease) or ruptured. Partial tears are treated by immobilisation in plaster. Complete acute tears are repaired surgically.

[52] Abnormal amount of valgus in slight flexion suggests less extensive involvement of the medial structures.

[53] Instability in extension suggests lateral ligament complex and maybe posterior cruciate damage. The lateral ligament often tears at the fibular attachment close to the common peroneal nerve. Complete tears are treated surgically.

[54] Sensory loss over the dorsum and lateral side of the lower leg and loss of ability to dorsiflex foot.

'The anterior drawer test is negative[55]. If there were any sign of rotational instability during the anterior drawer test this can be confirmed by the Macintosh test[56], Losee test[57] or pivot shift test[58].'

(The Lachman test[59] is an alternative to the anterior drawer test but more difficult with small hands!)

Now jerk tibia backwards.

'The posterior drawer test is negative[60] (see fig on pg 146). I would now like to examine the MENISCI[61]. I have already inspected for cysts[62] and palpated the joint line for tenderness earlier.'

Put your fingers and thumb along the joint line, palm on the patella. With knee flexed, sweep the foot around in a U shape. Extend the leg.

'I am listening for crepitus and feeling for clicks.'

Now perform the McMurray test.

'In the McMurray test for the medial meniscus (see fig on pg 146), the leg is flexed (1), the foot externally rotated (2) and the hip is abducted (3). Clicks and grating are felt for while leg is smoothly extended (4).

---

[55] If anterior displacement is >1.5 cm then anterior cruciate is almost certainly torn +/- medial ligament and capsule damage. If one condyle moves forward more than the other there may be antero-lateral or antero-medial instability (anterior cruciate plus lateral or medial ligament injury respectively). Anterior cruciate tears often occur after tears of medial meniscus that block full extension. Isolated anterior cruciate tears do not often need surgery. If acute or associated with instability surgery may involve a) adductor gracilis as dynamic replacement, b) tube pedicle from iliotibial tract or c) carbon fibre implants.

[56] **MacIntosh test (see fig on pg 146)**: fully extend knee. Hold foot in internal rotation (1). Apply valgus stress (2+3). Gradually flex knee (4), it will jerk at 30° as the tibial condyle reduces. It confirms rotatory instability.

[57] **Losee test**: as above but starting with leg flexed, pushing on fibular head, gradually extend it and hear clunk as tibial condyle subluxates.

[58] **Pivot shift test (see fig on pg 146)**: with foot tucked in under arm tilted in valgus (1) and internally rotated (2), hold lower leg firmly with both hands and flex knee (3). The femoral condyle should appear to jerk forward as tibial condyle reduces since the tibia is fixed, and jerk backwards as tibia subluxates when leg is extended.

[59] **Active Lachman's test (see fig on pg 146)**: relax knee in 10° flexion. Hold femur with one hand and pull tibia forward with the other.

Passive Lachman's test: knee rests on bolster flexed at 30°. Patient asked to extend leg that leads to anterior subluxation of tibia with posterior subluxation on relaxation. Indicates complete anterior cruciate tear.

[60] If displaces >1 cm rupture of the posterior cruciate ligament is likely. If one condyle moves more than the other there may be posterolateral rotatory insufficiency (posterior cruciate + lateral ligaments).

[61] **Lesions of the menisci**

1) Congenital discoid meniscus in childhood – D shaped meniscus extends towards tibial spines and blocks extension and causes clicking. Treatment is excision.

2) Meniscus tears in the young adult usually a sporting injury when flexed leg is twisted. Longitudinal split (bucket handle tear) goes towards centre of joint and causes locking and rupture of anterior cruciate eventually in the case of the medial meniscus. Treated by excisions in whole or in part, rarely repair of peripheral lesions.

3) Degenerative meniscus lesions in middle age – usually horizontal. May resolve, may need excision.

[62] **Meniscal cysts** lie in the joint line, feel firm on palpation and are tender on deep pressure. They may be associated with tears and are usually on the lateral side. Be suspicious of cysts on the medial side, they may be ganglions arising from the insertion of sartorius, gracilis and semitendinosus.

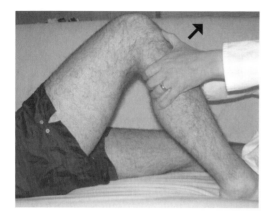

Anterior drawer test

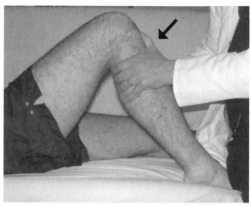

Posterior drawer test

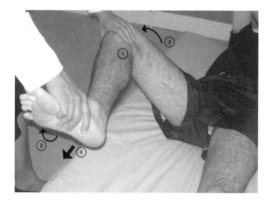

McMurray manoeuvre for the medial meniscus

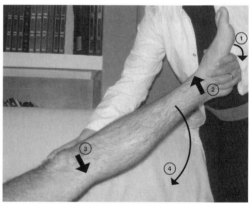

MacIntosh test

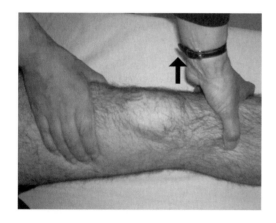

Active Lachman test

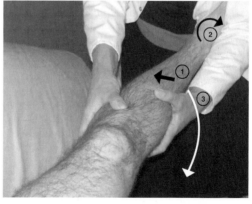

Modified pivot shift test

In the McMurray test for the lateral meniscus, the leg is flexed, the foot
internally rotated and the hip is adducted. Clicks and grating are felt for while
leg is smoothly extended. Now I would like to have a closer look at the
PATELLA. I examined the extensor apparatus earlier. I can palpate 2/3 of the
articular surface which may be diseased in chondromalacia patellae[63] and check
its mobility which may be restricted in retropatellar arthritis.'

*Displace the patella medially and laterally to palpate the under-surface. Move the
patella from side to side and up and down. Then do it pressing down on the
patella against the femur.*

'Is this sore? Pain is suggestive of chondromalacia patellae or retropatellar
arthritis. I would like to do the apprehension test.'

*Try to push the patella laterally while flexing the extended knee. Positive if patient
gets jumpy and tries to stop you.*

'A positive apprehension test indicates a tendency to recurrent dislocation[64]. I
would now like to examine the knee from BEHIND.'

Turn patient over, hold knee flexed.

'I am palpating the popliteal region with the knee flexed, and now looking for
bursae[65] with the knee extended.'

To the examiners:

'Finally I would like to examine this patient's GAIT and look for GENU VARUM[66]
or VALGUS[67] by observing her standing and then by requesting standing X-RAYS
of the knee with all the weight on each leg in turn. In a child I would measure
the INTER-MALLEOLAR GAP[68].'

---

[63] Chondromalacia patellae is common in girls. The articular surface of the patella becomes soft and spongy
giving rise to aching pain in front of the knee. It may follow recurrent dislocation of the patella and may lead to
retropatellar osteoarthrosis. Treatment: immobilise in plaster; may need surgical paring or even patellectomy.
Chronic anterior knee pain without changes of chondromalacia is common and just needs physiotherapy.

[64] **Recurrent dislocation of the patella** often follows a traumatic episode initially, often in a teenage girl. It may
spontaneously reduce or need manipulation, and thereafter may recurrently dislocate or be permanently
displaced laterally. Associated with knock-knees, hyperextension (genu recurvatum), a high patella,
underdeveloped lateral femoral condyle or abnormal attachment to quadriceps. Galeazzi repair is used before
epiphyseal closure using distal semitendinosus tendon. Hauser operation is used after epiphyseal closure. The
tibial tuberosity is transposed medially and distally to alter the line of pull of the patellar tendon.

[65] See pg 217. Cystic swelling in popliteal region. May cause pain worse on flexion. Commonly
semimembranosus bursa but can be other bursae. Treatment is excision. Prepatellar and infrapatellar bursitis also
occurs and can be aspirated or excised if recurrent.

[66] **Bowleg** is common in childhood and often resolves. May be caused by tibia vara or rarely by rickets and
treated by osteotomy. In adults osteoarthritis, rheumatoid arthritis or Paget's can be the cause.

[67] **Knock-knee** is seen in children, often with flat feet, and usually resolves by age 6. May contribute to recurrent
dislocation. In adults often occurs with rheumatoid arthritis, uncorrected tibial plateau fractures or neurological
disorders. Treatment is corrective osteotomy.

[68] In a child simply grasp the ankles while child is sitting or lying straight-legged. Rotate legs until patellae are
vertical then bring legs together until the knees just touch and measure the gap between the malleoli. Serial
measurements every six months.

EXAMINATION OF RHEUMATOID HANDS

'Hello, my name is Dr Parchment Smith. May I examine your hands please? Could you roll up your sleeves above the elbow? Do you mind if I talk about you to these doctors as I go along? Put both your hands on your lap/on this table.'

LOOK at the hands. To the examiners:

'On inspection there is a symmetrical deforming polyarthropathy of the small joints of the hand. There is spindling of the fingers due to soft tissue swelling at the proximal interphalangeal joints and metacarpal phalangeal joints but the distal interphalangeal joints are spared. There is wasting of the small muscles of the hands[69]. The skin looks thin and there is some bruising[70].'

Pick the hands up and look at the fingers individually.

'On closer inspection I can see that there is ulnar deviation of the fingers[71], radial deviation at the wrist, and swan neck[72]/boutonnière[73]/Z thumb deformities of these fingers.' (indicate which)

'I can see scars of previous surgery over the wrist[74]/thumb[75]/interphalangeal joints[76].'

'The nail beds are pale and there are/are no vasculitic lesions[77] in the nail folds or fingers. There is no nail pitting or scaly rash[78].'

To the patient:

'Could you turn the hands over and show me your palms?
On the palms I am looking for pallor in the palmar creases indicating anaemia[79], and palmar erythema[80]. I am now going to palpate the joints.'

---

[69] Disuse atrophy. Pain and deformity limit use.

[70] Due to steroid use.

[71] Due to subluxation and dislocation at the MCP joints.

[72] Swan neck – hyperextension of PIP joints with fixed flexion of MCP and DIP joints due to tendon prolapse (see pg 195).

[73] Boutonnière (English translation – 'button hook') flexion deformity of PIP with extension contracture of DIP and MCP joints (see pg 195).

[74] Usually arthrodesis for strength and stability.

[75] Usually arthrodesis in the MCP joint, again for strength and stability.

[76] Usually arthroplasty with silastic spacers for flexibility and pain relief.

[77] Nail fold infarcts caused by an associated vasculitis that can also cause chronic leg ulceration, purpuric rash and Raynaud's phenomenon. The vasculitis is immune complex induced and may affect small, medium or large vessels.

[78] **Psoriatic arthropathy** is an asymmetric arthropathy involving mainly the DIP joints with pitting of the fingernails, onycholysis and hyperkeratosis. There is a red and silvery scaly rash over the extensor surfaces and behind the ears (see pg 199).

[79] There are five causes of anaemia in rheumatoid arthritis (see pg 192).

[80] Redness around palm sparing the central area, associated with pregnancy, RA, liver disease.

FEEL each joint gently and quickly.

'There is evidence of bony destruction of the PIP and MCP joints with sparing of the DIP joints. I can't feel any rheumatoid nodules[81] **or Heberden's nodes**[82] **in the hand. None of the joints are tender or warm at present**[83]**.'**

Feel the wrist. Now grip the arm.

'I am now going to carry out a basic assessment of MOVEMENT and FUNCTION.'

To the patient:

'Can you move your wrist up and down? Now circle it. Can you grip my fingers? Harder! OK, can you touch each finger with your thumb like this? Now can you undo and do up the button on the front of your shirt?'

While they are doing this, say to the examiners:

'Both power grip and pincer grip are incomplete, and wrist function is impaired. Function is affected but pretty well preserved despite the weakness, pain and deformity.'

Touching first the little finger[84]*, then the index finger*[85]*, then the anatomical snuffbox*[86]*. To the patient:*

'Can you feel me touching you here? and here? and here? I am looking for SENSORY DEFICIT in the distribution of the median, ulnar and radial nerves.'

'Finally can I look at your ELBOW? There are two firm subcutaneous nodules lending support to my diagnosis of rheumatoid arthritis.'

To the examiners:

'To complete my examination I would like to see if any of the OTHER JOINTS are affected[87] **and look for EXTRA-ARTICULAR MANIFESTATIONS of rheumatoid arthritis**[88]**. I would also like to see the X-RAYS of these hands**[89]**.'**

---

[81] Firm subcutaneous nodules caused by immune complex deposition.

[82] Bony osteophytes which occur in osteoarthritis secondary to rheumatoid arthritis. Primary osteoarthritis of the hands tends to affect the thumb and distal interphalangeal joints of the fingers. In general it is not as mutilating or deforming as rheumatoid disease.

[83] Indicating 'active' arthritis.

[84] Ulnar nerve: typically affected by rheumatoid nodules on the elbows. Usually better to assess nerves by sensation rather than power since the hand may be too weak to assess motor supply.

[85] Median nerve: affected in carpal tunnel syndrome, associated with RA.

[86] Radial nerve: no specific associations, but bear in mind that sensation in any distribution may be affected by cervical spine disease.

[87] Typically knees, neck, elbows, shoulders.

[88] **Extra-articular manifestations of rheumatoid arthritis** (see pg 192).

[89] **X-ray signs of rheumatoid arthritis** (see pg 192).

EXAMINATION OF THE SHOULDER

'Hello, my name is Dr Parchment Smith. Would you mind if I examined your shoulder? Do you mind if I talk to these doctors as I go along? Will you take a seat in the centre of the room please?'

LOOK from the front, crouching down. To the examiners:

'I am inspecting for asymmetry and obvious deformity. From the centre out, I am looking in particular for a prominent sterno-clavicular joint[90], deformity of the clavicle[91], prominent acromio-clavicular joint[92] and deltoid wasting[93].'

Move to the side.

'From the side I am looking for swelling of the joint[94].'

Look from above.

'Now I am looking from above for swelling, asymmetry of the supraclavicular fossae or deformity of the clavicle.'

Move behind.

'Now I am inspecting the scapulae and the back, again for asymmetry, wasting, abnormally high or small scapula[95].'

To the patient:

'Can you stand up and push your hands against the wall? I am looking for winging of the scapula[96].'

---

[90] Indicates subluxation. **Dislocation of the sternoclavicular joint** is comparatively uncommon. There is always a history of trauma and joint asymmetry is obvious. Hard to see on X-ray, only rarely needs surgery.

[91] Indicates an old fracture.

[92] Indicates subluxation or osteoarthritis. **Acromioclavicular dislocation** may occur as a result of a fall on the outstretched hand. In major injuries the conoid and trapezoid ligaments are torn and clavicle is very unstable. Surgical fixation of the clavicle to coronoid may be needed. Normally only a sling is needed. Hard to see on X-ray.

[93] Disuse or axillary nerve palsy.

[94] Infection or inflammatory reaction e.g. from calcifying supraspinatus tendinitis or from trauma.

Calcifying supraspinatus tendinitis often accompanies degenerative changes in the shoulder cuff. The mechanism is local deposition of calcium salts that may be asymptomatic or may give rise to sudden incapacitating subdeltoid bursitis. Tender swollen warm acute joint relieved by aspiration, hydrocortisone injections or curettage.

[95] Occurs in Sprengel shoulder and the Klippel-Feil syndrome. There are several related congenital malformations affecting the neck and shoulder girdle. In the most minor cases one of the scapulae may be slightly smaller or higher than the other.

Sprengel shoulder: congenital malformation with one or both shoulders high, scapulae small, +/- webs of skin running from the shoulder to neck.

Klippel-Feil syndrome: high scapulae, short neck, multiple anomalies of cervical vertebrae including vertebral body fusions, spina bifida. Also associated with diasomatomyelia, cord tethering, lumbosacral lipomata and renal abnormalities.

[96] Due to weakness of serratus anterior (see pg 228).

Now FEEL. To the examiners:

'**I am now going to palpate the joint. Tell me if this is tender**[97]**. I am feeling the anterior and lateral aspects of the glenohumeral joint**[98]**. Lift your arm for me please, I am now feeling the humeral shaft and head via the axilla**[99]**. Now I will palpate the acromio-clavicular joint for tenderness or lipping**[100]**, and move the arm while palpating it, listening for crepitations**[101] **and for tenderness during movement**[102]**. Now I am feeling for local tenderness along the clavicle**[103] **and finally the sterno-clavicular joint.**'

Now go on to MOVE the joint – do the movements yourself to encourage the patient!

'**I would now like to assess the movements of the joint. Can you raise both arms slowly out to the side like this? Carry on right over your head. Can your shoulders touch your ears? Is it painful at all? Hold your arms there. Now release them slowly back down to your side, telling me if it's sore, thank you.**'

---

[97] **Infections around the shoulder**
Staphylococcal osteitis of the proximal humerus is the commonest infection in UK but still pretty rare.
TB of the shoulder is now rare; moist form: commonest in first two decades of life, shoulder swollen, abundant pus production, rapid destruction. Dry form: caroies sicca in older patients, slow progress, little destruction or pus formation.
Gonococcal arthritis of the shoulder is uncommon; there is moderate swelling of the joint and great pain that often seems out of keeping with the physical signs.
[98] Diffuse tenderness is suggestive of infection or calcifying supraspinatus tendinitis.
[99] Exostoses of the proximal humeral shaft are palpable via this route.
[100] Tenderness is found after recent dislocations and in osteoarthritis. Lipping is usually palpable in osteoarthritis. **Osteoarthritis** of the glenohumeral joint is rare and most frequently occurs secondary to aseptic necrosis of the humeral head which may be idiopathic, following high fractures or in deep-sea divers. Rheumatoid is more common. Osteoarthritis in the acromioclavicular joint gives rise to prolonged pain associated with shoulder movements. Usually obvious prominence of the joint with arthritic lipping and well-localised tenderness. Conservative treatment with local heat and exercises may be helpful but occasionally acromionectomy may be needed.
[101] In osteoarthritis.
[102] Sudden tenderness during a portion of the arc of movement is found in tears or inflammatory lesions involving the shoulder cuff and/or subdeltoid bursa. **Shoulder cuff tears** may result from sudden traction. It occurs most readily in the middle aged where degenerative changes in the shoulder cuff have become established. Most commonly the supraspinatus tendon is involved thereby causing difficulty initiating abduction of the arm. In other cases a torn or inflamed supraspinatus tendon impinges upon the acromion during abduction giving rise to a painful arc of movement. The range of passive movements is not initially disturbed but limitation of rotation may supervene leading to a 'frozen shoulder'.
[103] Tender in sternoclavicular dislocations, infections especially TB, tumours (rare) and radionecrosis (e.g. after treatment for breast cancer, which may be mistaken for mets). X-ray if local tenderness in seen.

To the examiners:

'In observing active ABDUCTION I am looking for initiation of abduction[104]**, painful arc during abduction**[105]**, and ability to hold the arm fully abducted**[106]**.'**

If the patient has restricted active abduction:

'Now I would like to test the passive abduction, rotating the arm externally first[108]**. Now I would like to test abduction with a fixed scapula**[109]**. Now I would like to test adduction**[110] **which should be around 50°.'**

Now look from the side.

'Can you swing your arms forward and right above your head? I am checking active FORWARD FLEXION, which is normally 165°. Now swing them back. Backward extension should be 60°. Could you put your arms behind your back as high up as you can, reaching for your shoulder blade? This is a screening test of internal rotation[111]**. Can you put your hands behind your head? This is a screening test of external rotation**[112]**. Keep your hands behind your head. I am just going to gently pull your elbows back to check for any difference.'**

'Now tuck your elbows into your sides, elbows bent, hands stretched out in front. Swing your hands out like a door (see fig on pg 153). This is EXTERNAL ROTATION in extension exclusively at the glenohumeral joint[113]**. Now swing your arms in across your stomach, keeping the elbows in to the side. That is INTERNAL ROTATION exclusively at the glenohumeral joint (see fig on pg 153). Lift your elbows out to the side to the level of the shoulders, forearms hanging down like a puppet.**

Now swing the arms up till you're standing like a weight lifter. This is a check of internal and external rotation in abduction (see fig on pg 153).'

---

[104] Difficulty in initiating abduction is suggestive of a shoulder cuff or supraspinatus tendon tear. These patients may use a trick movement to initiate abduction i.e. leaning over or 'flicking' the arm out. After initiation the deltoid takes over.

[105] A painful arc from 70°-100° is suggestive of a shoulder cuff lesion (e.g. tear, degenerative changes). A higher painful arc from 100–150° is suggestive of osteoarthritis of the acromio-clavicular joint.

[106] If the patient can hold the arm up in a vertical position, deltoid and the axillary nerve are likely to be intact.

[107] Restricted abduction will occur in the **frozen shoulder**. This is a clinical syndrome caused by various pathologies that can seldom be differentiated. Affects the middle aged whose shoulder cuffs are degenerative. Severe limitation of glenohumeral joint movement, especially internal rotation, and pain which disturbs sleep are characteristic. Frequently a history of minor trauma, immobility or myocardial infarct initiating symptoms. X-rays usually normal. Treatment includes graduated shoulder exercises, hydrocortisone injections or MUA.

[108] This delays the impingement of the greater tuberosity on the glenoid rim, thus increasing the gleno-humeral range of abduction to slightly over 90°.

[109] Fix the angle of the scapula with one hand; abduct the arm with the other. You should get 90° glenohumeral abduction unless this joint is restricted.

[110] Patient puts his hand on the opposite shoulder; you swing his elbow across his chest.

[111] Hand should reach top of scapula on opposite side. Screens internal rotation in extension. This movement is commonly affected in frozen shoulder.

[112] Should be able to get hands behind the neck. Screens external rotation at 90° abduction. This movement is compromised in frozen shoulder.

[113] The normal range is 70° external rotation (from forearms sticking straight out forward).

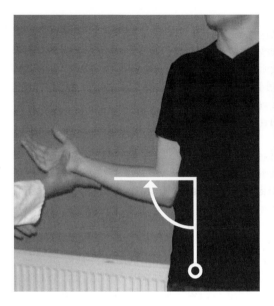

External rotation in extension

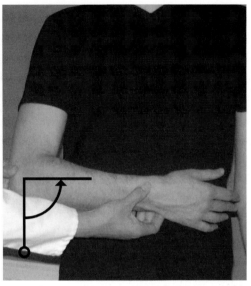

Internal rotation in extension

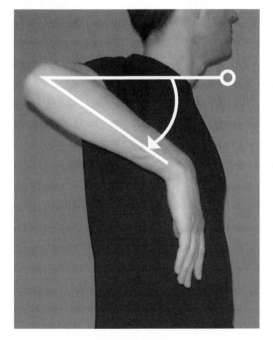

Internal rotation in abduction

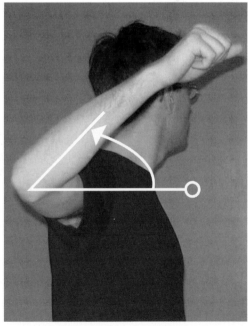

External rotation in abduction

To the examiners:

'I am just going to feel for CREPITATIONS.'

Place one hand over the shoulder, the middle finger lying along the acromio-clavicular joint. Abduct the arm, feeling and listening for crepitations[114].

'Now I would like to check for DELTOID POWER[115]. Lift your elbow out to the side. I'm going to feel this muscle. Keep your elbow there. Don't let me push it down. Can you feel me touching you here on the shoulder?'

To the examiners:

To complete my examination, I would like to examine the CERVICAL SPINE[116] and check SENSATION and REFLEXES in the arm.

Depending on the history there are certain special tests that may be appropriate, such as the DRAWER TESTS (of Gerber and Ganz)[117], for recurrent dislocation[118] or the test for RUPTURED LONG TENDON OF BICEPS[119]. Finally, I would like to see the X-rays.'

---

[114] This may indicate osteoarthritis of the acromioclavicular joint (common) or glenohumeral joint (less common).

[115] Traction injuries of the axillary nerve resulting in deltoid involvement and numb 'regimental badge' area are seen after dislocations of the shoulder.

[116] Shoulder pain or arm weakness can be due to problems with the cervical spine.

[117] **Drawer tests of Gerber and Ganz.**

For anterior dislocation (patient lying supine): hold upper arm relaxed in one hand, in 90° abduction, slightly flexed and in slight external rotation. Hold scapula in other hand with thumb on coracoid and fingers behind. Try to pull the humeral head anteriorly. Observe movements, clicks and patient apprehension (can use axial radiographs).

For posterior dislocation (patient supine): hold forearm in one hand. Elbow flexed, shoulder in slight flexion and 90° abduction. With other hand put thumb lateral to coracoid pressing humeral head backward with thumb while you internally rotate the shoulder and flex it to 80°. Feel for backward displacement with the thumb. Can use X-rays.

[118] **Recurrent dislocation of the shoulder** is seen in 20–40 age group. History of previous frank dislocations of the shoulder with less trauma each time. Repair advised if 4 or more dislocations. Beware **habitual dislocation of the shoulder** in a psychotic patient or one with joint laxity syndrome in which the patient painlessly voluntarily dislocates and reduces shoulder. X-ray changes may be absent.

[119] Support elbow; hold wrist with other hand and get patient to flex elbow against resistance. If the long tendon of biceps is ruptured, belly of biceps will appear globular in shape. Compare sides. **Rupture of the long head of biceps** may occur spontaneously or as the result of a sudden muscular effort, usually in a middle aged or elderly patient in whom degenerative tendon changes are present. No treatment is usually required (see pg 233).

EXAMINATION OF THE NECK

'Hello, my name is Dr Parchment Smith. May I examine your neck? Could you sit on a chair facing me? Would you mind if I talk to these doctors as I go along? I would like the neck and shoulders exposed if possible.'

Stand back and LOOK from the front, then move to inspect from behind.

'On inspection I am looking for asymmetry or obvious deformity, torticollis, scars, sinuses or muscle wasting. The head is held in a normal position. Now I would like to FEEL the neck. Is it tender anywhere?'

From behind feel gently in the midline from the occiput downwards.

'I am feeling for localised tenderness and any obvious step or deformity[121].

Now feel the lateral aspects of the vertebrae.

'I am feeling for masses and tenderness laterally.'

Now feel the supraclavicular fossae from behind.

'I am feeling for a prominent cervical rib[122], tumour masses, or enlarged lymph nodes and I am quickly feeling for obvious abnormalities in the anterior triangle of the neck such as the thyroid gland. Palpation is normal with no local tenderness, muscle spasm or increased temperature. I'd now like to assess MOVEMENTS[123].'

Look from the side.

'Could you put your chin to your chest please? I am assessing FORWARD FLEXION[124]. Now tip your head as far back as it can go – I'm assessing EXTENSION[125]. Touch your ear to your shoulder like this, good, now the other side. This is LATERAL FLEXION[126]. Now can you look backwards over your right shoulder? and your left? this is testing for ROTATION[127].'

---

[120] Note the most prominent spinous process is that of T1 not the so called 'vertebra prominens' C7.

[121] **Cervical spondylosis** (osteoarthritis of the cervical spine) is the most common condition affecting the neck. It can start in the third decade and usually affects the disc between C5 and C6. It is difficult to detect a restriction of movement clinically because of the compensating mobility of the other cervical vertebrae. Sharply localised pain centrally or to the side of the neck is felt, often radiating to the occiput or to the lower scapula. Nerve root involvement leads to pain or neurological signs of the arm in a dermatomal distribution. Infections such as TB causing **osteitis of the cervical spine** are rare in the UK but may produce localised pain or a 'step' due to vertebral collapse.

[122] See pg 319, *The Circulatory System*, Chapter 4.

[123] A **goniometer** is an instrument for measuring these angles accurately. Don't try to use one but know the principle (look through it and read off the angle using a spatula clenched in the patient's teeth as a marker).

[124] Normally the chin can touch the chest.

[125] The plane of the nose and the forehead should be nearly horizontal. Watch out for the lumbar spine and thoracic spine bending back to contribute.

[126] The ear should touch the shoulder with only slight shoulder shrugging (45°). If lateral flexion cannot be carried out without forward flexion this is indicative of atlanto-axial and atlanto-occipital joint disease. These two joints are responsible for about a fifth of the total range of lateral flexion. Loss is common in osteoarthritis.

[127] Normally the chin falls just short of the plane of the shoulder (80° to either side). About a third of this movement occurs in the first two cervical joints. Rotation is usually restricted and painful in osteoarthritis of the spine.

Spread your hands on each side of the neck and feel as the patient flexes and extends his neck.

'I am feeling for CREPITATIONS[128]**, can you bend your head forward and back as if you are slowly nodding?'**

Step away from the patient.

'To complete my examination I would like to check for the signs of a CERVICAL RIB[129]**, do a NEUROLOGICAL EXAMINATION of the arms**[130] **and view the lateral, AP and peg view**[131] **X-RAYS.**

---

[128] Facet joint crepitations are normally detected in this way and are a common finding in cervical osteoarthritis.
[129] See pg 319, *The Circulatory System*, Chapter 4.
[130] See pg 169.
[131] Anterior-posterior through the mouth views of C1-C3 showing the odontoid process.

Examination of a cervical spine X-ray

Is it complete? Can you see all 7 cervical vertebrae and the top of the first thoracic vertebra?

Lateral view
1. Cervical curve: normally convex anteriorly, can be:
    Reduced (positional error or spasm)
    Kinked (subluxation or intense local spasm)
2. General shape of the vertebrae noting:
    Vertebral fusion (congenital)
    Vertebral collapse (fracture, tumour, TB)
3. Position of each vertebra compared with those above and below it.
    Displacement occurs in dislocation, which may be unilateral (25% displacement) or bilateral facet dislocation (50% displacement).
4. Disc spaces and margins looking for:
    Disc space narrowing (osteoarthritis)
    Anterior and posterior lipping (osteoarthritis)
    Fusion (ankylosing spondylitis)
5. Fractures: Unstable fractures of C3–7 show one or more of the following signs:
- Disruption of the anterior and all of the posterior elements
- A fracture with the upper vertebra overriding the vertebra beneath it by more than 3 mm
- A fracture with angulation between two adjoining vertebra of more than 11°.
6. The position of the odontoid peg
- The anterior arch of the atlas should not lie more than 4 mm in front of the axis (rupture/laxity of transverse ligament)
- Upward migration of the odontoid peg is seen in rheumatoid arthritis.
7. The pharyngeal shadow
If this is not lying close to the vertebral bodies there may be a space-occupying haematoma, tumour or retropharyngeal abscess.
8. Flexion and extension views: to detect instability.

A-P view
1. Shape of vertebral bodies: lateral wedging may result from fracture, tumour or infection. A cervical rib may be seen.

C1–3 through the mouth (peg) views
1. Symmetry in alignment of the odontoid process with the atlas.
2. Fracture through odontoid peg (beware congenital failure of fusion of ossification centres which looks like a fracture.

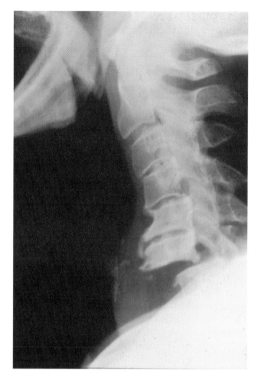

Lateral C spine X-ray showing anterior
dislocation of C6 on C7

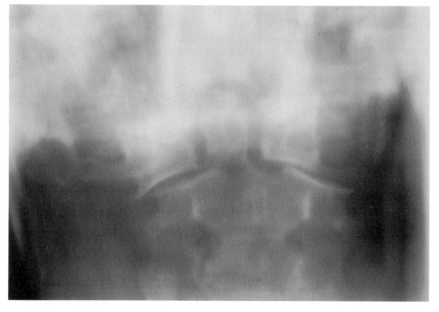

'Peg view' showing fracture of odontoid process

EXAMINATION OF THE BACK

'Hello, my name is Dr Parchment Smith. May I examine your back? Can you stand with your back to me with your trousers down? Is it OK if I talk to these doctors about you as I go along?'

Stand back and LOOK.

'On inspection from the back I am looking for any obvious scoliosis[132]. There are no obvious swellings[133], scars[134], abnormal pigmentation[135], hair[136], or café au lait spots[137].'

If there is a scoliosis, ask the patient to sit to exclude a compensatory scoliosis[138] and bend forward to exclude a postural scoliosis[139] before diagnosing a structural scoliosis[140].

Now look from the side.

'From the side I am looking for a kyphosis[141] or a gibbus[142] of the thoracic frame. I am also looking at the lumbar curvature[143]. I am now going to palpate the spine.'

FEEL from the prominent T1 vertebral spine down, palpating between the spines of the vertebrae, the muscles either side of the lumbar spine, and along the sacro-iliac joint.

---

[132] Scoliosis is a lateral curvature of the spine. The commonest cause for a scoliosis is a protective scoliosis secondary to a prolapsed intervertebral disc.

[133] A fat pad may indicate spina bifida.

[134] Previous thoracotomy or spinal surgery.

[135] May indicate spina bifida.

[136] May indicate spina bifida.

[137] May indicate neurofibromatosis.

[138] For example in a shortened leg.

[139] Occurs most commonly in adolescent girls and usually resolves spontaneously.

[140] In structural scoliosis there is alteration of vertebral shape and mobility, and the deformity cannot be corrected by alteration of posture, and on sitting forward a rib hump may be seen.

True structural scoliosis may be
    Idiopathic (the commonest)
    Congenital: (e.g.hemivertebra, fused vertebra, fused ribs)
    Paralytic (e.g. polio)
    Neuropathic (e.g. neurofibromatosis, cerebral palsy, spina bifida, syringomyelia, Friedreich's ataxia)
    Myopathic (e.g. muscular dystrophy, arthrogryphosis)
    Metabolic (e.g. Marfan's disease, rickets)

[141] **Kyphosis** is an increased forward curvature of the spine The commonest causes are senile kyphosis (worsened by osteoporosis, osteomalacia and pathological fracture) and ankylosing spondylitis. Scheurmann's disease (spinal osteochondrosis) is idiopathic vertebral wedging that often leads to osteoarthritis.

[142] **A gibbus** is an undue prominence of a spinous process often associated with an abrupt angular kyphosis. The commonest causes are fracture (traumatic or pathological), tuberculosis or a congenital vertebral abnormality.

[143] Flattened in prolapsed intervertebral disc, osteoarthritis of the spine, infected vertebral bodies and ankylosing spondylitis. Increased curvature is seen as a normal variant (especially in women), in spondylolisthesis or secondary to increased thoracic kyphosis or to a flexion deformity of the hip.

'Tell me if it's tender here... here... here. I am looking for tenderness over the lumbar spine[144], over the lumbar muscles[145] and along the sacroiliac joints[146]. *Slide the fingers down the spine.*
'I can't feel a step in the lumbar spine[147]. Bend forward please?'
Lightly tap the spine with your fist from the neck to the sacroiliac joint.
'There is no marked localised pain on percussion[148]. I am now going to test MOVEMENTS. Can you try to lean forward as far as you can? This estimates FORWARD FLEXION. The patient flexes to within 7 centimetres of the floor[149]. If his flexion is limited I can mark the spine to determine if the limitation is in the thoracic or lumbar spine[150]. Now can you stand with your hands on your buttocks and lean back slowly, letting your hands slide down the back of your leg? This is EXTENSION that is normally about 30° in total[151]. Now can you stand up straight with your hands resting against your thighs? Lean to the left, not leaning forward or back, and slide your hand down your left leg. Now to the right. I am checking LATERAL FLEXION that should be around 30°[152]. Now can you sit down, cross your arms and, without moving your bum on the seat, twist your shoulders as far round as you can ... to the left ... now the right. This is checking ROTATION which is normally up to 40°[153]. Could you lie down flat on your back please?'
To the examiners:
'I am now going to screen for a PROLAPSED INTERVERTEBRAL DISC.'

---

[144] Common in prolapsed intervertebral discs.

[145] Common in prolapsed intervertebral discs or mechanical back pain.

[146] Seen in mechanical back pain and sacroiliac joint infections.

[147] Due to spondylolisthesis where the vertebra (usually L5) slips forward on S1 due to a fracture or fatigue of the part of L5 anterior to the downward projecting inferior articular process (spondylolysis). Incidence increases with age. It causes low back pain radiating into the buttock and may need local spinal fusion, especially if associated with disc protrusion or stretching of the cauda equina or lumbosacral plexus.

[148] TB or other joint infections.

[149] This is the normal range. It is an indication of overall thoracic and lumbar movement but be aware that the hips play an important role in this action and may mask limitations in the spine or limit flexion in the presence of a normal spine. Actual normal range of flexion is 45° thoracic and 60° lumbar.

[150] To mark the spine use **Schrober's method**: Mark a point midline between the dimples of Venus and another point 10 cm above it. This approximates to the lumbar spine. Measure the distance between the two points when the patient is standing and when the spine is maximally flexed forward. The increase should be 8–10cm (<3 cm suggests severe restriction). Do the same for the thoracic spine marking the prominent T1 spinous process and a point 20 cm distal to that. The increase should be about 8 cm. Gross restriction of flexion is an outstanding feature of ankylosing spondylitis.

[151] Theoretically 25° thoracic, 35° lumbar but usually only 30° total. Pain on extension is common in prolapsed intervertebral disc.

[152] The contributions of the thoracic and lumbar spine are about equal.

[153] This is almost entirely thoracic with <5° contributed by the lumbar spine.

To the patient:
'Bend your knee with your foot in the air[154] **and let me move your foot out...
and in. This is a quick test to eliminate gross osteoarthritis of the hips that can
be confused with lower back pain (see fig on pg 162). I will now do a straight
leg raise test**[155]**. Can you straighten the leg and let me lift it? Stop me when you
feel pain.'**
Lift the leg by the heel keeping the knee straight.
**'Now? Is that pain along the back of your leg or in your back? What about if I
move your foot like this?'**
Passively dorsiflex the foot.
'If I suspected a high prolapse I could perform the reverse Lasègue test[156]**. If I
suspected functional overlay I could test for this also**[157]**.
I am now going to test the sacroiliac joint (see fig on pg 162). Can you bend the
knee? I'm just going to press it across your body**[158]**. Does that make the pain
worse? Now I'm going to grasp your hip bones**[159] **– does this make the pain
worse?'**

---

[154] The hip and knee should be flexed to 90°. You are doing a quick check for external and internal rotation at the hip.
[155] **The straight leg raise (see fig on pg 162) test for:**
    Nerve root irritation (usually by lateral disc prolapse)
    If paraesthesia or radiating root pains (sciatica) down the leg (must be distinguished from hamstring tightness)
    Raising the good leg can produce signs in the relaxed bad leg
    Passive dorsiflexion increases tension in the nerve roots.
    Central disc prolapse
    If pain is in the back.
[156] **The reverse Lasègue test for high lumbar disc lesions (see fig on pg 162)** (rare compared with L5/S1 and L4/L5 lesions)
    Lay the patient prone
    Flex each knee in turn
    This stretches the femoral nerve roots and gives rise to pain in high lumbar lesions
    Lifting the knee off the bed thus extending the hip will aggravate it.
[157] **Tests for functional overlay** (e.g. malingerers, Munchausen's)
    1. Sit them up after the straight leg raise and pretend to examine their back. If they can sit up with their legs straight they should have been able to straight leg raise to 90°.
    2. With the patient standing press firmly with both hands on the head, this should not exacerbate the pain in genuine cases.
    3. Pinch the skin at the side, such superficial stimulation should not influence the back pain.
    4. Make the patient stand with his arms straight firmly held by the sides and tell him to turn from side to side. Most of the rotation occurs in the legs so should not be restricted by back pathology.
    If three out of four of these tests are positive, surgery should be considered with caution and only in the presence of firm evidence of causative pathology.
[158] Flex the hip and knee and forcibly adduct the hip. Pain is very non-specific but may suggest early ankylosing spondylitis, tuberculosis and other infections, Reiter's syndrome or sacroiliitis.
[159] Hook the thumbs round the anterior superior iliac spines and try to 'open out' the pelvis. Pain suggests sacroiliac involvement.

Step back and say to the examiners:

'To complete my examination I would do a neurological examination of the legs[160], check the femoral pulses[161] and do an abdominal examination[162]. I would also check the ESR[163] and the AP and lateral thoracic and lumbar spine X-rays.'

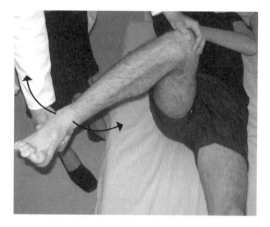

Screening hips

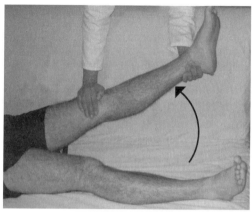

Straight leg raise

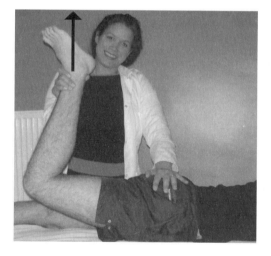

Reverse Lasègue test

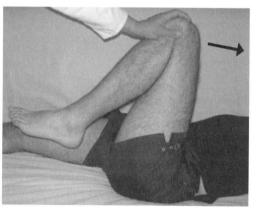

Test for sacro-iliac joint involvement

---

[160] See pg 177. Especially important are the ankle jerk (S1, 2) or knee jerk (L3, 4), power on dorsiflexion (L4, 5) and plantar flexion (S1, 2) and sensation at the lateral border of the foot (S1).

[161] Back, buttock and leg pain can be claudication due to iliac artery stenosis, especially if exercise related.

[162] Ensure no gross abdominal malignancy is causing the back pain by radiation (e.g. pancreatic), metastasis (e.g. prostate) or nerve involvement (e.g. colonic).

[163] Normal in prolapsed disc, mechanical back pain and Scheuermann's disease, but almost invariably elevated in ankylosing spondylitis, infections and neoplasms. False positives are common.

EXAMINATION OF THE OTHER JOINTS

If required to examine any joints other than those described in detail on previous pages, follow the principle of LOOK, FEEL then MOVE.

EXAMINATION OF THE ELBOW

LOOK
Valgus, varus, wasting, lumps, scars.
FEEL
Back and sides.
Warmth, nodules, synovium, fluid.
Palpate:
• Either side of olecranon
• Joint line by pronating and supinating forearm
• Ulnar nerve
MOVE
Flexion and extension (with arms outstretched level with shoulders)
Pronation and supination (with elbows to the sides, flexed at 90°)

THE ELBOW – COMMON CASES

Cubitus varus or cubitus valgus[164], rheumatoid arthritis[165], osteoarthritis,[166] tennis elbow[167], ulnar neuritis[168], olecranon bursitis (see pg 216), myositis ossificans[169].

---

[164] **Cubitus varus or valgus**: decrease or increase in the carrying angle of the elbow commonly after supracondylar fracture in childhood. Can be corrected by osteotomy.
Valgus = Lateral deviation of distal limb when in anatomical position. Remember there is an L in valgus and lateral.
[165] **Rheumatoid arthritis**: may be unilateral or bilateral. Characteristic RA of hands is often present. Look for rheumatoid nodules. Arthroplasty may be considered if functional disablement is severe.
[166] **Osteoarthritis**: primary in manual labourers, commonly secondary to old fractures. May have loose bodies causing locking of the joint.
[167] **Tendonitis of the common extensor origin**: is the commonest cause of elbow pain. Usually aged 35–50 years. Pain on lateral side of elbow, difficult to hold objects at arm's length. Ask about repetitive movements e.g. sweeping, painting and decorating. Relieved by injections of steroid and local anaesthetic. **Common flexor origin tendonitis** on the medial side of the elbow (golfer's elbow) is less common.
[168] **Ulnar neuritis**: irritation of the ulnar nerve after trauma or due to excess mobility as the nerve slips repeatedly over the medial epicondyle. Can be anchored or transposed.
[169] **Myositis ossificans**: most commonly occurs after supracondylar fractures or dislocated elbow. Due to calcification in the haematoma of the brachialis muscle. May also occur after inadequate immobilisation or aggressive passive physiotherapy. Leads to mechanical block to flexion. Treatment is prevention and delayed excision if necessary.

EXAMINATION OF THE ANKLE AND FOOT

LOOK
Standing
Legs, ankles, feet, arches, toes, obvious deformity.
Plantigrade foot (both heel and forefoot squarely on the floor), intoeing, genu valgum, flat foot, eversion, inversion, splaying, proportion.
Sitting
Heel: exostosis, bursitis, talipes, old fracture.
Dorsum: exostoses from 5th metacarpal head or base, cuneiform exostosis, dorsal ganglion – check dorsalis pedis pulse.
Big Toe: hallux valgus, bunion, gout, hallux rigidus, hallux flexus. Callous underneath?
Toenails: onychogryphosis, subungual exostosis, fungal infection, psoriasis.
Toes: length, clawing, hammertoe, mallet toe, quinti varus, corns.
Sole: hyperidrosis, athlete's foot, ulcers, callous, verruca, plantar fasciitis.
FEEL
Tenderness: heel (Sever's disease, exostosis, fasciitis, bursitis, pes cavus) forefoot, medial malleolus (tarsal tunnel syndrome) big toe.
Joint crepitations
Temperature
MOVE
Ankle joint: hold the shin still and grip the whole heel. Move the foot, there should be plantar flexion (55° from right angle), dorsiflexion (15° from right angle).
Subtalar joint: hold the ankle still and grip the lower heel. Move the heel – there should be inversion (10°); eversion (20°).
Forefoot (midtarsal and tarsometatarsal): hold the heel still and grip the forefoot. There should be inversion (15°); eversion (10°).
Now check plantar and dorsal flexion of the first, fifth and third metatarsophalangeal joints. Finally get the patient to curl their toes then extend them.

LIGAMENTS OF THE ANKLE AND FOOT

There are three main ligaments round the ankle.
1. Lateral ligament from fibula to talus and calcaneus. Feel for it below the lateral malleolus. Test for it by forcibly inverting the foot – if lax it will open up.
2. Medial (deltoid) ligament from the tibia to the talus, navicular, calcaneus and spring ligament. Very strong, rarely torn without a fracture.
3. The inferior tibio-fibular ligament. Feel for it just above the joint line on the dorsal surface of the ankle between the fibula and tibia. Test for it by dorsiflexing the foot (will produce pain) and trying to move the talus laterally (will displace laterally if ligament is disrupted).

THE ACHILLES TENDON

Palpate for a defect, then palpate while the patient plantar flexes against resistance (or stands on tiptoes).

ANKLE AND FOOT – COMMON CASES

Ankle

Diastasis/unstable ankle[170], ruptured Achilles[171], shortened Achilles[172], tenosynovitis[173], pseudogout (see pg xx- 65).

Forefoot

Pes cavus (see pg 227), gout (see pg 203), verrucas (see pg 68, superficial lesions), March fracture[174], Freiberg's disease[175], anterior metatarsalgia[176], Morton's neuroma[177], rheumatoid arthritis[178], tarsal tunnel syndrome[179], Hammer toe[180], mallet toe[181].

---

[170] **Diastasis**: usually as a result of fractures or ligamentous injury. The function of the ankle is reliant on the restoration of the mortice joint. If the lateral ligament is ruptured the talus can tilt in the mortice leading to chronic instability. If the inferior ligament is damaged, lateral displacement of the fibula and lateral drift of the talus (diastasis) may result.

[171] **Ruptured Achilles' tendon**: this is disrupted as a result of sudden plantar flexion and is commoner in a tendon weakened by degeneration in the middle-aged. Surgical repair or conservative management in plaster are often successful.

[172] **Shortened Achilles' tendon**: this results in plantar flexion of the foot and clumsiness of gait as the heel fails to reach the ground. Usually associated with congenital or neurological deformities such as polio, club-foot etc. but can be secondary to ischaemic contracture or be idiopathic.

[173] **Tenosynovitis**: associated with unusual activities (e.g. dancing), flat foot, rheumatoid arthritis or degenerative changes, this inflammation causes pain and puffiness behind either malleolus. Tibialis posterior and peroneus longus are most commonly affected and may rupture. Treatment is rest in plaster.

[174] **March fracture**: this fracture of the second metatarsal occurs in young adults after unaccustomed activity. It can also affect the third and fourth metatarsals. It usually settles within six weeks of union of the fracture.

[175] **Freiberg's disease** is osteochondritis of the second metatarsal head. Palpable deformity and pain may eventually necessitate excision.

[176] **Anterior metatarsalgia**: this is pain under the metatarsal heads often associated with splayfoot (a widening of the foot at that level). It is the commonest cause of forefoot pain, although other causes should be excluded. It typically occurs in middle-aged women and is associated with obesity, prolonged standing, flattened medial longitudinal arches, weak intrinsic muscles, claw toes and callouses on the sole. Shoe inserts and chiropody are the first lines of treatment.

[177] **Morton's neuroma**: this is a plantar or digital neuroma commonly affecting the plantar nerve running between the third and fourth metatarsal heads to the third web space. Any of the other digital nerves can be affected, usually just before the bifurcation at the toe clefts. It causes piercing pain in the foot. It typically occurs in women aged 25–45 years and is treated by excision.

[178] Deformities seen in the **rheumatoid foot** include pes planus, splay foot, hallux valgus, claw toes, anterior metatarsalgia and hammer toes. Surgical shoes with moulded insoles may alleviate symptoms. Fowler's arthroplasty of all the metatarsophalangeal joints and reconstruction of the metatarsal weight bearing pad is a surgical option for severe cases.

[179] **Tarsal tunnel syndrome**: caused when the posterior tibial nerve is compressed beneath the flexor retinaculum causing dysaesthesia in the sole of the foot and the toes. Flexor retinaculum division relieves tarsal tunnel syndrome.

[180] **Hammer toe**: flexion deformity of the proximal interphalangeal joint causing dorsal callous. Chiropody or joint fusion remedies the situation. May accompany hallux valgus in which case this should also be corrected.

[181] **Mallet toe**: flexion deformity of the distal interphalangeal joint. May cause nail problems or callouses. Treatment is chiropody, joint fusion or amputation of distal phalanx.

Big toe

Ingrowing toenail (see pg 205), hallux valgus (see pg 201), hallux rigidus, bunion, gout (see pg 203).

Dorsal and medial side of the foot

Flat foot[182], cuneiform exostoses (see pg 225)[183], Köhler's disease[184], osteoarthritis, rheumatoid arthritis.

Heel

Calcaneal exostosis (see pg 225), bursitis, plantar fasciitis[185].

In children

Club-foot[186], Sever's disease[187], intoeing[188].

---

[182] **Flat-foot** (pes planus) or the absence of the arches of the foot is normal in young children. It can persist in cases of knock-knees and deformities of the heel and tibia. Well fitting shoes, supportive insoles and occasionally physiotherapy are normally all that are required. Peroneal (spastic) flat-foot is a painful condition typically seen in adolescent boys due to spasm of peroneal muscles. The foot is everted and fixed and gait is disturbed. It may be related to ossification of a congenital cartilaginous bar that can be excised. Incipient flat-foot in adults is a gradual flattening of the arches due to obesity, prolonged standing and degenerative changes. Secondary arthritis may occur. Weight loss, physiotherapy and arch supports are the mainstays of treatment.

[183] **Cuneiform exostoses**: these can all cause blisters, callouses and difficulty with shoe fittings and can be treated by local excision.

[184] **Köhler's disease**: osteochondritis of the navicular occurring in children aged 3–10 years. It is self-limiting.

[185] **Plantar fascitis** is tearing of the calcaneal attachment of the plantar fascia. Usually in the middle-aged due to degenerative changes. Treatment is heel supports, physiotherapy or steroid injections.

[186] **Talipes equino varus (club-foot)** is the commonest major congenital foot deformity involving:
  Varus deformity of heel
  Adduction of forefoot
  Plantar flexion
  Inversion.
Treatment in order of severity of deformity may involve:
  Corrective stretching
  Splintage
  Corrective plasters
  Surgery to soft tissues (e.g. Achilles tendon and plantar fascia)
  Wedge excision of bone and fusion of the mid-tarsal and subtalar joints.
Talipes calcaneus is a much rarer condition in which the dorsum of the foot lies against the shin.

[187] **Sever's disease** is chronic heel pain in children aged 6–12 years arising from calcaneal epiphysis. Thought to be osteochondritis due to the pull of the Achilles tendon. Settles spontaneously.

[188] **Intoeing** is internal rotation of feet in toddlers causing tripping and falling usually corrects itself by the age of six. Deformity of the tibia is a rare cause in persistent cases.

EXAMINATION OF THE WRIST

LOOK
Scars, deformity
Swelling: diffuse, localised
FEEL
Warmth, tenderness, bony landmarks
MOVE
'Prayer' position (palms together) – dorsiflexion
Backs of hands together – palmar flexion
Radial deviation
Ulnar deviation
Pronation
Supination

THE WRIST – SPECIAL TESTS

For de Quervain's tenosynovitis,[189] Tinel's sign for carpal tunnel syndrome (see pg 207), neurological examination of hand (see pg 169).

THE WRIST – COMMON CASES

Ganglions (see pg 213), carpal tunnel syndrome (see pg 207), de Quervain's tenosynovitis,[190] rheumatoid arthritis,[191] carpometacarpal osteoarthritis of the thumb, complications of Colles' fracture (see pg 239).

---

[189] **Finkelstein's test**: ask the patient to make a fist with the thumb tucked in under the fingers. Now steady the wrist and move the hand into ulnar deviation. This is very painful in de Quervain's tenosynovitis.

[190] **De Quervain's**: this is tenosynovitis involving abductor pollicis longus and extensor pollicis brevis. Occurs in the middle-aged and leads to localised tenderness and swelling on the lateral aspect of the radius (just proximal to the anatomical snuffbox). There is weakness of grip. Treatment is rest or splitting lateral wall of the fibrous tendon sheaths.

[191] **Rheumatoid arthritis**: common. Gross swelling, local heat, pain and stiffness. Hands usually have typical rheumatoid features (see pg 193).

NEUROLOGICAL EXAMINATION OF THE UPPER LIMB

It is likely if you are asked to perform a neurological examination of the hand or arm in this station the abnormality will usually either be an ulnar nerve palsy (see pg 209), a radial nerve palsy (see pg 211) or a median nerve palsy with or without carpal tunnel syndrome (see pg 207). If it is immediately obvious which one it is, you should proceed with the appropriate examination. If it is not, you may need to do a more general neurological examination of the upper limb (see below); alternatively you may be asked directly to 'examine this patient's ulnar/median/ radial nerve.'

Vague instructions such as **'Examine this patient's arms'** test your flexibility – rise to the challenge! If nothing springs out at you and you have no idea which nerve or joint to examine start off with a logical, general upper limb examination and if a pathology becomes evident, move to a more specific examination as appropriate.

'Hello, I'm Dr Parchment Smith. Would you mind if I had a look at your arms? Could you take your shirt off please? Do you mind if I talk to the examiners as I go along?'

Take a step back.

To the examiners:

'On general inspection there are no obvious abnormalities to see regarding the patient himself, who looks healthy, or regarding his face[192] or neck.[193]'

To the patient:

'Put your arms out in front of you please? Lean forward so I can look at your back. The patient moves his arms easily and there are no obvious deformities,[194] scars, tremor, muscle wasting or swollen joints.'

Let him sit back again.

---

[192] Look for asymmetry (hemiplegia), nystagmus (cerebellar problems), wasting (muscular dystrophy), ptosis, small pupil (Horner's syndrome, syringomyelia).

[193] Enlarged lymph nodes or Pancoast's tumour (can invade brachial plexus), cervical spondylosis (common cause of arm neurology via cervical cord or nerve root compression).

[194] Look at: Shoulders (scars, winging of scapula, stiffness)

Elbows (psoriasis, rheumatoid nodules, scars over ulnar nerve)

Hands (tremor, swollen joints, pitting nails, clubbing, vasculitic lesions, claw hand)

Muscles (wasting, fasciculation, asymmetry).

'I am now going to examine the arms. Are the arms painful or stiff anywhere sir[195]? Relax your arm, sir and let me move your hand. I am just testing his TONE[196]. Now I am going to test POWER. Put your elbows out to the side; don't let me push them down (Deltoid, C5). Bend your elbows; don't let me pull them straight (Biceps, C5, C6). Push against me; don't let me bend your elbows (Triceps C7). Squeeze my fingers (C8, T1, gross, functional test). Hold your fingers out straight; don't let me bend them down (Radial nerve, C7 – finger extension). Make a fist and cock your wrists back. Don't let me pull your wrists forward or back (Wrist extension radial nerve C7). Spread your fingers, don't let me push them together (dorsal interossei – ulnar). Hold this piece of paper between your fingers, don't let me pull it out (palmar interossei, ulnar). Point your thumb to the ceiling; stop me pushing it down (Abductor pollicis brevis – median nerve).

I am now going to test CO-ORDINATION. Can you do this?'

Slowly pat the back of one hand with the palm of the other.

'Now flip your hand each time like this (continue in the same rhythm, pat with the palm then the dorsum of the active hand in turn)[197]. Now go faster. Try it with the other hand now. Touch my finger then your nose. Do it faster. Now keep going as I move my finger… keep going. Now with the other hand.'

To the examiners:

I need a tendon hammer to check REFLEXES[198]. Relax your hands on your lap, palms upward. I'm checking biceps, triceps and supinator[199].

---

[195] This is a gamble, but if you can't see anything obvious by now you need to go fishing without cheating. It is acceptable to check for pain before you touch the patient, and if you phrase it carefully you will seem considerate and may prompt the patient to say 'it's my arthritis in this left elbow' which will help you move on to a more targeted and appropriate examination.

[196] Take his hand as if you are going to shake it, and hold his elbow lightly in your other hand. Shake hand slowly and exaggeratedly, up and down and in gentle circles, moving whole arm forward and back at elbow simultaneously. Repeat with other hand to compare sides. Look for cogwheel rigidity (Parkinson's), increased tone/spasticity (upper motor lesion like CVA) reduced tone/flaccidity (lower motor lesion like plexus or nerve injury). Beware stiff joints or contractures in long-standing paralysis of any cause that may mimic increased tone.

[197] Inability to do this is dysdidokokinesis – try to chant it as you pat your hand when demonstrating the test in practice to help you remember – Dys-di-do-ko-ki-ne-sis! The test highlights defects in cerebellar dysfunction.

[198] They should have a tendon hammer if it is appropriate for this examination. If not, don't insist – take the hint – it's probably meant to be a joint examination!

[199] Biceps – strike your own finger resting on patient's antecubital fossa (C5, C6).
Triceps – strike just above the back of elbow (C7).
Supinator – strike your own finger resting on the base of the patient's thumb (C5, C6). These take practice to do impressively!

I am now going to test SENSATION[200]**. Close your eyes and tell me if you can feel me touch you here does it feel the same on the other side? Say yes when you feel me touch you.**

Stand up and say to the examiners:

'A full neurological examination includes JOINT POSITION[201] **and VIBRATION SENSE**[202]**. To complete the examination of the arm I would like to check the range of movement of the neck, shoulder, elbow and wrist and check the pulses**[203]**.'**

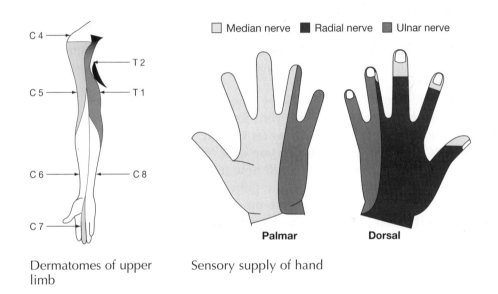

Dermatomes of upper limb

Sensory supply of hand

---

[200] Light touch and pinprick. Know your dermatomes or, alternatively, remember this list:
Neck (C3), collarbone (C4), shoulder (C5), at elbow laterally (C6), either side of the index finger (C6 radial side, C7 ulnar side), hypothenar eminence (C8), at elbow medially (T1), inner arm (T2), armpit (T3).

[201] It is unlikely that orthopaedic surgeons will want you to go this far, but it is part of a full neurological examination. so you should know how to do it. Hold the base of the thumb steady with one hand and, with the other, hold the sides of the terminal phalanx of the thumb. Moving it up, tell the patient 'this is up' and moving it down 'this is down'. Get the patient to close his eyes and tell you whether you are moving the thumb up or down.

[202] Similarly, vibration sense is rarely formally tested in a surgical exam, but in glove and stocking paraesthesia and peripheral neuropathies it is the first to go. Using a tuning fork, which they will have if needed. Strike the tuning fork firmly to set it buzzing and place it on the patient's sternum or forehead. 'Can you feel that buzzing? Tell me if it feels the same here on your wrist.' If yes, vibration sense is intact. If not, move up to elbow then clavicle to determine a level.

[203] If still completely stuck at least you will have gone through a sensible examination of the limb as requested. If the neurology, joints and circulation are all normal, say so. If you have done a thorough examination the examiners will have to agree. Maybe the case is not a particularly suitable one for the exam, or the arms are normal. In any case you will have taken a sensible, professional approach as you would in clinic to exclude any significant pathology. So long as you can show off your examination skills do not despair! Few candidates would have been as impressive if the case really is that obscure. See examinations for individual joints (shoulder pg 150, elbow pg 163, neck pg 155) and for vascular examination of the upper limb (pg 269).

EXAMINATION OF THE MEDIAN NERVE[204]

'Hello, my name is Dr Parchment Smith. Would you mind if I examined your hands? Would you roll up your sleeves and place your hands palm up on your lap/this table please?'

To the examiners:

'On INSPECTION I am looking for thenar wasting and a Simian thumb[205], decreased pulp of the index finger[206], cigarette burns or local trauma between the index and middle finger[207], wasting of the lateral aspect of the forearm[208], and the Benedictian sign[209].'

To the patient:

'Can you stretch both arms out please? I am looking for cubitus valgus or varus indicating an old supracondylar fracture, and scars around the elbow, forearm and wrist.[210]'

I would now like to PALPATE the nerve where it is superficial – can you bend your wrist pushing against me with your fist[211]? Is it tender? Do you feel any numbness or tingling in your hand when I feel it[212]? I would now like to test SENSATION. Can you feel me touch you here[213]? Here? Here? Does it feel the same as here on the other hand? I will now move on to test POWER. Lie your hand on the table, palm up please. I'm going to hold your wrist so you don't move your hand. Now lift your thumb up off the table to touch my finger[214]. Push against it! Keep the rest of your hand still! Now, can I hold your thumb

---

[204] **For roots, course and branches see pg 206.**

[205] Due to wasting of the thenar eminence – Simian means 'like a monkey.' The thumb lies in the plane of the hand instead of at right angles to it.

[206] Due to denervation of the lateral 2 1/2 fingers.

[207] Due to denervation.

[208] In high lesions.

[209] The Benedictian sign is the extended index finger (like that of a Benedictine monk giving a blessing) caused in high lesions of the median nerve. This is due to the paralysis of flexor digitorum profundus which normally holds the index finger partially flexed at rest.

[210] **Causes of damage to the median nerve see pg 206.**

[211] The nerve lies superficially between the prominent tendons of flexor carpi radialis and palmaris longus (sometimes absent) which are easily seen on the palmar side of the wrist when the fist is flexed against resistance.

[212] Note: this is not the fixed flexion test for carpal tunnel syndrome (see later), they are only flexing the wrist to demonstrate the position of the tendons you need for landmarks.

[213] Use a pin if one is provided (gently!), otherwise touch lightly with your finger. Do not stroke over a large area, and do not poke too hard. Compare with the other hand if sensation is present but altered. The deficit is present on the radial side of the palm and thumb and the radial 2 1/2 fingers on the palmar side and the radial 2 1/2 fingers and the tip of the thumb on the dorsal side.

[214] This tests **abductor pollicis brevis** that is invariably and exclusively supplied by the median nerve. If you have time to do only one test for the median nerve, this is it. As the patient resists, feel for the muscle in the thenar eminence and compare it with the other side.

and ask you just to wiggle the tip of it[215]? Finally I'm going to hold your hand like a handshake. Now can you twist against my hand while I feel your forearm[216]?

Turn to the examiners:

'The patient shows signs of a high/low median nerve palsy. There is no evidence of the cause/it appears to be caused by....

(If a low lesion) I would like to carry out some of the tests for carpal tunnel syndrome if time allows[217].'

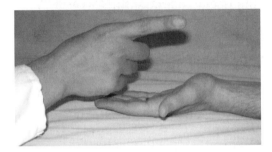 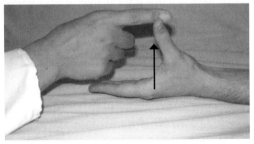

Testing for abductor pollicis brevis

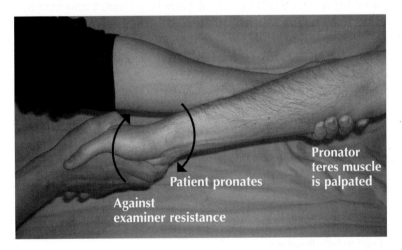

Testing pronator teres

---

[215] To test for **flexor pollicis longus** (affected in lesions proximal to the wrist or in injuries to the anterior interosseous branch) immobilise the proximal phalangeal joint of the thumb and ask the patient to flex the distal interphalangeal joint.

[216] This tests for **pronator teres**. The patient extends the elbow, hand supine. You hold his hand and resist as he tries to pronate. Feel for contraction medially and just distal to the elbow (try it on a friend and identify pronator teres). Pain and tenderness over pronator teres is found in the pronator teres entrapment syndrome.

[217] Diagnostic tests for carpal tunnel syndrome (see pg 206) include:
   Fixed flexion
   Tourniquet test
   Nerve conduction tests (not a bedside test).

EXAMINATION OF THE ULNAR NERVE[218]

'Hello, my name is Dr Parchment Smith. Would you mind if I examined your hands? Would you roll up your sleeves and place your hands palm up on your lap/this table please?'

To the examiners:

'On INSPECTION I am looking for a claw hand[219], ulceration of the skin[220], brittle nails[221], trophic changes. I am also looking for wasting of the hypothenar eminence[222], the dorsal first web space[223] and the medial forearm[224].'

To the patient:

'Can you stretch both arms out please? I am looking for cubitus valgus or varus indicating an old supracondylar fracture, and scars around the elbow, forearm and wrist.

I would now like to PALPATE the nerve first at the elbow – can you straighten and bend your elbow please[225]? Then at the wrist[226]. Is it tender? Do you feel any numbness or tingling in your hand when I feel it?

I would now like to test SENSATION. Can you feel me touch you here[227]? Here? Here? Does it feel the same as here on the other hand?

I will now move on to test POWER. Hold your hand out. Palm down, fingers together please. I'm just going to slide this card between your index and middle fingers. Keep your fingers straight! Can you grip the card between those fingers and stop me pulling it out? Now between your middle and ring fingers... and finally between your ring and little fingers. This tests the interossei muscles. (See fig opposite.)

---

[218] **For roots, course and branches see pg xx.**

[219] Due to flexed proximal interphalangeal (PIP) joints. If the distal interphalangeal (DIP) joints are also affected it paradoxically suggests a more DISTAL lesion – the deformity is more marked when the flexor digitorum profundus is intact (the ulnar paradox).

[220] Due to unnoticed trauma on the desensitised medial skin of the dorsum and palm and the medial (ulnar) 1 1/2 digits.

[221] Due to denervation.

[222] Due to denervation of the hypothenar muscles.

[223] Between thumb and index finger (see pg XX (fig)) due to wasting of the interossei muscles.

[224] Lesions proximal to the wrist only, due to denervation of the flexor carpi ulnaris and the flexor digitorum profundus.

[225] The nerve is palpable in the groove of the medial epicondyle (test this on yourself). If it snaps over the medial epicondyle while the joint is moved this may indicate a traumatic ulnar neuritis caused by a deficiency in the tissues which normally anchor it.

[226] Just lateral to the flexor carpi ulnaris which is visible on the medial palmar side of the wrist when the fist is flexed against resistance.

[227] Use a pin if one is provided (gently!), otherwise touch lightly with your finger. Do not stroke over a large area, and do not poke too hard. Compare with the other hand if sensation is present but altered. The deficit is most reliable on the ulnar side of the palm over the hypothenar eminence. There should also be loss of sensation over the ulnar 1 1/2 fingers. Loss of sensation on the ulnar side of the dorsum of the hand indicates a lesion proximal to the wrist.

Now put your hand, palm down on the table. Can you push your index finger against my finger? I'm testing abduction of the index finger that relies on the first dorsal interosseus. Now push your little finger out against my finger. Abduction of the little finger relies on the abductor digiti minimi.

Finally I would like to perform FROMENT'S TEST for adductor pollicis. Could you grab hold of this sheet of paper with your thumb on top of it holding it against the side of your index finger? Now stop me pulling the paper away. If the adductor pollicis is denervated the thumb will flex at the interphalangeal joint using the thumb flexors to compensate (see fig below).'

Turn to the examiners:

'The patient shows signs of an ulnar nerve palsy. There is no evidence of the cause/It appears to be caused by...[228] I could also test for flexor carpi ulnaris[229] and flexor digitorum profundus[230] which are both affected in a proximal lesion[231].'

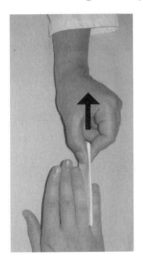
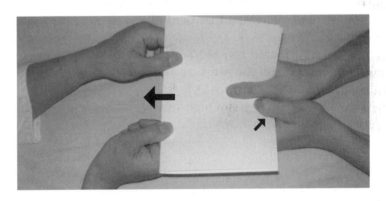

Testing the interossei

Froment's test for adductor pollicis. Note patient's affected left thumb is flexing at the interphalangeal joint.

---

[228] **For common causes of ulnar nerve palsy (distal to proximal) see pg 208.**

[229] Test for FCU: patient palmar flexes fist against resistance and the tendon is palpated on the medial palmar side of the wrist. It also helps abduction of the straight little finger.

[230] Test for FDP: hold little finger PIP joint still and ask patient to flex DIP joint. Loss of power indicates lesion at or above elbow.

[231] **Signs of a distal ulnar nerve lesion (e.g. at wrist)**
    Flexor carpi ulnaris intact
    Ulnar half of flexor digitorum profundusis intact (paradoxically <u>worse</u> claw hand)
    No muscle wasting of forearm
    Sensation of ulnar side of dorsum of hand intact.

Signs of a proximal ulnar nerve lesion (e.g. at elbow)
    FCU affected (decreased abduction of little finger)
    Ulnar half of FDP affected (decreased flexion of DIP joint of little finger)
    Muscle wasting of medial forearm
    Sensation of ulnar side of dorsum of hand affected.

EXAMINATION OF THE RADIAL NERVE[232]

'Hello, my name is Dr Parchment Smith. Would you mind if I examined your hands? Would you roll up your sleeves and stretch your arms out in front of you please?'

To the examiners:

'On INSPECTION I am looking for wrist drop,[233] forearm wasting[234] and triceps wasting[235]. I am now going to test POWER.'

To the patient:

'Can you bend your elbow in to your side and give me your hand, palm down? I will support your wrist. Can you extend your fingers? Straighten them. Don't let me push them down. Now make a fist. Try to cock the fist back. Don't let me pull it down. I am testing the EXTENSORS[236].

Now straighten your elbow. Can you turn your hand over? I'm going to hold your hand. Do it again, don't let me stop you. I am testing SUPINATOR[237].

Now with your fist in a neutral position, can you bend your elbow? Don't let me stop you. I am testing BRACHIORADIALIS[238].

Now try and straighten that bent elbow. Don't let me stop you. I am feeling for TRICEPS[239].

I would now like to test SENSATION. Can you feel me touch you here[240]? Here? Here? Does it feel the same as here on the other hand?

To the examiners:

'I think this patient has a high/low radial nerve palsy. There is evidence that this may have been caused by...[241].'

---

[232] **For roots, course and branches see pg 210.**

[233] Due to loss of extensors.

[234] Due to loss of extensors, the muscle bulk of which is in the forearm.

[235] In high lesions.

[236] Extensors of wrist and fingers are weakened in radial nerve palsy.

[237] Testing **supinator**. Straighten the elbow to exclude biceps that also supinates. Loss of supinator suggests a lesion proximal to the exit of the supinator tunnel.

[238] Look at and feel **brachioradialis**. Loss of power suggests a lesion above the supinator tunnel.

[239] **Triceps** weakness suggests a lesion at mid-humeral level. Loss of all triceps activity suggests a high (plexus) lesion.

[240] Use a pin if one is provided (gently!), otherwise touch lightly with your finger. Do not stroke over a large area, and do not poke too hard. Compare with the other hand if sensation is present but altered. The deficit is present just over the anatomical snuffbox (the dorsum of the wrist on the radial side) in lesions distal to the elbow. Loss of sensation along the back of the forearm suggests a higher lesion.

[241] **Causes of damage of radial nerve see pg 210.**

NEUROLOGICAL EXAMINATION OF THE LOWER LIMB

'Hello, my name is Dr Parchment Smith. Do you mind if I examine your legs? I'll talk to these doctors as I go along if that's OK. Could you take your trousers off and sit with your legs stretched out straight ahead of you on the couch please?'
To the examiners:
'On general inspection of the patient I'm looking for asymmetry[242], nystagmus[243], muscle wasting[244], fasciculation[245] and pes cavus[246]. I would like to examine the muscle TONE.'
To the patient:
'Relax the legs please if you can.'
Roll each thigh gently from side to side (hip) and lift the knee a couple of inches and let it drop (knee). Note resistance, jerkiness, spasm or lack of tone.
'I am now going to examine POWER. Lift the whole, straight leg up. Don't let me push it down (hip flexors, L2, L3). Now push your straight leg into the bed against my hand (hip extensors L4, L5). Bend your knee. Push it straight against resistance (knee extensors, L3, L4). Pull your heel in to your buttocks against my hand (knee flexors, L5, S1). Flex your foot, don't let me pull it down (Tibialis anterior and long extensors of the toes, L4, L5). Now point your toe against my hand (calf muscles, S1, S2). Now to examine CO-ORDINATION,[247] could you run your heel up and down your shin? Now the other side. Now to examine REFLEXES, could I have a tendon hammer please? Relax as I do these if you can.'
First support the knee and tap just above tibial tuberosity (L3, L4). Then, bend the knee and let it fall to the side, gently dorsiflex the foot and tap the Achilles tendon (L5, S1). Firmly dorsiflex foot in a sudden movement to try and elicit CLONUS (typical of an upper motor lesion). Scrape the lateral sole of the foot

---

[242] Typical of CVA (very common).
[243] Suggests cerebellar dysfunction.
[244] Typical of lower motor neurone lesions, but disuse atrophy will be evident even in upper motor lesions.
Typical patterns (old polio or infantile hemiplegia: unilateral muscle loss, one small leg)
    Charcot-Marie-Tooth disease: muscle wasting stopping partway up leg (champagne bottle leg)
    Diabetic amyotrophy: isolated anterior thigh
    Polymyositis: generalised proximal wasting
Wasted hands indicate motor neurone disease, Charcot-Marie-Tooth disease and syringomyelia.
[245] Lower motor neurone problem, almost always motor neurone disease.
[246] High arched foot with clawed toes (Friedreich's ataxia, Charcot-Marie-Tooth disease).
[247] Affected in cerebellar lesions.

with the sharp end of the tendon hammer (warn the patient: **'bit of a scratch'**) in an arc to elicit BABINSKI'S SIGN[248].
'I would now like to examine SENSATION[249]. Can you feel this pin as sharp on your foot? Does it feel different on the other side? Please say 'Now' when you feel the pin as I work my way up the leg. Now I'll repeat that with cotton wool.'
'A complete examination should include vibration and proprioception[250]. To examine VIBRATION I would use a tuning fork[251]. Now I would like to examine PROPRIOCEPTION[252]. Please close your eyes. I'm going to hold your big toe still with one hand and just move the tip up or down with my other hand.
Tell me if it's moving up or down... now... now... now.

---

[248] Normally the first movement of the great toe is plantar flexion (the toe points down). If the toes go UP (dorsiflex) this is a positive test indicating an upper motor neurone lesion, most commonly CVA.

[249] **Deficits in sensation and what they mean:**
Outer thigh (L2) Inner thigh (L3) Inner calf (L4) Outer calf (L5) Medial foot (L5) Lateral foot (S1).
Stocking distribution: Peripheral neuropathy. Most common sensory defect (causes: idiopathic, diabetes, B12 deficiency in alcoholics, drug toxicity, Charcot-Marie-Tooth).
Front of thigh, medial calf and foot: femoral nerve (and saphenous nerve, its terminal branch) Also look for reduced knee jerk, wasted quadriceps, reduced hip flexion. Causes of injury usually indirect e.g. iliacus muscle haematoma in haemophiliacs.
First web space, dorsum of foot and lower leg: common peroneal nerve. Also look for foot drop, abnormal gait. Causes of injury: trauma or pressure at fibular neck, compartment syndrome, ganglion.
Sole of foot: posterior tibial nerve or sciatic nerve. If posterior tibial nerve, look for clawing of toes, loss of toe flexion. Injuries caused by tibial fractures, compartment syndrome, trauma behind medial malleolus, tarsal tunnel syndrome. If sciatic nerve, look for extensive wasting and loss of power of hamstring and all compartments of lower leg, drop foot and loss of sensation on the sole, dorsum and entire lateral aspect of the lower leg. Injuries caused by hip dislocation, hip surgery, pelvic fractures.

[250] Most orthopaedic surgeons would stop you there! However you should know how to do these tests just in case!

[251] They will have a tuning fork if it is needed. Strike the tuning fork firmly to set it buzzing and place it on the patient's sternum or forehead. 'Can you feel that buzzing? Tell me if it feels the same here on your ankle.' If yes, vibration sense is intact. If not, move up to knee then iliac crest to determine a level. In most peripheral neuropathies vibration sense is the first to go.

[252] Explain to the patient what you mean by 'up' and 'down' before he closes his eyes. Hold the toe by the lateral aspects.

Finally I would like to see the patient WALK[253] and perform ROMBERG'S TEST[254].'

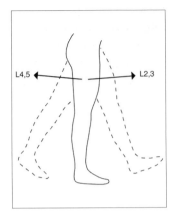
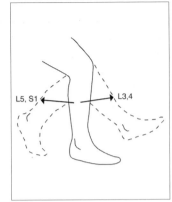
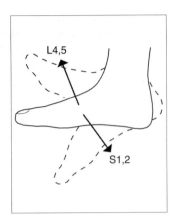
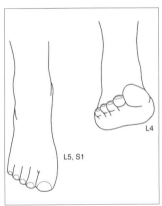
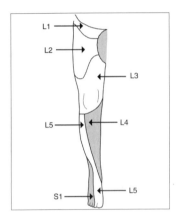
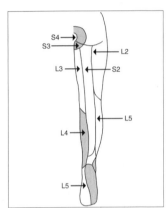

Myotomes and dermatomes

---

[253] If the examiners indicate or hint that you should examine the gait ask if the patient can walk without help. Then:

'Walk normally to that wall please and then back to us'

Wide based gait – cerebellar ataxia.

Stiff 'walking through mud' gait – spastic paraplegia.

Stamping gait – sensory ataxia (should have positive Romberg's test also).

Stooped, hesitant shuffling gait with no arm swing – Parkinson's.

High-stepping gait – foot drop (e.g after peroneal nerve injury).

One leg stiff with semicircular swing and ipsilateral arm flexed – hemiplegia.

Lumbar lordosis, swaying trunk and waddling gait – Duchenne muscular dystrophy and proximal myopathy.

Broad-based 'walking on ice' – gait apraxia, senile degenerative disease especially of frontal lobe.

'Walk in a line putting your heel to your toe like this' – exacerbates ataxia, which side do they fall to?

'Walk on tiptoes (S1). Now walk on your heels (L5). – cannot do it in footdrop.

[254] Romberg's test. 'Stand with your feet together and your hands outstretched. Good. Now close your eyes.' Positive if patient is more unsteady with eyes closed. Suggests ataxia, e.g. subacute combined degeneration, tabes dorsalis.

C   The Cases

Osteoarthritis of the hip

Top Five Case: seen by over a third of candidates in our survey. Examination of the hip accounted for 13.8% of cases in this bay.

[260] OA hip may develop in a relatively young adult as a sequel to congenital subluxation, Perthes' disease, coxa vara, acetabular deformities or injury. In the older patient it may also be secondary to rheumatoid arthritis (see pg xx, Rheumatoid arthritis of the hip), avascular necrosis (see below) or Paget's disease (see pg xx). When no underlying cause is present it is referred to as primary osteoarthritis.

[261] **Symptoms** are long-standing groin pain radiating to the knee after activity. It may become constant and disturb sleep. Stiffness is initially after rest but it increases until putting on socks and shoes is difficult. Ask about previous injury, illness or surgery (see above).

[262] **Radiological findings include**: decreased joint space, sub-articular sclerosis, cyst formation and osteophytes. **Treatment** is conservative (walking aids, analgesia, physiotherapy) and surgery (most commonly arthroplasty).

Trendelenburg test

A) Normal – Hip is higher on the side of the lifted leg (1)

Centre of gravity is over supporting leg (2)

When standing on a healthy leg, the hip abductors (gluteus medius and minimus) of the supporting leg contract to pull the pelvis down on that side (3).

The pelvis is tilted so the opposite hip is lifted (1) and the centre of gravity is brought over the supporting leg (2) so the patient can hold steady for 30 seconds.

B) Abnormal (positive Trendelenburg's test) – Hip is not higher on the side of the lifted leg (1), or position cannot be held for 30 seconds.

When standing on the affected side, the hip abductors of the supporting leg fail to pull the pelvis down on that side (3). The opposite hip cannot be lifted (1). Do not allow the patient's upper body to tilt in compensation (4). The centre of gravity will fall outside the supporting leg if the opposite hip does not drop, therefore a positive Trendelenburg's is either the opposite hip falling below the horizontal (1) or the patient is unable to hold the position.

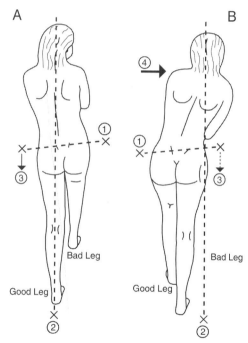

C

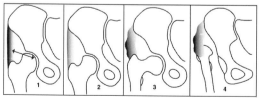

C) *Reasons for a positive Trendelenburg Test*

1) Pain arising in the hip joint inhibiting the gluteal muscles
2) Gluteal paralysis or weakness from polio or a muscle wasting disease
3) Gluteal inefficiency from coxa vara
4) Gluteal inefficiency from congenital dislocation of the hip
5) False positive due to pain, generalised weakness, poor co-operation or bad balance (10% of patients)

OSTEOARTHRITIS OF THE HIP[260]

Carry out a full examination of the hip (see pg 137).

'The affected leg lies in external rotation and adduction with apparent shortening. Thomas' test reveals fixed flexion. Mild muscle wasting is detectable. The greater trochanter is somewhat high and posterior and deep pressure elicits mild tenderness. There is marked restriction of all hip movements but movement is painless within this limited range. There is an obvious limp and positive Trendelenburg's test. I would like to ask the patient a few questions[261] and see the X-rays[262], but my diagnosis is osteoarthritis of the hip.'

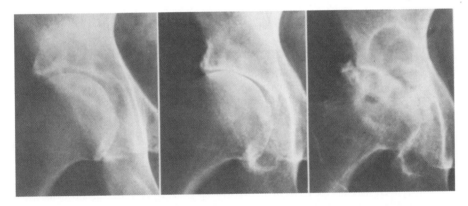

X-rays of osteoarthritis over a period of four years this patient developed progressive diminution of the joint space, subarticular sclerosis, cysts and peripheral osteophytes

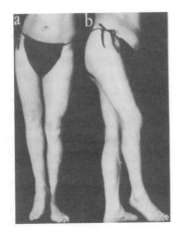

Osteoarthritic right hip showing apparent shortening with adduction and flexion deformities

Rheumatoid arthritis of the hip

[263] The hip joint is frequently affected by rheumatoid arthritis. The hallmark of the disease is progressive bone destruction on both sides of the joint without any reactive osteophyte formation. The patient complains of pain in the groin, which has come on insidiously, and a limp. When more severe, moving from sitting becomes difficult, and even movement in bed is painful.

X-rays

> <u>Early RA</u>: osteoporosis, loss of joint space
> <u>Later RA</u>: erosion of acetabulum and femoral head
> <u>Severe</u>: gross bone destruction. Perforation of acetabulum

Treatment

Once cartilage and bone are eroded, no medical treatment will influence the progression to joint destruction. Total hip replacement relieves pain and deformity and improves mobility. Even in young patients this tends to be undertaken as polyarthropathy limits activity so that the implants do not wear out rapidly.

<u>Total hip replacement</u>

Charnley low friction arthroplasty: this or one of its variants is the most widely used replacement. This prosthesis comprises a socket of high density polyethylene and a replacement femoral head of stainless steel. Both components are anchored with quick setting acrylic cement. If a lateral approach is used, the greater trochanter is usually detached and replaced at the end of the operation with stainless steel wires.

Other replacements. Many variations: some need no cement, some need no detachment of the trochanter.

<u>Hemiarthroplasty</u>. Where functional requirements are not expected to be very high (e.g. after intracapsular hip fractures in the very elderly) the femoral head is replaced with a stemmed prosthesis and the acetabulum is not replaced.

<u>**Surgical approaches to the hip**</u>

<u>Anterior approach</u>

Through the interval between sartorius and tensor fascia lata, detaching the tensor fascia lata, rectus femoris, anterior parts of gluteus medius and iliacus from hip so that upper and anterior parts of the joint capsule can be accessed. Structures to avoid: lateral femoral cutaneous nerve, femoral nerve, ascending branch of lateral femoral circumflex artery.

<u>Antero-lateral approach</u>

Between tensor fascia lata and gluteus medius. It involves partial or complete detachment of some or all of the abductor mechanism so that the hip can be abducted during reaming of the femoral shaft and so that the acetabulum can be more fully exposed. Beware of the femoral nerve as it is the most laterally placed structure in the neurovascular bundle in the femoral triangle, mostly compression neuropraxia from misplaced retraction results. The femoral artery and vein are at risk from retractors that penetrate iliopsoas. Beware of the ascending branches of the lateral circumflex femoral vessels which are deep to the tensor and gluteus medius.

<u>Posterior approach</u>

This approach involves splitting of the middle of gluteus maximus in the line of its fibres. Piriformis, obturator internus and the gemelli are divided at their femoral attachments to expose the joint. The sciatic nerve is retracted medially and protected by turning the cut ends of obturator internus and gemelli backwards over the nerve.

Postoperative complications

<u>Dislocation</u>: stability depends on 1) initial alignment, 2) time since surgery – gets progressively more stable, 3) degree of use/violence of trauma. Treatment is closed or open reduction, revision in severe cases.

<u>Component failure</u>: socket failure is rare, but the stem of the femoral prosthesis may fracture. Risk is increased in overweight patient or varus alignment. The wires around the greater trochanter may break, or the trochanter itself may fail to unite causing local discomfort and a Trendelenburg gait.

<u>Component loosening and infection</u>: this usually occurs at the interface of cement and bone in the area of the femoral stem. The loosening is seen on X-ray and is usually due to infection although often no causative organism is identified. Revision procedures are fraught and necessitate thorough débridement under antibiotic cover and reinsertion of a fresh prosthesis specially designed to accommodate migration or loss of bone stock. Antibiotic loaded cement may also be used, but in some cases the prosthesis has to be removed altogether with disastrous results for the patient's mobility.

RHEUMATOID ARTHRITIS OF THE HIP[263]

Carry out examination of the hip (pg 137).

'This patient (with extensive rheumatoid disease affecting many joints) has a painful hip. The buttock and thigh are markedly wasted with the limb held in external rotation and fixed flexion. All movements are restricted and painful. The diagnosis is rheumatoid arthritis of the hip. I would like to see the X-rays of this patient.'

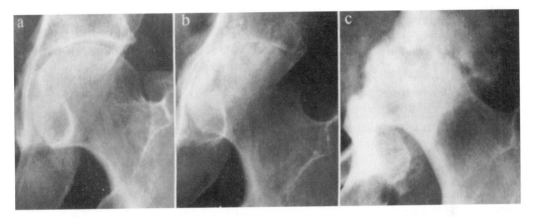

Rheumatoid arthritis. Three stages in the development of rheumatoid arthritis:

a) Loss of joint space
b) Erosion of bone after cartilage has disappeared
c) Perforation of the acetabular floor – such marked destruction is more likely to occur if the patient is taking corticosteroids.

Fractured neck of femur

[264] Two types of fracture:

1. Neck fracture (intracapsular) see fig (a) opposite
    subcapital, cervical or basal
    disrupt blood supply from diaphysis
    and risk retinacular blood supply so high risk of avascular necrosis
    classified Garden's stage I – IV (see fig below))
    <u>Management</u>
    undisplaced: internal fixation (2–3 screws)
    displaced: hemiarthroplasty, ORIF in younger patients

2. Trochanteric fracture (extracapsular) see fig (c) opposite
    intertrochanteric, basal or subtrochanteric
    classification based on number of fragments provided by fracture (e.g. two-part, three-part, four-part)
    <u>Management</u>
    Intertrochanteric and basal fractures: dynamic hip screw (DHS) – closed reduction using traction on fracture table. The main leg screw should be parallel to the femoral neck in all planes extending up to the subchondral bone within.
    Subtrochanteric fractures: ORIF

Complications of fractured neck of femur surgery

Usually elderly and frail patients so mortality is 14–36% at 1 year. Complications include infection, dislocation, femoral screws loosening, acetabular erosion, non-union, osteoarthritis, avascular necrosis.

Avascular necrosis following fractured neck of femur

There is a high incidence of avascular necrosis of the femoral head in Garden III or IV fractures due to the disruption of the nutrient artery in the shaft and the retinacular vessels in the capsule leaving only the vessel in the ligamentum teres which may not be sufficient to prevent ischaemia of the femoral head (see fig below). The bone dies and eventually collapses with distortion of the femoral head and irreversible damage to the joint. This causes pain and loss of function. The treatment is total joint replacement. Other causes of avascular necrosis of the femoral head include Perthes' disease, dislocation of the hip and slipped upper femoral epiphysis.

Other femoral injuries

Adolescents: slipped upper femoral epiphysis
Adults: hip dislocation as opposed to fracture
Elderly: fractured neck of femur

[265] These will reveal the operation she has had (see fig opposite) and may reveal avascular necrosis (see pg 186).

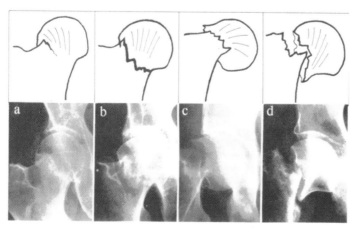

Garden's classification of femoral neck fractures. (a) Stage I: incomplete (so-called abducted or impacted). (b) Stage II: complete without displacement. (c) Stage III: complete with partial displacement – fragments still connected by posterior retinacular attachment; the femoral trabeculae are malaligned. (d) Stage IV: complete with full displacement – the proximal fragment is free and lies correctly in the acetabulum so that the trabeculae appear normally aligned.

FRACTURED NECK OF FEMUR[264]

Carry out examination of the hip, (see pg 137).

'There is (in this elderly lady) a scar over the right hip. The right leg is shortened and externally rotated with marked loss of range of movement at the hip. This patient has had a fractured neck of femur and has secondary osteoarthritis. I would like to see her X-rays[265]'

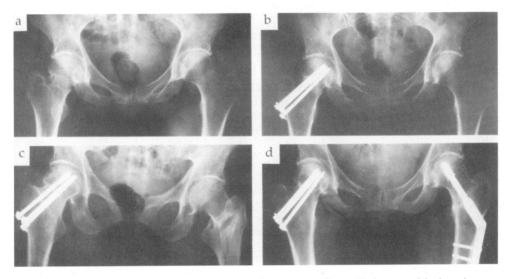

This elderly woman was osteoporotic but otherwise well, until she stumbled and fractured the right femoral neck (a). The fracture was fixed with three long screws (b) and united soundly. Then, a year later, she tripped and sustained an intertrochanteric fracure on the left side (c). This needed more extensive fixation – a large screw fitted to a plate attached to the femoral shaft (d).

Fractured neck of femur (continued)

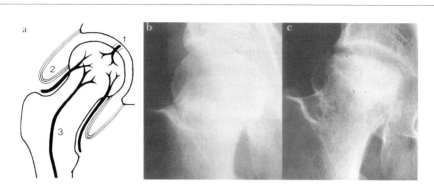

(a) The blood supply to the femoral head comes from (1) a vessel in the ligamentum teres, (2) the retinacular vessels and (3) the nutrient artery. Fracture of the femoral neck interrupts at least one source of supply and may seriously compromise the others. Even (b) an impacted fracture, if it is displaced in marked valgus, can lead to avascular necrosis (c).

Avascular necrosis as a result of femoral neck fracture

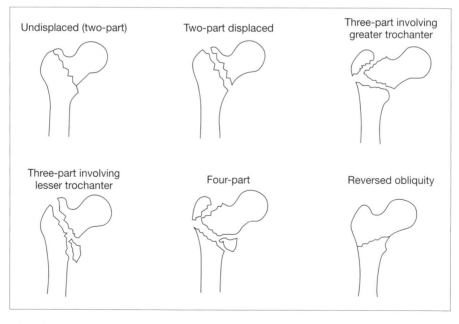

Classification of extracapsular fractures

OSTEOARTHRITIS OF THE KNEE[266]

Carry out full examination of the knee (see pg 141).

'There is an obvious deformity/scar of a previous operation (secondary osteoarthritis). There is swelling and deformity of the knee joints with development of varus (or valgus) deformity. There is wasting and weakness of the quadriceps. The presence of osteophytes distinguishes this from rheumatoid arthritis. There is little effusion and no warmth (except during an exacerbation). The synovial membrane is not thickened. Range of movement is reduced and there is crepitus in the knee. Pressure on the patella elicits pain. On a weight bearing X-ray I would expect to see diminished tibiofemoral joint space (often only in one compartment), subchondral sclerosis, osteophytes and chondrocalcinosis[267]. This patient has osteoarthritis of the knee[268].

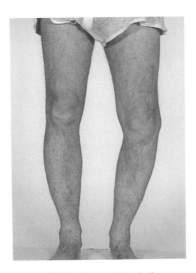

Varus deformity of the left knee

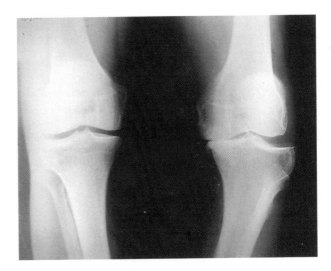

OA of the medial compartment causing a varus deformity

Top Five Case: seen by over a third of candidates in our survey. Knee examination accounted for 13.2% of cases in this bay.

[266] **Symptoms:** (if allowed to question patient) are pain after use (especially up stairs), stiffness after rest, swelling, giving way and locking. Ask what other joints are affected (hip and back are typical) and about childhood or past trauma and operations.

[267] Soft tissue calcification in the suprapatellar region or in the joint itself.

[268] **Treatment:**   Conservative especially quadriceps exercises.

Realignment osteotomy of tibia (in younger patients with only one compartment affected).

Knee replacement (in older patients where joint destruction is advanced).

187

Rheumatoid arthritis of the knee

[269] Occasionally, rheumatoid arthritis starts in the knee as a chronic monoarticular synovitis but is more often part of a polyarthropathy. An elderly patient with 'burnt out' chronic rheumatoid disease (Case 1) is far more likely to be found for examination than someone with an acute synovitis or flare-up of their monoarthritis (Case 2). Treatment of the acute flare-up involves systemic medication (e.g. non-steroidal anti-inflammatory drugs, steroids, immunosuppressants), local splintage and steroid injections with synovectomy reserved for severe or resistant cases. Treatment of the chronic disability depends on the degree of deformity, disability and loss of cartilage and bone. Femoral or tibial osteotomy may be considered to improve function and relieve pain, but joint replacement is advised once the joint is unstable.

[270] These factors determine whether the patient has an acute flare-up (see Case 2) or quiescent arthritis. The latter is more likely to come to the exam.

[271] Show periarticular osteoporosis, loss of joint space, marginal erosions and an absence of osteophytes distinguishing it from the sclerotic picture of osteoarthritis, in which osteophytes are a characteristic feature.

[272] It is possible to develop OA of the knee secondary to joint disease of the hip or ankle or previous trauma or surgery that put abnormal stresses on the joint.

RHEUMATOID ARTHRITIS OF THE KNEE[269]

Carry out examination of the knee (pg 141).

Case 1

'The patient has extensive rheumatoid disease affecting many joints, most obviously in his hands (and say where else). He has wasting of the quadriceps and painless restriction of the knee joint. There is no effusion or thickened synovium palpable, and the joint is not red or hot[270]. There is valgus/varus and fixed flexion deformities and instability of the joint. The diagnosis is chronic rheumatoid arthritis. I would like to see his weight-bearing X-rays[271], which would exclude osteoarthritis secondary to rheumatoid disease elsewhere (e.g. the hip)[272].'

Case 2

Alternatively (but not as likely in the examination)
'The patient (who may or may not have signs of rheumatic disease in other joints) has a painful, warm, swollen knee with a large effusion and a thickened synovium easily palpable. Movement and mobility are restricted by pain. The diagnosis is acute rheumatoid arthritis of the knee but septic arthritis and gout (see pg 203) should be excluded by careful history and aspiration if necessary.'

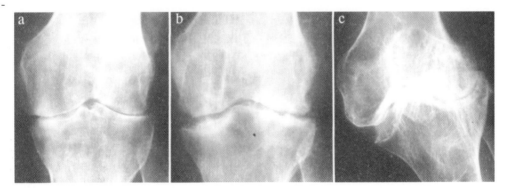

X-rays of Rheumatoid knees. (a) Early changes are cartilage erosion (giving a narrow joint space) and osteoporosis. (b) Later, joint destruction becomes more obvious, and (c) in severe cases gross deformity may result.

Dupuytren's contracture

Top Five Case: seen by more than half the candidates in our survey. Accounted for 17.1% of cases in this bay.

[255] **Definition**: nodular hypertrophy and contracture of the palmar aponeurosis

Causes:

Idiopathic

Familial (autosomal dominant)

Alcoholic liver disease

Trauma

Manual labour

Drugs (e.g. phenobarbitone)

Diabetes

AIDS

Peyronie's disease.

Epidemiology: 5% usually middle-aged men.

Differential diagnosis: skin contractures secondary to burns or scarring; tendon contracture (thickened cord moves on passive flexion of the finger).

Treatment (surgery): careful dissection and excision of the thickened part of the aponeurosis. 'Zed-plasty' is often needed to lengthen the wound and permit adequate skin closure. Postoperative splinting and physiotherapy are important. Recurrence may occur in progressive cases.

[256] Can affect the plantar aponeurosis.

[257] Alcoholism is associated with Dupuytren's and can produce a large fatty liver.

[258] The knuckle pads of the hands are often thickened.

[259] Fibrosis of the corpus cavernosum causing curvature of the penis may be associated with Dupuytren's. The examiners are unlikely to expect you to confirm this so choose a tactful way of telling them you know about the association!

DUPUYTREN'S CONTRACTURE[255]

Spot diagnosis.

'There is a painless, bilateral (or unilateral) nodular thickening of the palm especially on the ulnar side extending distally to involve the ring/little finger. It is causing a fixed flexion deformity of the little (+/– ring) finger(s) at the metacarpophalangeal (+/– proximal interphalangeal) joints. There is evidence of previous surgery over this area/on the other palm. This is Dupuytren's contracture.'

Common examiner's question: 'What else would you like to examine?'

Answer: 'The soles of the feet[256], the liver[257], the dorsal knuckle pads[258]. Dupuytren's is also associated with Peyronie's disease[259].'

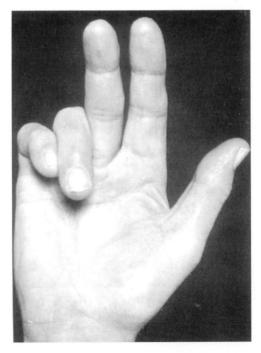

Dupuytren's contracture

Rheumatoid arthritis of the hands

Top Five Case: seen by over a third of candidates in our survey. Accounts for 11.2% of cases in this bay.

[273] **A very common case.** If there is time, or if this is your first case in the bay, you should go through the examination described on pg 148 for maximum marks. If the examiners are rushing you or hint that you should be quick i.e. 'a quick spot diagnosis please' or 'one last quick one before the bell' this is an alternative.

[274] There are five causes of anaemia in rheumatoid arthritis.

1. **Anaemia of chronic disease.**
2. **GI bleed** due to NSAIDs use.
3. **Bone marrow suppression** by gold, phenylbutazone, indomethacin, penicillamine.
4. Associated **pernicious anaemia** leading to megaloblastic anaemia.
5. **Felty's syndrome** – rheumatoid arthritis, neutropaenia and splenomegaly. Occurs in 5% of older patients with long-standing RA.

[275] **X-ray signs of rheumatoid arthritis** depend on the stage of disease. Features include soft tissue swelling, periarticular osteoporosis, narrowing of joint space, marginal bony erosions (especially around the wrist), articular destruction and joint deformity.

Extraarticular manifestations of rheumatoid arthritis from the top down:

Eye signs: episcleritis, cataracts due to chloroquine or steroids, scleromalacia perforans, Sjögren's syndrome.

Chest signs: pleural effusion, fibrosing alveolitis, rheumatoid nodules, Caplan's syndrome (rheumatoid nodules in lung fields associated with massive fibrotic reaction), obliterative bronchiolitis (due to penicillamine therapy).

Cardiac signs: pericarditis (40% at autopsy but rarely apparent clinically), granulomatous infiltration (rarely causing myocarditis, conduction defects and valvular incompetence).

Abdominal signs: splenomegaly in Felty's syndrome. Hepatosplenomegaly in secondary amyloidosis.

Neurological signs: peripheral neuropathy, mononeuritis multiplex, carpal tunnel syndrome.

Skin signs: leg ulceration, vasculitis, pyoderma gangrenosum.

Other autoimmune disorders: vitiligo, myasthenia gravis, hypothyroidism, primary biliary sclerosis.

Treatment of rheumatoid arthritis

1. Stop the synovitis. Anti-inflammatories (symptomatic not disease modifying).

Disease modifying drugs (gold, penicillamine, immunosuppressive drugs. Side-effects on liver, kidney, bone marrow so monitor and use sparingly).

Corticosteroids (during flare-ups, many side-effects).

Rest and splintage.

Intraarticular injections.

Synovectomy (last resort).

2. Prevent deformity. Surgery (joint replacement, tendon repair etc.)

Physiotherapy (passive and active)

3. Reconstruct. Arthrodesis, osteotomy, joint replacement.

4. Rehabilitate. Physiotherapy, keep active, treat comorbidity.

Swan neck – hyperextension of PIP joints with fixed flexion of MCP and DIP joints due to tendon prolapse. The two lateral slips of the extensor tendon usually rupture or stretch, and so cannot extend the distal phalanx, while the pull of the central tendon hyperextends the middle phalanx. Can be corrected by check-rein procedure that shortens and reimplants the lateral slips of the extensor tendons.

RHEUMATOID ARTHRITIS OF THE HANDS[273]

Carry out examination of rheumatoid hands, (see pg 148).

'There is symmetrical deforming polyarthropathy of the joints with spindling of the fingers, affecting the MCP and PIP joints but sparing the DIP joints. There is wasting of the small muscles of the hand. Typical features are seen, such as ulnar deviation at the MCP joints with radial deviation at the wrist, swan neck/boutonniere/'Z' thumb deformities (say where). There is thin skin, bruising pale nail beds[274] and vasculitic lesions. The palms show pale palmar creases and palmar erythema. I can feel joint destruction and rheumatoid nodules. This patient has rheumatoid arthritis. I would like to look at the elbows, assess function and neurology and see the X-rays[275].'

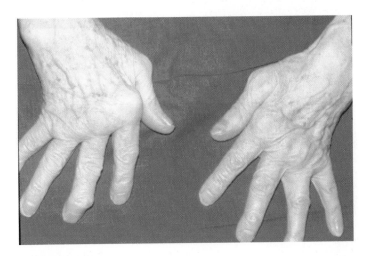

Rheumatoid hands

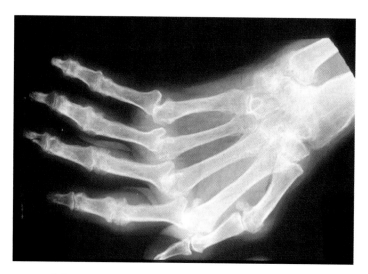

X-ray of rheumatoid hand

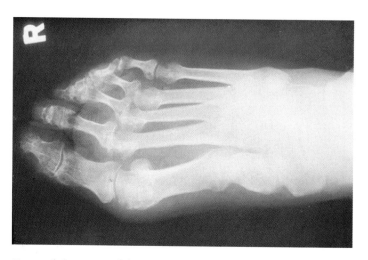

X-ray of rheumatoid foot

Note soft tissue swelling, periarticular osteoporosis, narrowing of joint space, marginal bony erosions, articular destruction and joint deformity.

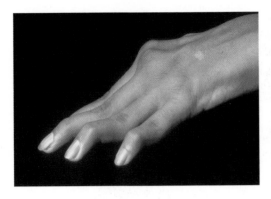

Swan neck deformity

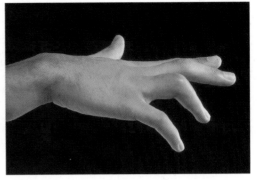

Rheumatoid hand showing Boutonnière deformity most marked in the ring finger

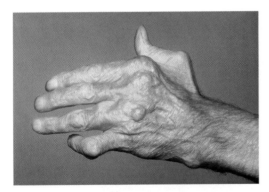

Rheumatoid hand showing deforming polyarthropathy affecting MCP and PIP joints sparing DIP joints. Note the Z thumb, Boutonnière deformity of the little finger, wasting of the small muscles of the hand and rheumatoid nodules

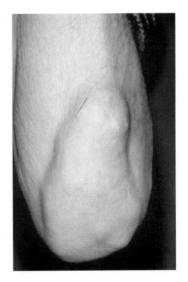

Rheumatoid nodules on elbow

Osteoarthritis of the hands

[276] **Definition:** a disease process of synovial joints characterised by focal areas of loss of hyaline articular cartilage associated with increased activity in marginal and subchondral bone.

Sites affected: knees, hips, hands, spinal apophyseal joints.

Aetiology: secondary OA associated with a clear abnormality (e.g. old injury to hip leading to OA of that knee) or primary/idiopathic. Risk factors include previous trauma, repetitive occupation, obesity and hypermobility.

Epidemiology: 1% overall, up to 10% of over-sixties.

X-ray findings: joint space narrowing, osteophyte formation, subchondral sclerosis, subchondral cysts.

Management: Conservative: prevention, walking aids, physiotherapy to avoid flexion deformity and wasting
          Analgesia: non-steroidal, joint injections.
          Surgery: arthroplasty of knee and hip

[277] Bony swellings in distal interphalangeal joints which form insidiously or from a hyaluronate-filled cyst that may be painful and warm. Nodal disease is more common in women and runs in families.

OSTEOARTHRITIS[276] OF THE HANDS

Carry out a full examination of the hands as for rheumatoid hands (see pg 148) if there is time. If not, spot diagnosis should mention these points:

'There are Heberden's nodes[277] present at the bases of the distal phalanges and Bouchard's nodes at the proximal interphalangeal joints. There is a 'square hand' deformity due to subluxation of the base of the first metacarpal. The patient has osteoarthritis of the hands.'

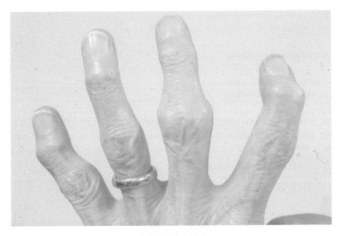

Osteoarthritis of hands showing Heberden's nodes and Bouchard's nodes

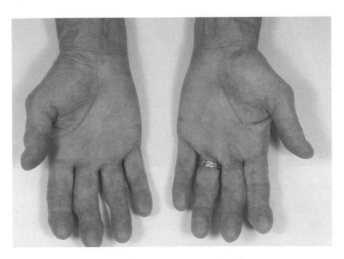

Osteoarthritic hand showing 'squared off' appearance and multiple Heberden's nodes

Psoriatic arthritis of the hands

[278] **Other forms of psoriatic arthropathy** include:

Arthritis mutilans

Arthritis clinically indistinguishable from rheumatoid arthritis but consistently seronegative

Asymmetrical oligo- or mono-arthropathy

Ankylosing spondylitis occurring alone or in conjunction with any of the other forms.

[279] Loosening or separation of nail from nail bed.

[280] Thick scale under nails.

[281] Psoriatic arthropathy can occur with minimal skin involvement. Other areas affected are typically the knees and other extensor aspects, the scalp, behind the ears and in the navel.

[282] **Incidence:**   1–5% of Caucasians in NW Europe and USA

Rare in Japanese, African Americans, American Indians.

Radiological findings

Soft tissue swelling (sausage digit)

A symmetrical destruction of distal interphalangeal joints

'Pencil in cup' deformity – erosions with adjacent bone proliferation

Ankylosis

Sclerosis of terminal phalanx (ivory phalanx)

Other joints affected

Feet, especially first toe interphalangeal joint

Lower cervical, thoracic, upper lumbar spine

Sacroiliac joint

Treatments: Sunlight, u.v. light, coal tar, dithranol, local steroids, PUVA (psoralen drugs and u.v. light). Systemic steroids and antimetabolites rarely used, chloroquine contraindicated. Analgesia, anti-inflammatories and intra-articular steroid injections alleviate symptoms.

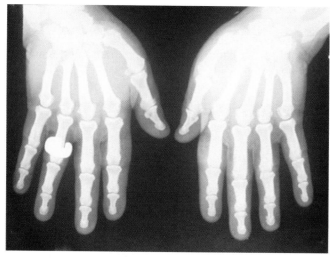

X-ray of psoriatic hands

PSORIATIC ARTHRITIS OF THE HANDS

Carry out a full examination of the hands as for rheumatoid hands (pg 148) if there is time. If not, mention the following features in a spot diagnosis.
'There is an asymmetrical arthropathy involving the terminal interphalangeal joints of the hands[278]. The fingernails are pitted with onycholysis[279] thickened nail plates and hyperkeratosis[280]. There are patches of psoriasis at the elbows[281]. The plaques are red with a silvery scaly surface and tend to be circular with well-defined edges. This patient has psoriatic arthritis[282].'

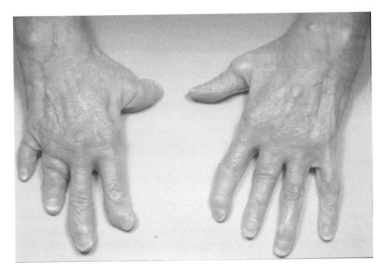

Psoriatic arthritis of hands

Hallux valgus

Top Five Case: seen by over a quarter of the candidates in our survey. Great toe accounted for 9.2% of cases in this bay.

[283] **Definition**: the commonest of the foot deformities, the underlying deformity is usually metatarsus primus varus (splaying of the forefoot) which predisposes to a lateral angulation of the big toe in people who wear shoes.

Causes:	Congenital metatarsus varus (often hereditary)
	Loss of muscle tone in the forefoot in old people
	Rheumatoid arthritis
	Worsened by narrow or pointed shoes (especially in women). In people who have never worn shoes (e.g. developing countries) the big toe remains in line with the first metatarsal retaining the fan-shaped appearance of the forefoot
Epidemiology:	Usually bilateral
	Most common in the sixth decade
	Most common in females
	Familial variety presents in adolescence
Symptoms:	Deformity
	Pain usually due to complications such as:
	Inflamed bunion (protective bursa over first metatarsal head)
	Hammer toe
	Metatarsalgia
	Secondary osteoarthritis of the first metatarsophalangeal (MTP) joint

X-ray findings: should be weight bearing. Shows degree of metatarsal and hallux angulation and subluxation or osteoarthritic changes of the first MTP joint.

Conservative treatment: wide shoes with soft uppers; padding to protect bunion/hammer toe; foot exercises; anterior platform support to relieve metatarsalgia.

Surgical treatment: (see diagram on pg opposite)

a) Corrective osteotomy of first metatarsal +/- bone graft insertion: in adolescents correction of the deformity may prevent the condition worsening.

b) In older people or more severe deformities Mitchell's osteotomy or

c) Wilson's osteotomy are the operations of choice.

d) Basal osteotomy and capsulorrhaphy: in adults between 20–50 years with moderate deformity an adductor hallucis tendon release on the lateral side of the big toe with trimming of the metatarsal head and tightening of the medial capsule may give adequate correction. A metatarsal osteotomy is also required in more severe cases.

e) Keller's operation is the simplest solution for elderly patients.

Postoperative complications: redistribution of stresses on weight bearing can lead to aching forefoot or even stress fractures of the metatarsal bones especially in osteoporotic patients.

Other conditions of the great toe:

Hallux rigidus: Primary osteoarthritis of the first metatarsophalangeal joint results in stiffness and pain. There is thickening due to circumferential exostosis formation. This affects walking, which normally involves considerable dorsiflexion at this joint. The toe may be held flexed (hallux flexus). It is common in men and is treated by fusion or Keeler's arthroplasty. A rocker-soled shoe relieves symptoms.

Bunion: A protective bursa formed at pressure areas e.g. hallux valgus.

Gout (see pg 203).

Ingrowing toenail (see pg 205).

HALLUX VALGUS[283]

Spot diagnosis.

'There is marked hallux valgus bilaterally with prominence of the first metatarsal head, worse on the left/right. Typical associated features seen here include widening of the forefoot, bunions, crowding and deformity (?overlapping) of the second toe, medial rotation of the hallux, and hammer toes (say which toes).'

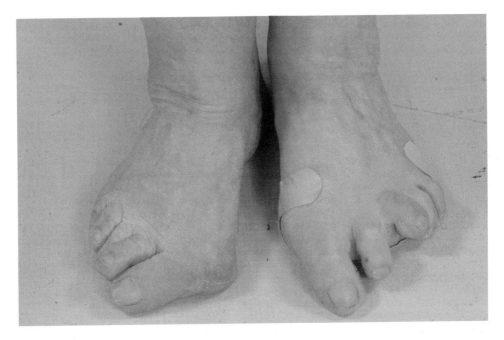

Hallux valgus

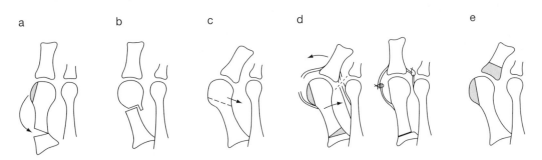

Surgical treatment of Hallux valgus (see footnote opposite)

Gout

[284] **Definition:** hyperuricaemia associated with recurrent attacks of acute arthritis triggered by crystallisation of urates in joints with asymptomatic intervals. In severe cases there is eventual development of tophaceous gout with aggregates of urates in and around joints and chronic often crippling gouty arthritis.

Aetiology: 90% primary (mostly idiopathic due to increased uric acid production or decreased excretion). 10% secondary to diuretics (thiazides especially), myeloproliferative/lymphoproliferative disorders and chronic renal failure.

Distribution: 90% big toe, also instep, ankle, heel, knee, small joints of the hands.

Pathological features:

1. <u>Acute arthritis</u>: acute inflammatory synovitis stimulated by monosodium urate crystals (long, needle-shaped, birefringent on microscopy). Leucocytes and macrophages release cytokines.

2. <u>Chronic arthritis</u>: urate precipitates in the synovial membrane following acute attacks stimulating a pannus (inflammatory overgrowth) over the synovium and cartilage degrading cartilage and bone. Leads to proliferation of marginal bone and bony ankylosis.

3. <u>Tophi</u>: urate deposition in periarticular tissues surrounded by intense inflammatory reaction involving white cells, fibroblasts and giant cells. Typical chalky exudative deposits may cause overlying skin necrosis and exude a paste of monosodium urate crystals (hence the unlikely story of the patient who kept the darts score on the pub blackboard with his gouty hands having no need of chalk!)

4. <u>Kidney disease</u>: acute uric acid nephropathy, nephrolithiasis, chronic uric nephropathy.

Associations: obesity, type IV hyperlipidaemia, hypertension, diabetes and ischaemic heart disease.

Treatment:

1. <u>Treat acute attack</u>: anti-inflammatories e.g. NSAIDs e.g. indomethacin or, rarely, colchicine.

2. <u>Prophylaxis</u>: reduce precipitating factors (alcohol, obesity, diuretics); decrease uric acid production (allopurinol); increase uric acid secretion (uricosurics e.g. probenecid).

Beware: altering uric acid metabolism can precipitate an attack, so do not start allopurinol during an acute attack, and cover introduction of prophylactic long term therapy with non-steroidal.

Pseudogout

Acute and chronic inflammatory joint disease caused by the deposition of either crystals of calcium pyrophosphate or basic calcium phosphates in the articular cartilage and menisci usually involving knees, ankles, wrists, elbows, hips or spine. Aetiology: hereditary (autosomal dominant); metabolic (hyperparathyroidism, haemochromatosis, hypothyroidism); idiopathic; post-surgical/trauma. Pathology is similar to gout but with short rhomboid water-soluble crystals. X-rays show calcification in soft tissues and linear densities in articular cartilage parallel to subchondral bone. Serum calcium is normal. Treatment involves rest, aspiration and steroid injections. Not as easy to control as gout.

[285] Typically the ulnar surface of the forearm, olecranon bursa, the Achilles tendon and other pressure points. Tophi can also occur in the patella bursa, kidneys, aorta and myocardium.

[286] Septic arthritis is excluded by joint aspiration. Microscopy shows typical crystals. Blood uric acid may or may not be raised.

Radiological findings: typically seen late (>6 years after first attack)

1. <u>Soft tissue swelling</u>

2. <u>'Punched out'</u> erosions. These start near joint margins and have a classic overhanging sclerotic margin. They are mostly set back from the articular surface.

3. <u>Eccentric soft tissue masses</u> in a periarticular location in tophaceous gout (rarely do these calcify).

4. <u>Cartilage destruction</u> (and hence joint space narrowing) is not typical except in very late cases and there is not typically osteoporosis (differentiating it from rheumatoid).

5. <u>Chondrocalcinosis</u> occurs in 5% of cases.

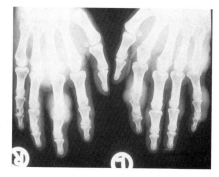

X-ray of hand with gout

GOUT[284]

Spot diagnosis or examine these hands (rheumatic hands examination pg 148).

'There is an asymmetrical swelling affecting the small joints of the hands with tophi formation in the periarticular tissues. The joints are (in some cases) severely deformed. There are tophi on the helix of the ear and in some of the tendon sheaths[285]. This is chronic tophaceous gout.'

Alternatively:
'There is swelling, redness and heat over the metatarsophalangeal joint of the big toe. It is exquisitely tender, but the patient shows no signs of systemic sepsis such as fever, sweating or rigors. This looks typical of acute gout, but if the patient had no previous history, septic arthritis would have to be excluded.[286]

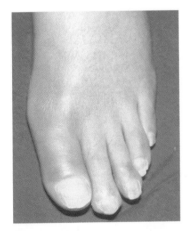 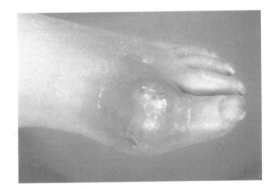

Gout of great toe

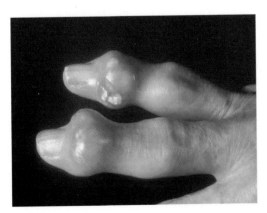 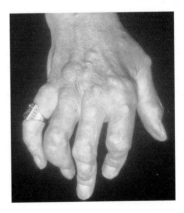

Tophaceous gout

Ingrowing toenail

[287] Beware the easy spot diagnosis. What a waste to simply say 'ingrowing toenails' and move on to a more complicated case when you can milk this gift of a case for every point. Make sure you know your facts on the simple cases and take them as seriously as the more obscure ones; each case is worth the same number of marks and it's hard to give top marks for a quick spot with nothing else offered.

[288] Encourage correctly fitting footwear and horizontal nail cutting.

[289] In the presence of gross sepsis or as a first line of treatment, **avulsion of the nail** may allow things to settle. However, recurrence should be expected and a definitive operation planned in case of this. Avulsion is easily carried out under local anaesthetic ring block with the nail simply pulled out leaving the entire nail bed to grow a new nail.

[290] In young patients who wish to conserve a toenail for cosmesis, **wedge excision** is the treatment of choice. The procedure is carried out after gross infection has settled, under general or ring block local anaesthesia with a rubber tourniquet applied at the base of the toe. The toenail is divided longitudinally one-third of the width of the nail from the affected margin with a scalpel held blade uppermost, and the ingrowing portion is avulsed leaving the central portion of the nail intact. The exposed strip of nail bed, granulation tissue and a margin of healthy skin are excised in a deep wedge extending proximally to the base of the distal phalanx. The wedge must be deep and wide enough to ensure complete removal of the lateral portion of the germinal matrix, since inadequate excision is followed by regrowth of a troublesome nail spike. If there is doubt about the removal of the corners, curette with a Volkmann spoon or phenol ablation (applying a cotton bud impregnated with phenol for 120 seconds to the corner) of the corners are both recognised methods. If phenol is used the surrounding skin is protected with petroleum jelly and the residual phenol is carefully rinsed with saline as soon as the time is up to prevent continued necrosis. The wedge is closed by suturing the skin margin to the cut edge of the nail with a non-absorbable suture such as nylon 2/0 on a cutting needle. For both the wedge excision and Zadik's procedure the toe is dressed with paraffin gauze, bulky gauze and crepe. The tourniquet is removed. The foot is elevated for 24 hours and firm bandaging treats any postoperative bleeding. The sutures are removed after 14 days. The patient should wear open-toed sandals (+/- socks in winter) until the wounds are healed.

[291] Zadik described **radical excision of the nail root** in 1950. This is more suitable in older patients with recurrent disease. The patient must be warned that the nail will never grow back after this procedure. Under general or local ring block anaesthesia with a tourniquet applied, the entire nail is first avulsed. Two oblique incisions are made from the corner of the nail bed to the crease of the distal interphalangeal joint. A skin flap is then raised with a scalpel from the proximal and lateral flaps thus formed. These are retracted to expose the underlying germinal matrix. A distal transverse incision in the nail bed is made at the level of the lunula and the entire germinal matrix is dissected proximally off the periosteum taking care to include the lateral and medial corners of the matrix from which spikes of nail may grow if left behind. The whole 'nail bed' or germinal matrix is removed as an 'envelope' of tissue and the corners of the resected specimen can be inspected to ensure complete removal. The skin flaps are sutured to the nail bed using 3/0 nylon sutures without tension.

[292] It is important to exclude peripheral vascular disease as, if present, the implications of sepsis are more severe, wound healing is likely to be compromised, and the minimal procedure likely to be useful should be selected (e.g avulsion).

[293] Ingrowing toenail surgery is usually suitable for day case surgery if the patient is fit. **Ring block** using a local anaesthetic such as 1% lignocaine provides adequate regional anaesthesia but the procedure can be performed under GA if the patient prefers. To achieve a ring block, the needle is introduced through the dorsal skin at the base of the digit and is advanced just to one side of the phalanx until it can be seen tenting the thick plantar skin (do not palpate for this as you risk needle stick injury). 2–3 mls of local anaesthetic are injected (the digital nerves run nearer the plantar than the dorsal surface) and the needle is withdrawn. The procedure is repeated on the other side. Local anaesthetic with adrenaline should not be used due to the risk of digital ischaemia (the end digital arteries run with the nerves).

[294] Intraoperative hazards: damage to extensor hallucis longus tendon. Opening the distal interphalangeal joint. Failure to excise the nail root.

Postoperative complications: infection of soft tissues (common) and osteomyelitis (rare). Bleeding. Recurrence or growth of nail spike.

INGROWING TOENAIL

Spot diagnosis[287].

'The patient has ingrowing toenails on the lateral and medial sides of both great toes. There is evidence of recurrent infection, worse on the lateral side of the right great toe (for example) which is currently infected with erythema, tenderness and a seropurulent discharge. The treatment options for ingrowing toenails include conservative measures[288], avulsion of the nail[289], wedge excision[290] and Zadik's procedure[291]. Since this patient is young, foot pulses are good[292], the nail obviously symptomatic, and the current sepsis not severe, I would suggest wedge excisions on the medial and lateral sides of both great toes (or whichever margins are affected) to preserve the central nail for cosmesis. I would discuss the benefits of general and local anaesthetic[293], explain the procedure and the possible complications[294], and suggest a course of antibiotics and open footwear for two weeks preoperatively to minimise the infection of that right toe.'

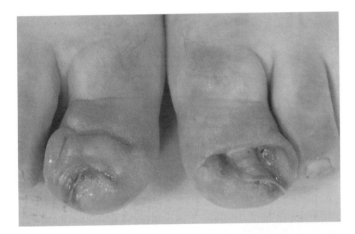

Bilateral ingrowing toenails with severe sepsis. It is important to check the peripheral circulation before undertaking surgery. Simple nail avulsions may be required to allow the sepsis to settle before the definitive operation is performed – probably bilateral Zadik's procedure if the patient is elderly and does not mind about the cosmetic result.

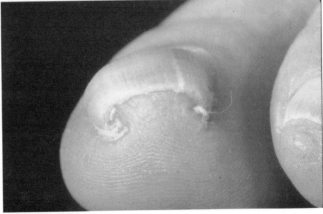

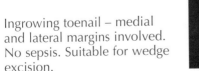

Ingrowing toenail – medial and lateral margins involved. No sepsis. Suitable for wedge excision.

Median nerve palsy and carpal tunnel syndrome

Very Common Case: either carpal tunnel syndrome or median nerve palsy were seen by over 1 in 10 of the candidates in our survey.

[295] **Facts about the median nerve:**

Nerve roots: lateral and medial cords of brachial plexus C (5), 6, 7, 8, T1.

Course: The medial root crosses in front of the third part of the axillary artery to join the lateral root. It runs downwards on the lateral side of the brachial artery, crossing to the medial side halfway down the upper arm. It is superficial but is crossed at the elbow by the bicipital aponeurosis (?). It passes between the two heads of pronator teres separated from the ulnar artery by the ulnar head of pronator teres. It runs down behind flexor digitorum superficialis and is attached to its deep surface by connective tissue. It rests posteriorly on flexor digitorum profundus. At the wrist the median nerve emerges from the lateral border of the flexor digitorum superficialis muscle and lies behind the tendon of the palmaris longus. It enters the palm by passing behind the flexor retinaculum and immediately divides into lateral and medial branches, each of which gives muscular and cutaneous terminal branches.

Branches supply:

Near the elbow	In the forearm (via anterior interosseous branch)
Flexor digitorum superficialis	Flexor pollicis longus
Flexor carpi radialis	Half of flexor digitorum profundus
Palmaris longus	Pronator quadratus
Pronator teres	

In the hand

Motor: The 'LOAF' muscles of the thenar eminence: **L** ateral two lumbricales
O pponens pollicis
A bductor pollicis
F lexor pollicis brevis

Sensation of the lateral palm and lateral 2 1/2 fingers.

Causes of damage to the median nerve:

1. Carpal tunnel syndrome: may occur after wrist fractures
2. At the wrist: especially from lacerations here
3. In the forearm: (anterior interosseous nerve) from forearm bone fractures
4. Distal to the elbow: pronator teres nerve entrapment syndrome
5. At the elbow: e.g. after dislocation

[296] Definition of carpal tunnel syndrome: compression and/or ischaemia of the median nerve due to swelling of the flexor retinaculum.

[297] The patient is typically obese, middle-aged and female. The story is characteristic – pain, numbness or paraesthesia worse at night. Patient hangs arm out of bed, shaking it. Knitting or holding a newspaper may bring the pain on in the day. The discomfort may be referred beyond the cutaneous distribution of the median nerve in the hand up over the whole forearm, but the sensory signs are confined to the distribution of the median nerve.

[298] **Diagnostic tests:** be prepared to carry out any of the first three.

Tinel's test: percussion over the carpal tunnel producing tingling in the distribution of the nerve (Tinel's sign).

Phalen's test: the patient flexes both wrists for 60 seconds and this reproduces symptoms. Symptoms relieved when wrists relaxed. Positive in 50%. Symptoms may be induced by hyperextension of the wrist in some patients.

Tourniquet test: apply sphygmomanometer just above systolic pressure for 1–2 minutes to reproduce symptoms.

Nerve conduction tests: Not a bedside test but a diagnostic investigation. Differentiates from cervical spondylosis involving C6 and C7.

[299] **Causes of carpal tunnel syndrome:**

Can occur in healthy people	Can be a sign of underlying disease
idiopathic	myxoedema
pregnancy	acromegaly
obesity	rheumatoid arthritis
occupational	diabetes
previous trauma	
contraceptive pill, unaccustomed activity (e.g. housepainting)	

MEDIAN NERVE PALSY AND CARPAL TUNNEL SYNDROME

Carry out median nerve examination (see pg 172).

'There is sensory loss over the palmar aspects of the first three and a half fingers and wasting of the thenar eminence. There is weakness of abduction, flexion and opposition of the thumb. The diagnosis is median nerve palsy[295].

The flexor muscles of the forearm are not involved, suggesting carpal tunnel syndrome[296], so I would like to question the patient[297], perform some diagnostic tests[298] and look for an underlying cause[299].

Alternatively:
'The symptoms you describe are suggestive of carpal tunnel syndrome. Tinel's test/Phalen's test (or the tourniquet test) are positive but the median nerve shows no deficit. The diagnosis is carpal tunnel syndrome[300].

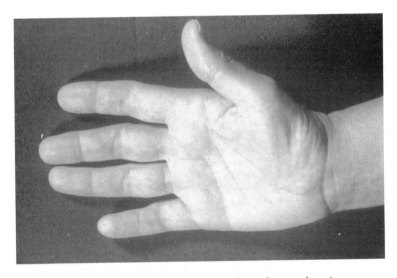

Median nerve palsy due to carpal tunnel syndrome showing wasting of the thenar eminence

Ulnar nerve palsy
Common Case: ulnar nerve palsy was seen by more than 1 in 20 of the candidates in our survey.
[301] **Facts about the ulnar nerve:**
<u>Nerve Roots</u>: Medial cord of brachial plexus C8 T1
<u>Course</u>: Descends between axillary artery and vein and then runs down on the medial side of the brachial artery as far as the middle of the arm. Here, at the insertion of the coracobrachialis, the nerve pierces the medial fascial septum, accompanied by the superior ulnar collateral artery and enters the posterior compartment of the arm. It descends behind the septum covered posteriorly by medial head of triceps. At the elbow it lies superficially behind the medial epicondyle of the humerus on the medial ligament of the elbow joint. It enters the forearm between the two heads of origin of the flexor carpi ulnaris (FCU). It runs down the forearm between FCU and flexor digitorum profundus (FDP) medial to the ulnar artery. At the wrist the ulnar nerve becomes superficial and lies between FCU and FDS tendons entering the palm in front of flexor retinaculum, lateral to the pisiform base and divides into a superficial branch which ends in muscular and cutaneus branches, and a deep branch which runs backward between the abductor digiti minimi and the flexor digiti minimi, piercing the opponens digiti minimi and winding around the hook of the hamate. It passes laterally in the deep palmar arch giving off muscular branches.

<u>Branches in the forearm supply</u>:
<u>Muscles</u>   flexor carpi ulnaris
          50% of flexor digitorum profundus
<u>Skin</u>   dorsal cutaneous branch
          medial skin of dorsum of hand
          medial 1x digits
<u>Joints</u>   elbow joint

Branches in the hand supply:
<u>Muscles</u>   hypothenar muscles
          the interossei
          two medial lumbricals
          adductor pollicis
<u>Skin</u>   superficial palmar branch
          palmar 1x digits
          palmar cutaneous branch
          medial skin of palm

Common cause of ulnar nerve palsy (distal to proximal):
1. <u>Ulnar tunnel syndrome</u> where the nerve passes between the pisiform and the hook of the hamate (e.g. due to a ganglion or fractured hook of the hamate). The most distal lesions affect the deep palmar branch and are entirely motor.
2. <u>At the wrist</u> from lacerations, occupational trauma and ganglia.
3. <u>Distal to the elbow</u> by compression as it passes between the two heads of flexor carpi ulnaris.
4. <u>At the level of the medial epicondyle</u> where it is very superficial due to trauma, local friction, pressure or stretching e.g. in cubitus valgus or osteoarthritis.
5. <u>After supracondylar fractures</u> or other fractures around the elbow.
6. <u>In the brachial plexus</u> due to trauma.

ULNAR NERVE PALSY[301]

Carry out examination of the ulnar nerve (pg 174).

'The hand shows generalised muscle wasting and weakness sparing the thenar eminence with features of a claw hand. There is loss of sensation over the fifth finger, the ulnar half of the fourth finger and the ulnar side of the hand on both dorsal and palmar surfaces. There is weakness of the interossei and abductor digiti minimi. Froment's test is positive indicating weakness of adductor pollicis. The diagnosis is ulnar nerve palsy. I would like to look for scarring at the wrist/elbow.'

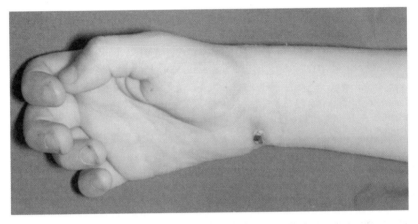

Ulnar nerve palsy with claw hand (note injury at the wrist)

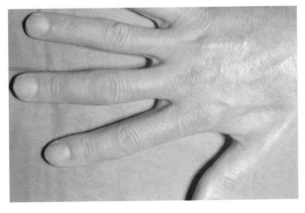

Ulnar nerve palsy showing lst web space wasting

Radial nerve palsy

[302] **Facts about the radial nerve**:

Nerve roots: posterior cord of brachial plexus C5, 6, 7.

Course: Arises posterior to axillary artery. Runs with profunda brachii artery between long and medial heads of triceps. Runs in spiral groove of humerus between medial and lateral heads of triceps (where it is susceptible to injury in humerus fractures). Lies deep to brachioradialis.

Branches supply:

Above the elbow:

Muscles: triceps, brachialis (lateral part), brachioradialis, extensor carpi radialis longus.

Skin: posterior cutaneous branch, to back of arm and forearm.

Joint: elbow.

Below the elbow: enters lateral cubital fossa. Divides into:

1. Posterior interosseous branch:

(runs between 2 heads of supinator passing into posterior compartment).

Supplies supinator and all extensors

2. Superficial radial nerve: (under brachioradialis and lateral to radial artery). Supplies skin of dorsum of radial side of hand and lateral three and-a-half digits.

Causes of damage of radial nerve:

In axilla

* 'Saturday night' palsy – neuropraxia from sleeping with arm over back of the chair.
* Ill fitting crutches.

Mid-humerus

* Fractures of humerus
* Tourniquet palsies

At and below elbow

* Elbow dislocations
* Monteggia fractures
* Ganglions
* Surgical trauma

[303] **Supinator tunnel**: The fibres of the supinator muscle are arranged in two planes, between which the deep branch of the radial nerve lies. The supinator arises from the lateral epicondyle of the humerus, the elbow joint and superior radial ulnar joint and the supinator crest and fossa of the ulna. It inserts into the posterior, lateral and anterior aspects of the neck and shaft of the radius as far as the oblique line.

RADIAL NERVE PALSY[302]

Carry out radial nerve examination (pg 176).

'There is wrist drop and sensory loss over the first dorsal interosseous. This is radial nerve palsy.' Weakness of the supinator and brachioadialis muscle suggest a lesion above the supinator tunnel[303]. Weakness of the triceps suggests a lesion at or above the midhumerus.'

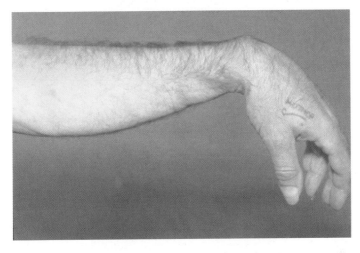

Wrist drop in radial nerve palsy

ERB'S PALSY[304]

Carry out neurological examination of the upper limb (pg 169).

'The arm hangs at the side, internally rotated at the shoulder, with the elbow extended and the forearm pronated in the 'waiter's tip' position[305]. There are/are not scars of trauma and surgery around the shoulder. Shoulder abduction and elbow flexion are not possible. The biceps and brachioradialis reflex jerks are absent. Sensory loss affects the lateral aspect of the shoulder and upper arm and the radial border of the forearm. The diagnosis is Erb's palsy.'

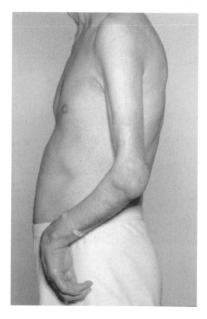

The elbow is usually extended but in this case some trauma has fixed it in flexion

---

Erb's Palsy

[304] Traumatic lesion of the **upper** portion of the brachial plexus (C5 and C6 roots or upper trunks).

Causes: traction injuries e.g. birth trauma (classical Erb's palsy), shoulder hits an obstacle when the patient is thrown from a vehicle (typically a motorcycle).

Prognosis and management: in birth injury, full recovery occurs in one-third of cases with residual weakness of shoulder abduction and elbow flexion in two-thirds. Sensory loss seldom persists. Prevention of contractures is a priority. Prognosis is worse if more of the brachial plexus (i.e. lower portions too) is involved.

Klumpke's paralysis is a rarer birth injury than Erb's palsy involving the cords of the **lower** brachial plexus (C8, T1) following traction with the arm extended. It results in paralysis of the intrinsic muscles of the hand with a claw hand deformity, weakness of the medial fingers and wrist flexors and a sensory loss over the medial forearm, hand and medial two fingers. Cervical sympathetic paralysis, giving rise to Horner's syndrome, is frequently associated.

[305] There is paralysis of deltoid, biceps, brachialis, brachioradialis and (if the roots are avulsed from the cords) rotator cuff muscles, serratus anterior, levator scapulae and the scalene muscles.

GANGLION[306]

Spot diagnosis. If in doubt, carry out examination of a lump (see pg 29).

'There is a smooth 2 cm subcutaneous lump on the extensor aspect (typically) of the wrist which is well-defined, cystic and (occasionally) seems to move with the extensor tendons. It is more obvious when the wrist is flexed. This is a ganglion.'

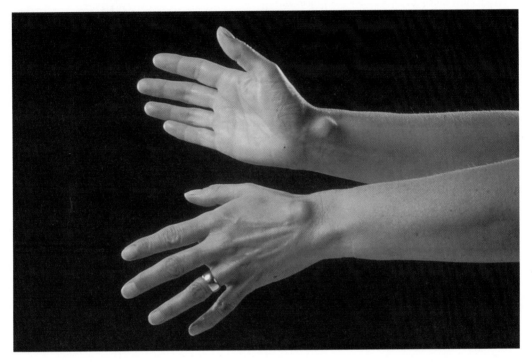

Ganglia on the wrists

Ganglion
Very Common Case: seen by over 1 in 10 of the candidates in our survey.
[306] **Definition**: a cystic degeneration in the joint capsule or tendon sheath resulting in a distended sheath containing fluid.
Clinical presentation: usually arises from the radiocarpal joint of young adults as described above. Tiny ganglia of this type may occur in the fingers. Fluctuations in size and rupture from trauma are common (the old fashioned home treatment of a ganglion was to hit it with the family bible!).
Treatment: patients may want it removed for cosmetic reasons or because it causes a persistent pain, ache or nuisance. It can be aspirated or excised, both carrying a risk of recurrence (especially the former). Excision may reveal a surprisingly deep root continuous with the underlying synovial joint so is often done under general or regional, rather than local anaesthetic. Injection of the aspirated ganglion sac with hyaluronic acid has been shown to reduce recurrence.
Compound palmar ganglion: a chronic inflammatory condition affecting the flexor tendon sheath. Large cystic mass is palpated proximal and distal to the flexor retinaculum and can be shown to be continuous with cross fluctuation.

External fixators

Very Common Case: seen by more than 1 in 10 of candidates in our survey.

[307] **Principle**: A fracture is held by transfixing screws which pass through the bone above and below the fracture and are attached to an external frame.

Indications

1. Fractures with severe soft tissue damage

   Where the wound can be left open for inspection, dressing or skin grafting.

2. Fractures associated with nerve vessel damage

3. Severely comminuted and unstable fractures

4. Fractures of the pelvis

   Which often cannot be held by any other method.

5. Infected fractures

   Internal fixation may lead to infected plates or nails.

Complications of external fixation

1. Pin track infection

   Especially if fixator is present for over 6 weeks.

2. Delayed union

   due to a) healing ends being held apart by fixator

   b) reduced load transmission through the bone (stress shielding) which is avoided by special fixators allowing axial loading or removing fixator at 6–8 weeks and replacing it with a splint allowing bone loading.

EXTERNAL FIXATORS[307]

'There is an external fixator on the lower right leg of this patient. There is a healing open wound over the mid shaft of the tibia on the anterior aspect of the leg. The quadriceps and calf muscles on the left look wasted/do not look wasted when compared with the right leg. The pin tracks look clean. This was probably an open fracture of the tibia which has been held externally due to the need for wound care and risk of infection. I would like to examine the distal neurology and circulation.'

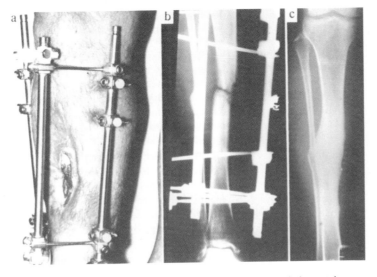

(ab) This patient had an open fracture with loss of skin. After debridement the fracture was held by external fixation; it went on to solid union (c).

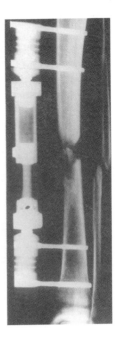

The bone is transfixed above and below the fracture. Stability is provided by the rigid external frame.

OLECRANON BURSITIS[308]

Spot diagnosis or carry out examination of the elbow (see pg 163).

'There is (in this young, otherwise healthy patient) a red hot tender fluctuant lump in the subcutaneous tissues over the extensor surface of the elbow. The range of movement of the joint is not affected. This is olecranon bursitis. I would like to look for signs of rheumatoid arthritis[309], gout[310] and infection[311], and ask the patient his occupation[312].'

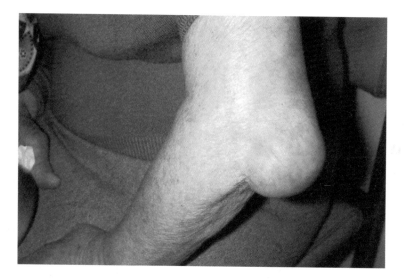

Olecranon bursitis

Olecranon bursitis
Common Case: seen by over 1 in 20 of the candidates in our survey.
[308] The small subcutaneous bursa over the olecranon process of the ulna can become enlarged by repeated minor trauma. A more acute, painful bursitis can be caused by infection, gout or rheumatoid arthritis.
[309] Such as polyarthritis especially of the joints of the hands (see pg 148).
[310] Such as bilateral bursitis, tophi, or calcification of the bursa on X-ray.
[311] Such as fever, rigors, reduced range of movement of the elbow. Septic bursitis is difficult to diagnose except by aspiration of pus. Local drainage is the treatment.
[312] Occupations at risk of olecranon bursitis include miners, carpet fitters or students – the condition is also known as 'scholar's elbow' (your examiners should be impressed if you display this sign yourself!).

BURSAE[313] OF THE KNEE AND BAKER'S CYST[314]

Spot diagnosis, or carry out examination of the knee (see pg 141).

Case 1

'There is a fluctuant swelling lying directly over the patella (or distal to the patella overlying the patellar ligament) but the joint itself is normal. The lump is not red or hot but (may be) tender. This is prepatellar/infrapatellar bursitis.'

Case 2

'There is (in this patient with chronic arthritis) a fluctuant swelling in the popliteal fossa. It is non-tender, non-pulsatile[315] and is/is not associated with an effusion of the knee joint. This is either a Baker's cyst (popliteal cyst) or a semi-membranosus bursa[316] (if medially placed with no associated arthritis).'

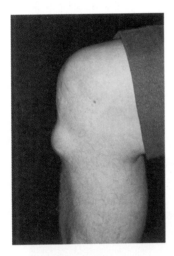

Infrapatellar bursa

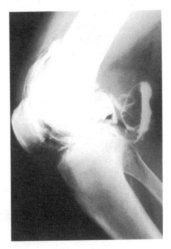

Arthrogram showing a Baker's cyst

Bursae of the knee and Baker's cyst

[313] The two commonest sites for symptomatic bursae (other than over a hallux valgus) are prepatellar and infrapatellar. These bursae become inflamed by constant friction, leading to a tender and swollen bursitis. A **prepatellar bursitis** (Housemaid's knee) is common in miners and carpet layers lying directly over the patella. An **infrapatellar bursitis** (clergyman's knee) is exacerbated in people who kneel more upright and lies superficial to the patellar ligament. Other sites for bursitis include the olecranon (scholar's elbow), Achilles tendon, hallux and shoulder. Treatment is to avoid the exacerbating activity, firm bandaging and occasional aspiration. In chronic cases the lump can be excised.

[314] A **Baker's cyst** or popliteal cyst usually develops in patients with chronic arthritis of the knee. It is a synovial sac bulging from the back of the joint. Occasionally it can leak or rupture into the calf causing pain and swelling difficult to distinguish from a deep vein thrombosis. Joint aspiration and intraarticular injection of corticosteroid will reduce the effusion and relieve discomfort.

[315] It is important to differentiate these swellings from a popliteal aneurysm.

[316] The bursa between the semi-membranosus muscle and the medial head of gastrocnemius may become enlarged. It presents as a painless lump in the medial part of the popliteal fossa. It is fluctuant but fluid and cannot be pushed between the muscles back into the joint. Unlike Baker's cyst, the knee is usually normal. If the lump aches it can be excised.

Trigger finger

[317] Thickening of the fibrous tendon sheath (usually after local trauma or unaccustomed activity) leads to narrowing of the sheath. A flexor tendon may become trapped at the entrance to the sheath until in forced extension; it passes the constriction with a snap (triggering). Rheumatoid tenosynovitis may cause a similar activity. Treatment is to stop aggravating activity if possible, but injection with prednisolone into the tendon sheath (but not into the tendon itself) is usually successful. In refractory cases surgery is required in which the fibrous sheath is incised allowing the tendon to move freely.

Related conditions

De Quervain's disease (stenosing tenovaginitis)

The sheath containing the extensor pollicis brevis and abductor pollicis longus becomes inflamed and thickened as a result of excessive or unaccustomed activity such as pruning roses or wringing out clothes. Typically women aged 30–50 years complain of pain on radial side of wrist +/- swelling. The tenderness can be pinpointed to the tip of the radial styloid. **Finkelstein's test** confirms diagnosis: Pain on passive adduction of thumb across palm and pain on active extension of thumb against resistance. Treatment as for trigger finger. Occasionally splintage of the wrist enforces rest.

Mallet finger/baseball finger

From injury to extensor tendon of terminal phalanx (e.g. by a cricket ball or baseball which forcibly ruptures the tendon). Patient cannot actively straighten terminal interphalangeal joint, so when all the fingers are extended the affected finger is bent at the TIP joint, although it can be passively straightened with ease. Treatment is by splintage for six weeks with the distal joint extended and the proximal interphalangeal joint flexed to allow tendon to reattach. K-wire fixation is another option.

Ruptured extensor pollicis longus

The long thumb extensor may rupture where it crosses the wrist (e.g. after a Colles' fracture or in rheumatoid arthritis). If the patient puts hands on a table, palm down, they cannot lift the thumb into the air (diagnostic test). Direct repair is unsatisfactory and a tendon transfer using the extensor indicis is needed.

Dropped finger

Sudden loss of finger extension at the metacarpophalangeal joint due to tendon rupture at the wrist (e.g. in rheumatoid arthritis). If direct repair is not possible, the distal portion can be attached to an adjacent finger extensor.

[318] Can be any digit, but typically the middle or ring fingers. The thumb may be affected in children.

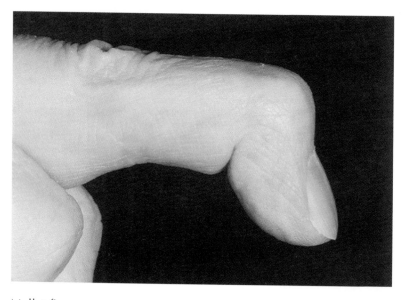

Mallet finger

TRIGGER FINGER[317]

Spot diagnosis.

'This patient's middle (or ring[318]) finger remains flexed when he tries to open his hands from a fist. On further effort, or with help from the other hand, it suddenly straightens with a snap. The finger clicks when he bends it and a tender nodule is felt in front of the affected sheath. The diagnosis is stenosing tenovaginitis or trigger finger.'

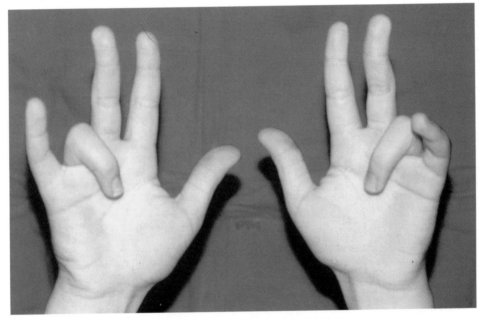

The patient has just clenched his fists then opened his hands. Both ring fingers have remained flexed until they straighten with a snap on further effort.

Ankylosing spondylitis

[319] **Definition**: idiopathic inflammatory disease mainly localised to the spine.

Epidemiology: young men (M: F/5: 1), age of onset 15–25 years. More common in Western Europe.

Cause: unknown. 90–95% have HLA B27. 1/4 of relatives affected.

Distribution: sacroiliac joints typically affected; vertebral joints often affected. Hips and shoulders sometimes involved. May present as an asymmetrical peripheral arthritis usually of the large, weight bearing joints. Small joints of hands and feet very rarely involved. May complain of painful heels at the site of insertion of the tendo-Achilles.

Pathological process: inflammation of ligamentous insertions → granulation tissue formation → erosion of articular cartilage and bone → replacement by fibrous tissue → ossification of fibrous tissue → ankylosis (fusion).

Clinical features: low back pain (differentiated from mechanical low back pain because it is typically worse in the morning and eases with exercise whereas mechanical back pain is brought on by exercise).

Stiff spine (decreased movement in all directions especially extension).

Deformity (as described in main text above).

The Wall test: if a healthy person stands with his back against the wall, the heels, buttocks, scapula and occiput should all be able to touch the wall simultaneously. If spine extension is diminished this is impossible.

Associated diseases: (also associated with HLA B27: Inflammatory bowel disease, Reiter's syndrome, Yersinia arthritis, acute anterior uveitis, psoriatic arthritis.

Extraskeletal manifestations: iritis (30%), aortitis (4%), apical pulmonary fibrosis, cardiac conduction defects (10%). Neurological complications (due to atlanto-axial dislocation or traumatic fracture of a rigid spine may result in tetra/paraplegia). Sciatica is also common and secondary amyloidosis.

Investigations: ESR is elevated, HLA B27 +ve in 90%

Treatment: analgesia (non-steroidal)

> Exercise and intensive physiotherapy – this is the mainstay of preventing deterioration
> Postural training
> Joint replacement e.g. hips – may be necessary but have a very poor outcome
> Vertebral osteotomy – severe flexion deformity of the spine can be partially corrected.

[320] **Beware**, this condition may be completely undetected if the patient is propped up in a hospital bed. Get them to try and look at the ceiling.

[321] In an attempt to keep the visual axis horizontal (otherwise they are looking at their feet).

[322] Because the patient breathes by increased diaphragmatic excursion.

[323] **X-ray features**: Typical loss of lumbar lordosis, increased thoracic kyphosis and compensatory c/spine extension seen on lateral views.

> Fuzziness or erosion of sacroiliac joints is typical.
> Ossification of the intervertebral discs – syndesmophytes bridge the intervertebral space giving a typical bamboo spine appearance on AP/PA views.

ANKYLOSING SPONDYLITIS[319]

Spot diagnosis[320] or candidate may be asked to examine the patient's back (see pg 159), neck (see pg 155) or gait.

'This young man has loss of lumbar lordosis and a fixed kyphosis compensated for by extension of the cervical spine[321] producing a stooped 'question mark' posture. When I ask the patient to turn his head he turns his whole body. The range of movement of the spine is reduced in all directions, especially extension. Chest expansion is reduced and there is a prominent abdomen[322]. The diagnosis is ankylosing spondylitis. I would be interested in this patient's lumbar and thoracic spine X-rays[323].'

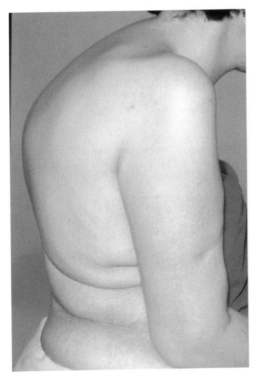

Kyphosis in ankylosing spondylitis

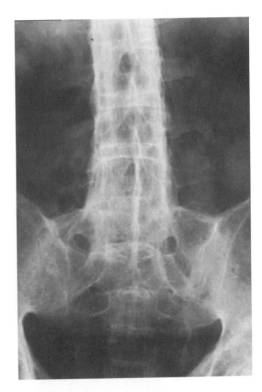

Lumbar spine X-ray of ankylosing spondylitis showing bamboo spine and sacroiliac fusion

Paget's disease

[324] Paget's disease is a noninflammatory derangement of bone metabolism occurring in up to 10% of British people over 70 years, most of whom are asymptomatic. The bone is enlarged and thickened but because of the abnormal internal architecture, is unusually brittle. The cause is unknown but may be post-viral.

Pathology: Initial osteolytic stage

Mixed osteolytic/osteoblastic stage

Final burnt out quiescent osteosclerotic stage

Clinical presentation: Incidental finding on X-ray

Pain, dull, constant, worse at night

Pathological fracture or non union of a fracture

Deformity (e.g. bowing of tibia/femur, kyphosis)

Headaches, nerve root pain

Deafness (as a result of progressive closure of skull foramina and involvement of the ossicles)

Sarcoma in the elderly is rare and where it happens is often secondary to Paget's. It carries a poor prognosis.

Rarer complications of Paget's (optic atrophy, brainstem signs, urolithiasis, high output cardiac failure).

X-rays: <u>General features</u> – the bone is thick and dense with increased cortical thickening. The trabeculae are coarse and widely separated, giving a streaky or honeycomb appearance.

<u>Skull X-rays</u> – in the lytic stage osteoporosis circumscripta (sharply defined lytic areas) starts in the lower parts of the frontal and occipital regions and can cross suture lines to involve large areas of the skull vault. In the sclerotic stage the skull vault thickens and 'cotton wool' areas of sclerotic bone are seen. The facial bones are not commonly affected.

Diagnosis: raised plasma alkaline phosphatase and hydroxyproline. Raised urinary hydroxyproline.

Treatment: is not indicated except in specific circumstances, when drugs such as calcitonin, diphosphonates and mithramycin suppress bone turnover.

Indications for treatment: Persistent bone pain

Repeated fractures

Neurological complications (excluding deafness)

High output cardiac failure

Hypercalcaemia due to immobilisation

Before and after bone surgery where there is a risk of excessive haemorrhage

[325] Paget's disease is the only cause of true bowing of the tibia apart from rickets.

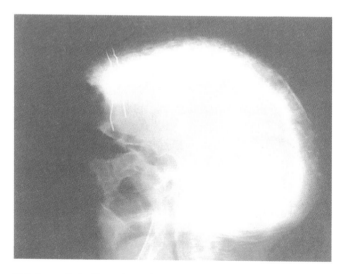

Thickened skull vault and cotton wool areas of sclerotic bone in skull X-ray of patient with the sclerotic stage of Paget's disease. The hairclip is an artefact.

PAGET'S DISEASE[324]

Spot diagnosis or look at these X-rays.

There is (in this elderly patient) enlargement of the skull. There is also bowing of the tibia[325] (and more rarely the femur) which is warmer than the unaffected leg. The patient is kyphotic. I note the hearing aid. The diagnosis is Paget's disease. I would like to see the X-rays of the skull.

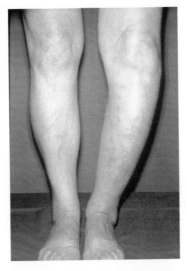

Bowing of the tibia in Paget's disease

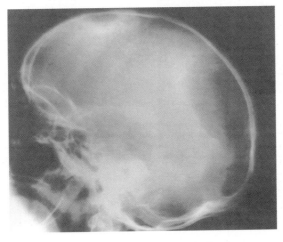

Osteoporosis circumscription seen in the occipital and frontal regions of the skull X-ray of a patient with the lytic phase of Paget's disease

Exostosis or osteochondroma

[326] This is the most common tumour of bone. It starts, usually in adolescence as a cartilaginous overgrowth at the edge of the epiphysial plate and has usually ossified by the time it is palpable. On X-ray it is well-defined; often it looks smaller than it feels because the cartilage cap is invisible.

[327] **Calcaneal exostosis**: prominence of the calcaneus above and to the sides of the Achilles tendon insertion causes blisters, calluses and difficulty in shoe fitting.

Cuneiform exostosis: formed by lipping of the first metatarsal and medial cuneiform.

Fifth metatarsal head: often associated with a varus deformity of the fifth toe (quinti varus).

Fifth metatarsal base: often unduly prominent in the narrow foot but seldom requires excision.

Subungual exostosis: commonest in the great toe and requires excision. May also occur under fingernails.

Tibial or femoral exostosis: seen at the diaphysis (around the knee).

Can also occur in other sites (e.g. humerus), typically arising from the epiphysial plate.

[328] Due to friction against footwear in which case it may be tender.

[329] Exostoses may be multiple, especially in the familial form (hereditary multiple exostoses *aka* diaphyseal aclasis)

[330] Exostosis is a benign tumour that continues to grow as long as the parent bone grows: any further growth after that is suggestive of malignant change. If, as an adult, the lump becomes suddenly bigger or painful then excision is urgent – it may have become malignant. Otherwise excision is only necessary if the lump is troublesome.

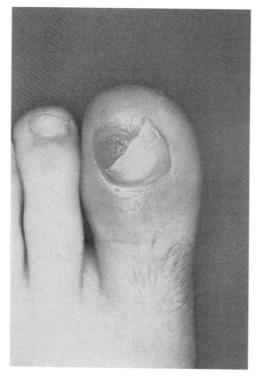

Subungual exostosis

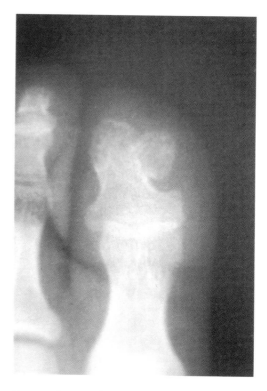

X-ray subungual exostosis

EXOSTOSIS[326]

Spot diagnosis or examination of the foot (see pg 164).

'There is (in this young person) a (1–2 cm) bony hard non-tender lump arising from the (say which typical site)[327]. It has (may have) a bursa overlying it[328]. There are no other similar lumps evident[329]. This is typical of an osteochondroma also known as a cartilage capped exostosis. I would like to ascertain from the patient that he has had it since adolescence and that it has not enlarged significantly since then[330].'

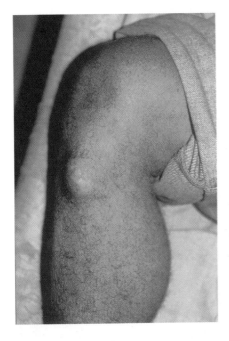

Exostosis of the tibia

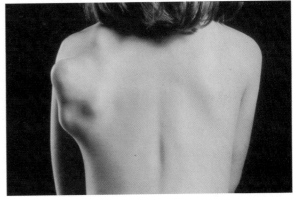

Multiple exostosis on scapula

Pes Cavus

[331] Abnormally high longitudinal arches produced by muscle imbalance. Usually associated with spastic diplegia, Friedreich's ataxia, Charcot-Marie-Tooth disease, polio or spina bifida. A neurological cause should always be sought if not obvious. In mild cases no treatment is required but special shoes may be required. Aims of surgery are to relieve symptoms and prevent skin breakdown in these areas. Options include correcting varus deformity of the heel, wedge osteotomy of the tarsus or metatarsal bases, fusion of PIP joints and flexor to extensor tendon transplants. Complex surgery should be deferred until the patient is over 16 years.

[332] **Friedreich's ataxia:** a progressive hereditary autosomal recessive ataxia with onset in childhood or adolescence. It is caused by spinocerebellar degeneration and is characterised by pes cavus, kyphoscoliosis, a clumsy, lurching broad-based gait and intention tremor affecting the lower limbs, upper limbs, trunk and head. Knee and ankle jerks are absent and the plantar response is extensor. Position and vibration sense are diminished in the feet. Co-ordination tests such as rapid alternate motion, finger-nose and heel-shin tests are impaired (see neurological examination of the lower limb pg 177 and upper limb pg 169). There may be nystagmus and dysarthria. Corrective foot or spinal surgery may be needed but death usually occurs before the age of 50.

[333] **Charcot-Marie-Tooth disease** is a hereditary motor and sensory neuropathy that usually presents in childhood or adolescence with difficulty in walking and pes cavus. There is muscle wasting restricted to below the knee, giving rise to an 'inverted champagne bottle' appearance and a high stepping gait due to foot drop. The tendon reflexes become depressed and there is a variable degree of sensory loss. Affected individuals may be helped by the use of orthotic appliances and sometimes by surgical correction of the foot deformity or tendon transfer.

[334] **Spastic paraparesis** has many causes including multiple sclerosis, cord compression, trauma to spinal cord, birth injury (cerebral palsy) and motor neurone disease. The patient is usually wheelchair bound. The tone in the legs is increased and they are weak with contractures and disuse atrophy. There is bilateral ankle clonus and the plantar responses are extensor.

[335] **Polio** may affect only one leg that will be short, wasted, weak, flaccid with absent reflexes and a normal plantar response. The affected leg may show true shortening due to growth impairment if the limb was affected in childhood.

PES CAVUS[331]

Spot diagnosis. Examination of the ankle and foot (see pg 164) may be useful, as may be neurological examination of the lower limb (see pg 177).

'The feet are markedly deformed with a high arch and clawed toes. There is first metatarsal drop, varus deformity of the heel, decreased subtalar mobility, weakness of intrinsic muscles, and callouses under the metatarsal heads and heel. This is pes cavus. Although it can be an isolated, familial problem, neurological problems such as Friedreich's ataxia[332], Charcot-Marie-Tooth disease[333], spastic paraparesis[334], polio[335], and spina bifida should be excluded.'

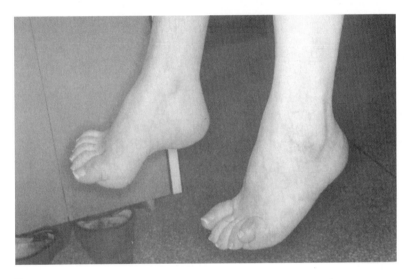

Pes cavus

WINGING OF SCAPULA

Spot diagnosis or examination of shoulder (see pg 150).

'There is winging of the (left or right) scapula evident when the patient, viewed from behind, extends his arms, puts his palms against the wall and pushes. There is/is no evidence of previous trauma or surgery. Winging of the scapula is a sign of weakness of the serratus anterior which may arise from damage to the long thoracic nerve, injury to the brachial plexus, injury or viral infections of the 5th, 6th and 7th cervical nerve and certain types of muscular dystrophy[336].'

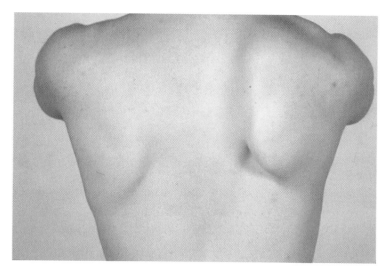

Winging of scapula

Winging of scapula

[336] Disability is usually slight and is best accepted. If function is markedly impaired the scapula can be stabilised by tendon transfer.

CHARCOT'S JOINT[337]

Spot diagnosis or examination of a knee (see pg 141) or ankle (see pg 164).

'This knee is markedly deformed and swollen, with a large effusion, gross instability and an abnormally increased range of movement accompanied by loud crepitus. Despite this the joint is painless which suggests a neuropathic arthritis or Charcot's joint. I would like to carry out a neurological examination of the leg (see pg 177) or ask the patient a couple of questions about his medical history[338].'

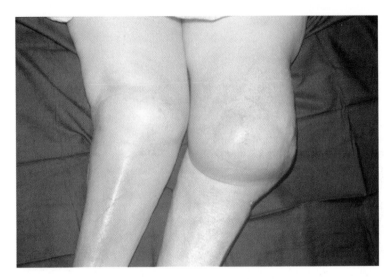

Charcot's joints of both knees

Charcot's Joints

[337] Charcot's disease or neuropathic arthritis is a rapidly progressive degeneration in a joint that lacks position sense and protective pain sensation. There is marked destruction of articular cartilage and the underlying bone, and microscopic spicules of bone become embedded in the synovium. Ligaments and capsule are lax and at the joint periphery there is florid new bone formation. X-rays show obvious gross bone destruction. The joint may be subluxated or dislocated. There are irregular calcified masses in the capsule. Treatment is of the underlying cause, but the affected joint can only be stabilised (e.g. with a calliper). Surgery is not usually useful or successful.

[338] Ask **'have you ever suffered from any of the following: diabetes, syphilis, leprosy, spinal cord injury, hereditary neuropathy?'** In the lower limb the underlying causes include diabetes and other peripheral neuropathies, tabes dorsalis, leprosy and cauda equina lesions. In the upper limb, syringomyelia.

Acromegaly

[339] This is a rare condition caused by excess of growth hormone, usually due to a hypersecreting pituitary adenoma. The mean age of onset is 27 years but the mean age of presentation is over 40 years due to the vague and insidious nature of the symptoms. These patients will not become giants unless the hormonal imbalance begins before epiphysial closure (i.e. adolescence). After this no further lengthening of the long bones is possible. The orthopaedic implications in this case are limited (a predisposition to osteoarthritis and carpal tunnel syndrome), but this is the neurological bay too, and apart from the signs (visual field disturbance, median nerve palsy, third nerve palsy) the treatment is often surgical.

Symptoms: sweating, increased size of gloves, shoes, hats, dentures and rings. Paraesthesia of hands and feet. Digital pain and stiffness. Arthralgia, hypogonadism, headache, visual field disturbance.

Clinical signs: as listed in main text plus goitre, gynaecomastia, galactorrhoea, small gonads (all due to hypopituitarism due to space occupying adenoma in pituitary), greasy skin, acne, prominent superficial veins of extremities, cardiomegaly, third nerve palsy.

Other features: diabetes mellitus, hypertension, hypercalciuria, hypercalcaemia, diabetes insipidus, osteoporosis.

MEN Type 1: acromegaly caused by a pituitary tumour may be sporadic or may be part of the Multiple Endocrine Neoplasia syndrome type I (Werner's syndrome) which involves two or more of:

> Pituitary tumour
> Islet cell tumour
> Primary hyperparathyroidism
> Adrenocortical adenoma

Investigations: comparative study of old photographs of the patient; skull X-ray; glucose tolerance test (normal growth hormone levels are nearly nil 60 minutes after 75g oral glucose, but are elevated in acromegalics). CT/MRI of pituitary.

Treatment: Trans-sphenoidal hypophysectomy, transfrontal hypophysectomy, external beam irradiation, radioactive implants, bromocriptine.

[340] **Features of acromegalic X-rays** (see pg 232)

Skull:	Enlargement and erosion of the pituitary fossa
	Prognathism (increased angle of mandible)
	Enlarged paranasal air sinuses and mastoids
	Enlargement of the occipital protuberance
Vertebrae:	An increase in AP and transverse dimensions
	Posterior scalloping
	Kyphosis
Hands:	'Spade like' with broadening of the fingers
	Terminal tufts ('oak trees')
	Widening of metacarpophalangeal joints due to cartilage hypertrophy
Joints:	Premature osteoarthritis and chondrocalcinosis

Soft tissues: Increased heel pad thickness (>25 mm)

[341] This gives him the appearance of a circus giant (many of whom were acromegalic). Don't say this in front of the patient in case it gives offence! Think of 'Jaws,' the villain in the James Bond movie.

[342] Due to proximal muscle weakness, arthralgia and osteoarthritis.

[343] Typically peripheral field defect due to enlargement of the pituitary mass pressing on the medial aspects of both optic tracts at the optic chiasma causing bitemporal hemianopia. Get the patient to cover each eye in turn, looking straight ahead and tell you when he can see your finger coming around from the periphery of his vision in each of the four quadrants. He should show marked delay in seeing the finger coming in from the lateral side (as if he were wearing blinkers).

ACROMEGALY[339]

Spot diagnosis/examine this patient's hands/X-rays[340].

'This patient's hands are large, doughy and spade-shaped and the skin over the back of them is thickened. There is (may be) loss of the thenar eminence bilaterally which is evidence of carpal tunnel syndrome (offer to carry out the carpal tunnel syndrome/median nerve examination on pg XX if so). The patient's face has some unusual characteristics, with a large lower jaw, full lips and prominent supraorbital ridges. There is poor occlusion of the teeth, the lower teeth overbiting in front of the upper. The nose, tongue and ears are enlarged[341]. He is kyphotic, with bowed legs and a rolling gait. He has difficulty standing from his seat[342]. He has a deep husky voice and is hirsute. The diagnosis is acromegaly. I would like to ask the patient if he finds he is sweating more than normal and if he has noticed any change in his vision[343].'

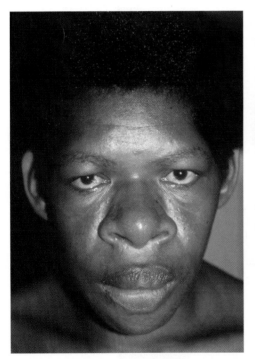

Acromegalic face

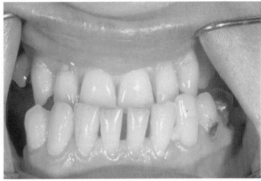

The teeth in acromegaly showing interdentate separation

231

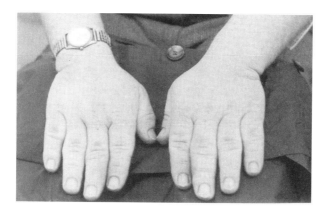

Acromegalic hands

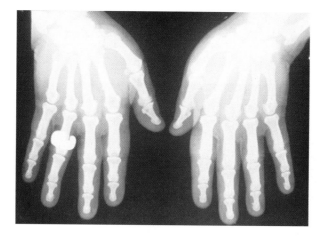

X-ray of acromegalic hands

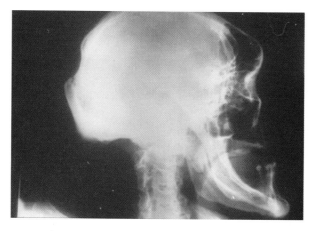

X-ray of acromegalic skull

RUPTURED BICEPS TENDON[344]

Spot diagnosis.

This (middle-aged or older) patient has good function of his shoulder and elbow but when the elbow is flexed actively against resistance the belly of the biceps muscle contracts into a prominent lump which is abnormal compared with the other side. The diagnosis is a tear of the long head of biceps. I would like to ask the patient when and how it happened[345].

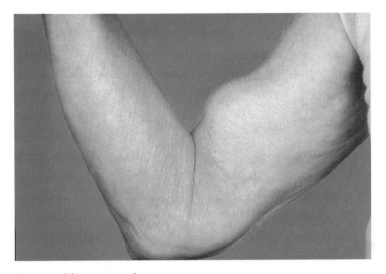

Ruptured biceps tendon

Ruptured biceps tendon

[334] Usually preceded by degeneration and fraying, tears of the long head of biceps normally require no surgical treatment. Related conditions:

Bicipital tendonitis: usually occurring together with rotator cuff impingement or after unaccustomed shoulder activity. Sharp localised tenderness in the bicipital groove worse on flexion against resistance. Rest or occasionally steroid injections usually settle it.

Tears of the distal biceps tendon: rare. Follow an acute flexion strain of the elbow rather than after degeneration. The tendon tears cleanly or is avulsed from the radial tuberosity. Difficult to diagnose; clues include suggestive history, pain in lower forearm, local bruising and loss of power in elbow flexion and supination. The tendon should be repaired to preserve full function.

[345] Usually while lifting, the patient feels something snap. The shoulder and upper arm ache for a while but then feel normal. Function usually returns to normal when the tenderness has settled.

D   Practical Stations

ASPIRATION OF JOINTS

You may be asked to explain how you would aspirate a joint. Say you would use full aseptic precautions in all cases (sterile trolley, instruments, gloves, suitable skin preparation and draping).

Knee
- Leg extended
- Local anaesthetic (LA) infiltrated into skin just above and lateral to the patella
- Infiltrate local anaesthetic more deeply into level of synovial membrane of suprapatellar pouch
- Squeeze fluid from upper limits of suprapatellar pouch to float patella before inserting needle
- Squeeze superior aspect and sides of joint to empty it into needle
- Apply sterile dressing
- Wool and crepe compression bandaging

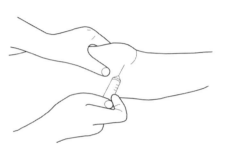

Shoulder
- Patient supine
- Follow clavicle laterally to acromioclavicular joint
- 5 cm obliquely below is the **coracoid**
- Rotate the arm: you can feel the head of the humerus
- LA into this point
- Large bore needle directly backwards into joint just below and lateral to the coracoid
- Sub deltoid bursitis presents a more superficial swelling to aspirate
- Sterile dressing

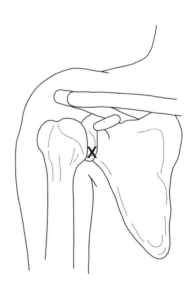

D   Practical Stations

Hip

- Lateral approach: needle passed in just above greater trochanter (1)
- Anterior approach: needle passed in just below the inguinal ligament and lateral to the femoral artery (2)
- Identify landmarks and infiltrate LA
- May be carried out under general anaesthetic

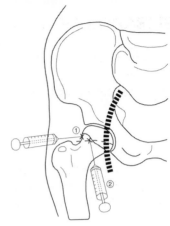

Elbow

- From the lateral side
- Flex elbow 90°
- Locate radial head by pronating and supinating forearm
- LA infiltration
- Introduce needle in area of palpable depression between the proximal part of the radial head and the capitulum
- Sterile dressing

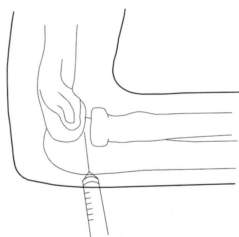

Wrist

- Dorsum of wrist medial to snuffbox
- Feel for depression at the back of the wrist between distal end of the radius and the scaphoid
- This is between the extensor carpi radialis brevis and extensor digitorum communis
- Infiltrate skin with LA
- Aspirating needle directed cranially inclined at 60°
- Sterile dressing

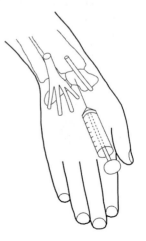

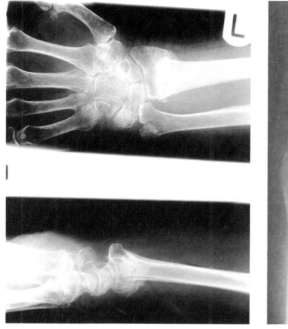

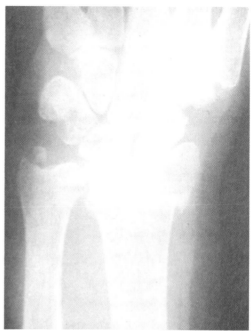

Lateral X-ray of a Colles' fracture showing anterior angulation, dorsal displacement and impaction

AP X-ray of a Colles' fracture showing radical displacement, ulnar angulation and impaction

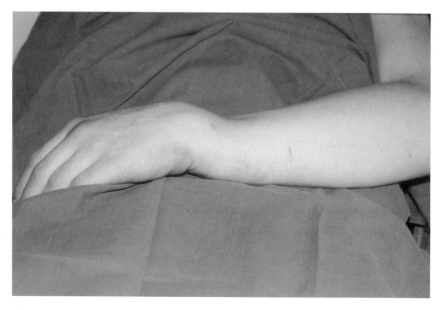

The dinner fork deformity of a Colles' fracture

REDUCTION OF A COLLES' FRACTURE

A practical station where discussion of common trauma cases and demonstration of practical techniques is possible. One case that would lend itself to this is Colles' fracture.

What is a Colles' fracture?

A fracture of the radius within 2.5 cm of the wrist with a characteristic deformity if displaced. It is the commonest of all fractures and is most typically seen in an osteoporotic woman falling onto an outstretched hand.

What are the 6 characteristic displacements?

1. Dorsal displacement
2. Dorsal tilt (aka anterior angulation. The radius is normally tilted 5° forward)
3. Radial displacement
4. Radial tilt (aka ulnar angulation)
5. Impaction
6. Rotational deformity
(See X-rays on opposite pg)

How would you make the diagnosis clinically?

This is usually evident by the classical dinner fork deformity. The ulnar styloid is 1 cm proximal to radial styloid in the normal wrist and this relationship is disrupted. It is important to clinically exclude coexisting injury by examining the scaphoid, elbow and shoulder.

What are the indications for reduction?

1. Displaced ulnar styloid (indicates serious disruption of inferior radioulnar joint)
2. Dorsal tilt of 10° or more (except in the old and frail)

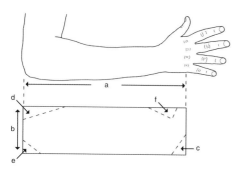

1. Cut the plaster backslab to shape
a) length = olecranon to the metacarpal heads
b) width = 15 cm in an adult (backslab should be 8 layers thick)
c) Cut to allow for ulnar deviation
d) Cut to allow for elbow flexion
e) Corner may be trimmed
f) Cut to allow for the first web space

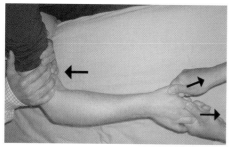

2. Disimpacting distal radial fragment

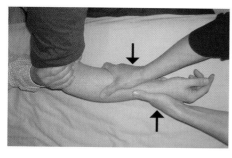

3. Reducing dorsal tilt and displacement

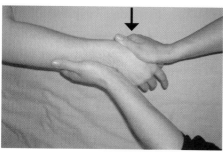

4. Correcting radial tilt and displacement

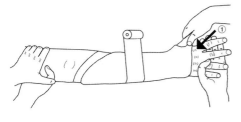

5. Lay backslab over stockinette on dorsal surface of forearm and secure with gauze bandage
Slab should cover anterior, lateral and posterior Surfaces of the arm. Turn the flap of plaster into the palm (1)

How would you reduce a Colles' fracture?

1. This can be done under local (haematoma block), regional (Bier's block) or general anaesthetic. Prepare the plaster backslab first (fig opposite).
2. Traction: this is done with elbow flexed. Disimpaction is confirmed by palpating the distal fragment (fig 2).
3. Reduce dorsal tilt and displacement (by pressing wrist in a volar direction and arm in a dorsal direction) (fig 3).
4. Correct radial tilt and displacement (by pushing distal fragment into ulnar deviation) fig4. Plaster in a below elbow back-slab. Hold position while plastering by holding the patient's thumb extended in one hand and her fingers extended in your other hand. Her elbow should be extended during plastering. The patient's wrist is held pronated, in full ulnar deviation and slight palmar flexion (fig 5).
5. Collar and cuff.

What about follow-up?

24 hours: check circulation, sensation, movement and swelling. Discharge if admitted.
5 days fracture clinic: complete plaster if swelling has subsided. Check position is adequate. Encourage elbow and finger mobilisation.
2 weeks fracture clinic: check X-rays on arrival. Check plaster and finger/elbow mobility.
5 weeks fracture clinic: remove plaster on arrival, assess union. If tender continue in plaster and reassess in 2 weeks. If non-tender, tubi-grip and mobilise.
7 weeks fracture clinic: discharge or physiotherapy depending on grip strength, wrist movements, finger 'tuck in', patient's occupation.
Normal supination 85°, pronation 70°.

What are the potential complications of a Colles' fracture?

1. Persistent deformity or malunion
2. Delayed rupture of extensor pollicis longus
3. Sudeck's atrophy
4. Carpal tunnel syndrome
5. Comminution of radial fragment
6. Persisting stiffness
7. Associated scaphoid fracture

Kocher's method of reducing a dislocated shoulder

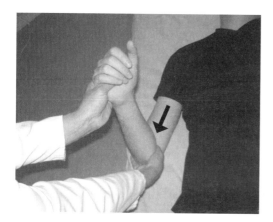

Traction

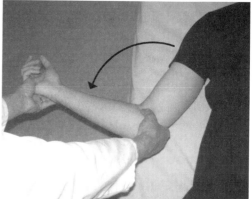

External rotation

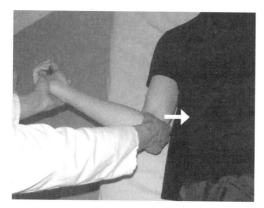

Adduction

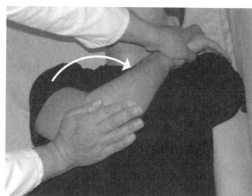

Internal rotation

REDUCTION OF A DISLOCATED SHOULDER

Another clinical skill you may be expected to demonstrate or explain is reduction of a dislocated shoulder.

What happens when you dislocate your shoulder?

Anterior dislocation is the most common and usually results from a fall forcing external rotation of the shoulder, or fall onto a backward stretching arm. The head of the humerus is driven forward and lies in front of the glenoid below the coracoid process.

Associated injuries include:
- Capsule torn from glenoid anteriorly (true Bankart lesion)
- Labrum torn (commonly referred to as Bankart lesion)
- Tearing of subscapularis
- Fracture of greater tuberosity
- Damage to axillary artery or brachial plexus

What should you look for on examination?

Pain is usually severe with no movement permitted. The patient supports the arm with the opposite hand. The lateral outline of the shoulder is flattened. A small bulge may be seen and felt just below the clavicle. It is important to check the sensation over the regimental badge area for axillary and radial nerve damage, as well as distal circulation, sensation and movement as usual.

What X-rays would you request and what would you look for on them?

Anteroposterior – a standard view but may be misleading. The humeral head lies below and medial to the socket in typical cases. The shadows of the humeral head and glenoid overlap.
Axial lateral – especially to exclude posterior dislocation if subluxation is suspected. Apical oblique – if possible.
Translateral – normal parabolic curve between the humerus and the scapula is disrupted.

How would you reduce this dislocation?

I would choose Kocher's method. It can be carried out under sedation or general anaesthesia. For sedation, adequate analgesia (usually opiates), sedation (usually midazolam given in 2 mg increments at least two minutes apart and not exceeding 6 mg in a 70 kg man unless an anaesthetist is available) and monitoring (one dedicated nurse, continuous pulse oximetry, regular observations, anaesthetist in the building) are mandatory. I would manipulate the joint as follows:

(Remember the TEAR mnemonic) see figs pg 240.
T raction: holding above flexed elbow with an assistant providing countertraction
E xternal rotation: Rotate upper arm slowly to at least 75° and up to 90°. Patient needs to be relaxed; this takes patience.
A dduction: moving flexed elbow firmly forward and deliberately across chest.
R otation (internal): rotate arm back to broad arm sling position.

Are there any other methods?

The **Hippocratic method** involves simple manual traction with the body stabilised (traditionally the surgeon's heel against the side of the patient's chest but a colleague can provide countertraction!) with the arm in slight abduction. **Gravitational reduction** may be effective in recurrent cases. It involves lying the patient prone with a sandbag under the clavicle and hanging the arm over the edge of the bed holding a weight.

What would you arrange for post-reduction care?

Reduction must be confirmed with a check X-ray. Patients are all discharged with a broad arm sling. Young patients should be advised that there is up to a 50% recurrence rate within two years, and if this is the first dislocation body strapping is recommended and the sling should be worn for at least three weeks. In the elderly, by contrast, stiffness is the main problem and early mobilisation (within two weeks) is vital. If the proximal humerus is fractured it may need surgical fixation. If the glenoid labrum is damaged or detached, recurrent dislocation is likely and anterior capsule reconstruction surgery may be required.

What about posterior dislocation?

This is technically a fracture-subluxation rather than a true dislocation. It is rarer than anterior dislocation and more frequently missed. It is usually caused by a direct blow or forced internal rotation of the abducted arm (e.g. during an epileptic fit). The arm is held in medial rotation and is locked in that position, making the clinical diagnosis fairly straightforward. Diagnostic mistakes occur because the AP X-ray may be misleading: the humeral head may seem to be in contact with the glenoid. The humeral head has a globular appearance because it is medially rotated. A lateral film is essential and shows posterior subluxation and sometimes indentation of the humeral head. Reduction is by traction and lateral (external) rotation while the head of the humerus is pushed forwards. Post-reduction management is as for anterior dislocation. Recurrent posterior dislocation is rarer and more difficult to treat surgically than recurrent anterior dislocation.

TRAUMA RADIOGRAPHS (X-RAYS)

It is possible that you will be shown an X-ray of a trauma case or complication of a fracture. There are too many possibilities to be covered in this book, but nothing can replace experience in a busy accident and emergency or orthopaedics post. To refresh your memory, I recommend the book *Practical Fracture Management* by Ronald McRae (Churchill Livingstone) which has an excellent overview of all the common fractures and their management and includes many X-rays of the commoner injuries. If in doubt, follow the guidelines below for looking at an X-ray.

Looking at an X-ray

1. Check the label

'This is the X-ray of Edward Burns who is 35, taken on the 5th of April 2001.'

2. Name the bone or joint, side and the view

'It is an anterio-posterior view of the left femur.'

3. Describe the obvious abnormality if there is one

How to describe a fracture on an X-ray:

You need at least two views and should be able to see the joint above and below the fracture.

If shown only one film ask if there are any other views

1. **Site**: side, bone and level (divide long bones into proximal, middle and distal thirds).
2. **Pattern**: hairline, greenstick, transverse, oblique, spiral, impacted, compression
3. **Comminuted**/non comminuted: how many parts?
4. **Special features** of fracture e.g avulsion fracture, depressed, involving the articular surface.
5. **Displacement** (estimate % of fracture surface in contact) and shortening
6. **Angulation** or tilt[346].
7. **Axial rotation**: you need to see the joint above and below the fracture.
8. **Associated features**: dislocation, soft tissue swelling, obvious compound (not easy to determine on X-ray unless dramatic), foreign bodies, pathological fracture.

---

[346] DO NOT USE THE TERM ANGULATION unless you have read it up and fully understand it. It means the opposite to what most people think: i.e 'fracture of the mid-shaft of the tibia with 20° of medial angulation' means that the distal end of the distal fragment has swung LATERALLY! Use the word TILT instead: i.e.; 'the distal fragment is tilted laterally by about 20°' – this means what it says and is safer during exam stress!

PRINCIPLES OF FRACTURE MANAGEMENT

Again, you should be familiar with the management of the common fractures; individual discussion of each is beyond the scope of this book. If asked to discuss management of any fracture keep in mind the following six principles. It may be worth starting your discussion with the words:

'In managing any fracture, 6 aspects need to be considered:
1. Initial emergency measures
2. Does the fracture require reduction?
3. If yes, how to reduce it?
4. What support is required while union is achieved?
5. Is the fracture open?
6. Does the patient need to be admitted?'

This will allow you time to organise your thoughts, give you a frame for discussing your answer and allow the examiners to steer you to the points they want you to discuss without the feeling that you have missed out any important principles. You can then address the fracture you have been asked to assess with reference to each relevant principle in greater detail.

1. **Initial measures:** ATLS guidelines for all major trauma
   Temporary splint (e.g. sandbags or inflatable splints)
   Reposition fragment immediately if overlying skin at risk
   If open, take pus swab, cover with sterile dressings and give antibiotics and tetanus
   Assess clinically and radiologically

2. **Does the fracture require reduction?**
   NO if undisplaced
   NO if displacement is likely to be corrected by remodelling (e.g. in children)
   NO if risks of anaesthesia outweigh disadvantage of deformity (e.g. some elderly)
   YES if slight displacement in functionally vital area e.g. articular surface
   YES if significantly displaced, angled or rotated (criteria vary for each fracture)

3. **If yes, how to reduce it?**
   Closed Manipulation under anaesthesia (MUA)
   Open reduction
   > if fracture is open anyway
   > if internal fixation is required
   > if MUA has failed

   Continuous traction (rarely used except in c/spine and femur)

4. What support is required while union is achieved?

Non-rigid, e.g. broad arm slings (for elevation of distal limb where support of the fracture is needed e.g. clavicle fractures).
Collar and cuff (for elevation of distal limb where traction is desirable e.g. shaft of humerus).

Plaster casts (commonest – usually one-sided slabs completed when swelling subsides).

Internal fixation: (e.g. screws, nails, plates see fig on pg XX) indicated where:
- closed reduction impossible (e.g. tissue between bone ends)
- holding closed reduction impossible (e.g. neck of femur)
- accuracy vital (e.g. articular surfaces)
- patient multiply injured: to reduce pain, immobility and risks of fat embolus and respiratory distress

Preferred but not absolutely indicated to achieve:
- high quality reduction
- earlier mobilisation of joints
- earlier discharge from hospital

Problems with internal fixation include:
- infection
- skill needed
- instruments and fixation devices needed
- lengthy anaesthetic

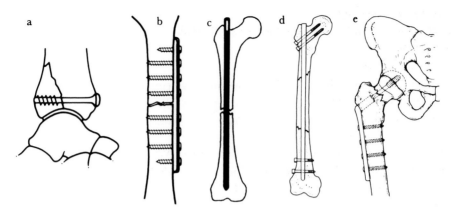

Internal fixation. The method used must be appropriate to the situation: (a) screws – interfragmentary compression; (b) plate and screws – most suitable in the forearm; (c) intramedullary nail – for the larger long bones; (d) interlocking nail and screws – ideal for the femur and tibia; (e) dynamic compression screw and plate – ideal for the proximal and distal ends of the femur.

External fixation: especially in open fractures with poor skin cover or risk of infection (see pg 215).
Disadvantages: cumbersome, can lead to pin track infection.

Continuous traction
- skeletal via pins or skin via adhesive strapping
- used mainly in femoral shaft or cervical spine fractures
- patient immobilised for many weeks

Cast bracing: after first few weeks of conservative fracture management. Hinged cast allows support and mobility.

5. Is the fracture open?

Initial measures as above (Swab, dress, antibiotics, tetanus)

Needs débridement under GA

Assess skin cover

Avoid large implants if badly soiled (external fixation often preferred)

Beware postoperative compartment syndrome (>30 mmHg pressure)

Beware neurological and vascular damage (high-energy injury)

Amputation a risk in crush injuries

MESS score (Mangled extremity severity score) of >7 suggests an amputation should be considered. MESS takes into account:

- energy of injury
- limb ischaemia
- shock
- age of patient

6. Does the patient need to be admitted?

GA or other inpatient treatment required

Observation e.g. co-morbidity, multiple trauma

Nursing care (bed bound, bilateral limb fractures)

Mobilisation

Social (e.g. elderly)

Child abuse suspected

ORTHOPAEDIC APPLIANCES

The MRCS syllabus says specifically that a discussion of walking aids is possible. Try to frame your answer: Introduction, Principles, Structure, Indications, Fitting and Use.

Introduction

Walking aids fall into three categories: sticks, crutches and frames and have three main functions: increasing extrinsic stability; providing propulsive force; enhancing intrinsic stability.

Principles of prescribing walking aids

- Each patient should be assessed individually for the correct walking aid.
- The equipment should always be checked before issuing.
- The patient's weight-bearing status must be ascertained (full, partial, total, none).
- The patient's premorbid mobility and any prior aids should be ascertained.
- Clear simple instructions and a demonstration are mandatory.
- Be realistic in your expectations and err on the side of safety for the patient.

Sticks

Structure

Wooden or lightweight metal. Handles are either 'crook' (usually wooden) or flat (usually plastic covered metal) 'Fischer' handles.
A **ferrule** is the rubber or plastic low friction 'shoe' at the base of the walking aid. Some ferrules are multi-ringed and depressed to form a vacuum in contact with the ground. Ferrules should always be checked for damage, should fit well and should have a metal washer inside to prevent the tip of the aid from piercing the ferrule.

Indications

Sticks give the lowest level of assistance. They provide increased extrinsic stability by enlarging the support area and supply some propulsive force. They are used when full or partial weight bearing – not for non-weight bearing.

Fitting

Correct length allows slight bend (15° flexion) of the arm at the elbow when the patient is upright. Measurement is taken from the floor to wrist crease.

Use

If using **one stick** it should be held in the opposite hand to the affected leg. The sequence is disabled leg and stick forward together, followed by sound leg and free arm swinging forward together. Patients often insist on using the stick on the same side as the disabled leg, usually when there is severe pain.

If using **two sticks** they can be both brought forward with the injured leg, then the sound leg is brought through (**three and one** pattern). An alternative which is more difficult for patients to pick up, but which maintains the normal walking pattern ready for discarding the aid, is the true **four-point** walking system: right stick, left leg, left stick, right leg.

When going up stairs the patient walks close to the bottom step, takes the good leg up first, then the disabled leg up to the same step then crutch/stick up last. When going down stairs the patient walks close to the top step, takes the stick/crutch down first then the disabled leg down, then the good leg down last onto the same step. Some patients may need to shuffle up and down stairs on their bottom – but can they get up from a sitting position at the top of the stairs?

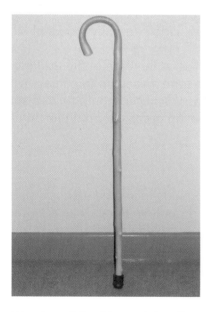

Wooden stick with crook handle and rubber ferrule

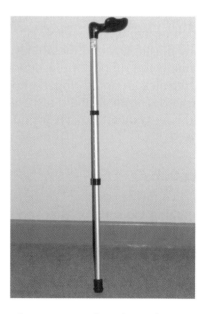

Aluminium stick with Fischer handle, adjustable shaft and rubber ferrule

Crutches

Structure

Crutches provide support across at least one joint in the arm. There are three main types: axillary, elbow and gutter crutches. **Axillary crutches** have one foot and two struts which end in an axillary cushioned pad, **Canadian crutches** are similar but end in a ring encircling the upper arm. Both have a handle between the struts for supporting the weight. **Elbow crutches** have only one strut and also have a handle, with a plastic band just above it that should sit just below the elbow joint. **Gutter crutches** are a type of elbow crutch, which end in a padded gutter in which the patient can rest the forearm. The forearm is kept in place with an adjustable strap. They are used when weight-bearing through the hand is not possible.

Indications

Axillary and Canadian crutches cross the wrist and elbow joints and give greater stability than elbow crutches which cross only the wrist joint. Crutches are usually grounded at points further from the body than sticks, and thereby give larger support areas. The degree of external stabilisation, intrinsic stabilisation and propulsion (via latissimus dorsi) are greater than with sticks.
Elbow crutches are used for full, partial, touch or non-weight bearing. Although not as stable as axillary crutches, they are more practical for long term use, as the crutch can be let go (e.g. to open a door) without dropping it. Axillary crutches are used for non-weight bearing, and sometimes for partial weight bearing patients. It is useful for patients with a full length P.O.P.

Fitting

Axillary crutches: contrary to its name, the axillary pad must not push into the armpit as it can cause neuropraxia. It should sit 5 cm below the armpit. The handle should allow a slight bend at the elbow.
Elbow crutches: correct length allows slight bend at the elbow, and the plastic band should sit below the elbow joint.
Gutter crutches: the forearm rests along the gutter with the elbow at a right angle.

Use

The elbow crutches can be used singly (as a stick) or in pairs. Axillary crutches are used in pairs and can be difficult to use. The patient should squeeze the axillary pads between the upper arms and chest wall and push down through the hand pieces.

In **three-point swing-to** walking (for non-weight bearing patients) the crutches start in front of the supporting leg. They are lifted and placed further in front, weight is taken on them and the sound leg is bent and swung to just behind the crutches. The disabled leg should be held clear of the ground and in front of the body. Stronger patients can use the **three-point swing-through** which is similar to the swing-to but the sound leg is swung through the crutches and the foot is put down in front of them. Partial weight bearing patients can use the **three and one pattern** in which the crutches and partial weight bearing leg go forward together and then rest on the ground while the able leg moves forward alone.

NB. If the patient's feet are in line with the crutches they will be unstable. A triangular base should always be maintained. Bolts must be checked and tightened before each episode of walking.

Crutches should never be used when transferring from standing to sitting or vice versa. If the patient falls, they will not be able to save themselves, and are at risk of hurting their arms.

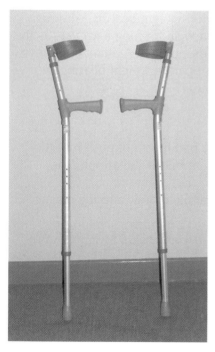

Elbow crutches with only one handle and a plastic band which should sit just above the elbow

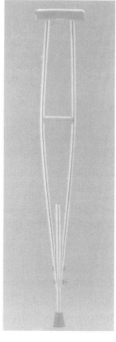

A metal axillary crutch length and handle adjustable

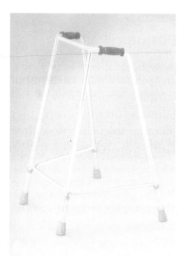

A pick up 'Zimmer' frame with three fixed sides and ferrules on leg

Frames

Structure

These are essentially large-based frames having four points and two or three sides. The common (Zimmer) frame has three fixed sides. There are usually ferrules on every leg, but there can be wheels on two legs to increase propulsion at the expense of stability. Another variation is a **gutter frame** that allows weight bearing through the forearm and gives support. The **pulpit frame** allows a lot of weight bearing through the upper limbs when the patients are particularly weak or injured.

Indications

These devices provide a large support area and are the most effective aids for increasing extrinsic stability. They can improve intrinsic stabilisation by allowing the patient to suspend himself or herself in the frame. The good contact points and addition of wheels make it excellent for propulsive force. They are good for patients with reasons other than their injury for being unstable e.g. the frail or elderly, but crutches are more useful for younger active patients with good intrinsic stability who may want to cover large distances.

Fitting

They come in three standard sizes all of which are adjustable. The frame should be measured with the patient upright with elbows slightly flexed.

Uses

A frame is used by picking it up, moving it forwards, putting it down, leaning upon it and walking into the frame. As normal a gait as possible should be encouraged; i.e. taking at least two small steps into the frame so the feet alternate. If one leg is injured, it should be moved forwards first, then the frame leant on while the good leg is brought level (**three-point walking** in total or partial weight bearing patients). If the patient is non-weight bearing **two-point walking** should be performed, with the affected leg off the floor at all times, the frame moved forward and the good leg hopping forward while pushing down through the arms. The frame should not touch the patient's abdomen – encourage big movements with the frame and small steps. A frame should not be used while transferring from standing to sitting or vice versa, as it is not fixed and is likely to move. The patient should be standing before they grip the frame and should let go of it before they try to sit.

Thanks to Rebecca Hunter, Physiotherapist at St. James Hospital, for her assistance with this section. Thanks also to Heather Harford for taking all the original photographs in this chapter.

E   Detailed Results of Questionnaire

ORTHOPAEDIC AND NEUROLOGY

Total of 152 cases reported in the survey.

TOP 5 CASES (accounted for 64.5% of all Orthopaedic and Neurology cases)

Type of case	Number seen in survey	Breakdown and details of cases
Dupuytren's contracture	26	8 from the Superficial Lesions Bay. Questions included causes, treatment options, anatomy, skin grafts, related features.
Hip	21	3 Examine hip ?diagnosis 7 Osteoarthritis 4 Avascular necrosis 6 Postoperative 1 Bilateral congenital 'problems' (not specified) Questions included preoperative assessment, Garden classification, features of Paget's disease, surgical approaches to the hip, screws and complications. Three candidates were shown hip X-rays.
Knee	20	11 Osteoarthritis, one with total knee replacement 2 Rheumatoid arthritis 2 Effusion 2 Anterior cruciate injury 1 Paget's disease 1 Seronegative arthritis (+ inflammatory bowel disease?) 1 Apparently normal knee Questions included history, examination, anterior drawer test, arthroscopy scars, X-ray changes of osteoarthritis, problems associated with rheumatoid disease.
Rheumatoid hand	17	3 in Superficial Lesions bay. Standard questions on features of rheumatoid hand
Great toe	14	9 Hallux valgus 2 Rheumatoid arthritis 2 Hallux rigidus 1 Claw toes Questions included causes and treatment options of hallux valgus, features of rheumatoid arthritis

OTHER CASES

Type of case	Number seen in survey	Breakdown and details of cases
Upper limb neurology	8	4 Ulnar nerve palsy (1 with cervical rib, 1 with elbow trauma) 2 radial nerve palsy (1 causing hyperaesthesia, 1 at the level of the brachial plexus) 1 posterior brachial plexus cord injury 1 examination of median nerve (also see carpal tunnel)
Carpal tunnel	7	3 cases with thenar muscle wasting. Questions included treatment and operative details.
Wrist	7	2 Colles'fracture 2 Rheumatoid arthritis 1 Avascular necrosis of scaphoid 1 Carpometacarpal osteoarthritis 1 Examine extensor tendons pathology not specified Questions included how to manipulate Colles' fracture, anaesthetic methods used, complications, wrist arthrodesis in rheumatoid disease for volar subluxation.
External fixators	6	2 Wrist, 1 with carpal tunnel decompression 3 Tibia 1 Femur Questions included complications of external fixation, surgical anatomy of the hip, median nerve supply, X-rays of radius and ulnar fracture.
Ganglion	6	3 Wrist 1 Thumb 2 Not specified 3 Seen in Superficial Lesions bay.
Shoulder	3	1 Rheumatoid arthritis 1 Decreased range of movement ?cause 1 Old scar and atrophy of muscles ?radical dissection Questions included examine movements, take short history.
Elbow	3	All olecranon bursa. 2 in Superficial Lesions bay
Trigger finger	2	1 in Superficial Lesions bay. Asked about treatment options
Ankylosing spondylitis	2	Questions included cervical spine examination, hip and knee examination, X-ray features.
Paget's disease	2	Both tibia. Questions included complications and X-ray features.
Gout	1	Tophi on finger, asked differential diagnosis. In Superficial Lesions bay.
Winged scapula	1	In Superficial Lesions bay.
Ankle	1	Arthritis after tibial fracture (with X-ray)
Ingrowing toenail	1	In Superficial Lesions bay
Lower limb neurology	1	
Bone graft	1	
Exostosis	1	
Osteochondrosarcoma of chest wall	1	In Superficial Lesions bay

CHAPTER FOUR
CLINICAL BAY 3
THE CIRCULATORY SYSTEM

CONTENTS

THE CIRCULATORY SYSTEM

A   The Bay

In the MRCS (Eng) examination the circulatory system or 'vascular' bay lasts 10 minutes, during which time candidates are expected to see about three patients. This will be extended to 15 minutes after December 2002 (see pg 5 for details of the changes). For each patient a potential 5 marks can be achieved, 3 for the clinical approach and 2 for the discussion and investigations. The MRCS (Eng) syllabus gives the following guidelines on this bay:

'Aim: to determine the ability of a candidate to assess the circulatory system and determine profiles of investigation in order to assist a differential diagnosis. A detailed knowledge of the surgical treatment is not required but an indication that the candidate knows the principles of treatment is required.

One of the examiners will be a vascular surgeon and one will be a non-vascular surgeon.'

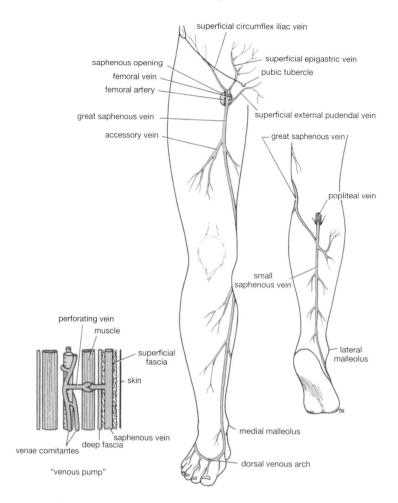

superficial circumflex iliac vein

saphenous opening
femoral vein
femoral artery

superficial epigastric vein
pubic tubercle

great saphenous vein

superficial external pudendal vein

accessory vein

great saphenous vein

popliteal vein

perforating vein
muscle

superficial fascia

skin

small
saphenous vein

lateral
malleolus

venae comitantes

saphenous vein
deep fascia

"venous pump"

medial malleolus

dorsal venous arch

Superficial veins of the right lower limb

[3] **The course of the long (or great) saphenous vein** is as follows: draining the medial end of the dorsal venous arch of the foot, the long saphenous vein passes directly in front of the medial malleolus (the best place for a cut-down or to start a vein harvest for cardiac surgery) and ascends with the saphenous nerve (of which you have to beware in vein harvest) in the superficial fascia over the medial side of the leg. It then passes behind the knee and curves forward around the medial side of the thigh. It passes through the lower part of the saphenous opening in the deep fascia and joins the femoral vein 4cm below and lateral to the pubic tubercle. The tributaries of the long saphenous vein are shown above. The common sites where the superficial long saphenous vein communicates with the deep venous system via perforators are shown in fig on pg 263.

The course of the short (or small) saphenous vein is as follows: draining the lateral part of the dorsal venous arch of the foot the short saphenous vein ascends behind the lateral malleolus and runs with the sural nerve following the lateral border of the Achilles tendon. It then runs up the middle of the back of the leg (like a stocking seam) and pierces the deep fascia passing between the two heads of gastrocnemius in the lower part of the popliteal fossa. It drains into the popliteal vein, but an anatomical variant is seen where it (or a branch of it) joins the long saphenous vein. The tributaries of the short saphenous vein are shown above.

B   The Examinations

EXAMINATION OF VARICOSE VEINS

'Hello, my name is Dr Parchment Smith. Would you mind if I examined your legs? Could you stand up with your trousers off please[1]? Do you mind if I talk about you as we go along?'

Crouch down and LOOK at the legs systematically but briskly[2]. To the examiners:
'On inspection I am looking for visible dilated or tortuous subcutaneous veins[3]. I am also looking for venous stars[4] and any sign of venous insufficiency in the gaiter area[5] such as oedema[6], haemosiderin deposition[7], lipodermatosclerosis[8], eczema[9] and ulceration[10]. Turn around please.'

Have a look at the back of the legs.
'I'm just going to FEEL the veins. Now I'm going to press for a second on your ankle.'

Palpate any obvious varicose veins, then check for pitting oedema. Turn the patient back around to face you and palpate behind the medial border of the tibia for tender defects in the deep fascia[11].

---

[1] On a platform or step if provided.

[2] Look from the feet up to the groin on both legs, concentrating on the gaiter area and the medial aspect of the leg, then turn the patient around and repeat the inspection from behind. The veins are often easier to feel than to see, and take a while to fill up, so if there are no obviously distended veins, start by pointing out the skin changes and then look for varicosities by gently feeling along the course of the long and short saphenous veins (see below).

[3] **See figures and footnote opposite.**

[4] These are tiny intradermal blue patches consisting of minute veins radiating from a single feeding vein.

[5] **Gaiter** *(n)* old fashioned leather covering for lower leg or ankle – the term 'gaiter area' refers to the lower medial one third of the leg and is the area typically first affected with visible skin changes in chronic venous insufficiency.

[6] Typically pitting especially in the earlier stages.

[7] This is caused by the loss of red blood cells into the tissues, a consequence of raised venous pressure.

[8] A term given to the skin and subcutaneous tissue changes of chronic venous hypertension; a progressive sclerosis of the skin and subcutaneous fat by fibrin deposition, tissue death and scarring.

[9] Which can lead to ulceration.

[10] See pg 283 for typical features of a venous ulcer.

[11] See fig on pg 263.

To the patient:
'Is it tender anywhere?
I am looking for evidence of perforator incompetence[12].'
To the patient:
'Do you mind if I feel in the groins? I'm palpating the saphenofemoral junction just medial to the femoral pulse. There is a varix here[13]. Cough please. I can feel a strong cough impulse suggesting an incompetent saphenofemoral junction. I'm just going to tap it and feel lower down.'
Rest a hand on the medial calf just below the knee and tap the saphena varix.
'I can feel the tap impulse[14] distally, indicating incompetent valves below the saphenofemoral junction.
I would like to perform the TOURNIQUET TEST[15]. Could you lie down please? I'm going to lift your ankle gently and rest it on my shoulder[16]. Keep your leg straight if you can, please.'
Lift the leg, put the ankle on your shoulder and stroke the leg firmly.

---

[12] The sites of communication between the deep and superficial venous systems (see fig opposite) are often the areas where varicose veins start. With exercise, the pressure exerted upon the deep venous system by the calf pump can result in blood being forced out into the superficial system at these sites if the valves are incompetent, thus reducing the efficiency of venous drainage of the leg, increasing intravenous pressure (venous hypertension) and dilating the superficial system (varicose veins). Disconnecting the two systems at the site of these incompetent perforators will restore the calf pump to correct functioning only if the deep system is patent and has functioning valves. If the deep system is also incompetent, operating on the superficial veins will make the matter worse.

[13] A swelling over the saphenofemoral junction with a cough impulse indicates an incompetent valve at that junction between the deep and superficial system. When the intra-abdominal pressure is suddenly raised by a cough the pressure in the deep venous system increases as well, but normally functioning valves would protect the superficial venous system from expanding.

[14] Normally functioning valves prevent the backflow of blood down the vein, so a fluid wave would be interrupted at the first valve. This wave is transmitted down the leg if the valves are incompetent. This sign is in practice difficult to elicit and unreliable, and like many of the other tests in this traditional varicose vein examination, have been superseded in clinical practice by Doppler ultrasound testing (see later).

[15] **Trendelenburg's test** is a version of the tourniquet test whereby the saphenofemoral junction is controlled by a finger firmly placed over it. It is notoriously unreliable as it is difficult to maintain complete occlusion of the junction with your finger while the patient struggles to her feet. Only the most sadistic of examiners would refuse to accept the tourniquet test as an alternative which works on the same principle. The principle is that if the superficial system does not fill then the varicosities are controlled at the level of the tourniquet (i.e. the saphenofemoral junction). Thus disconnecting this junction would improve the varicosities. On the other hand, if the superficial system does fill, this indicates that the incompetence is occurring below the level of the tourniquet (usually one of the perforators), so disconection of the saphenofemoral junction is not the whole answer.

[16] Although now replaced by Doppler in most modern clinics, examiners ask hapless candidates to perform this test time and time again. This is probably because, as you can imagine, it quickly sorts out the wheat from the chaff. It takes practice to do smoothly, professionally and elegantly. Try it on your flatmate today, and on three obese inpatients on your ward tomorrow. You will regret it in the exam if you don't!

'I'm just emptying the veins[17].'
Put the tourniquet around the upper thigh.
'Stand up please.'
Do the veins fill immediately?
If not:
'The varicosities are controlled at the level of the saphenofemoral junction'
If they do fill immediately:
'The varicosities are not controlled at the level of the saphenofemoral junction suggesting incompetence lower down.

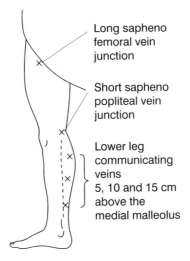

Long sapheno femoral vein junction

Short sapheno popliteal vein junction

Lower leg communicating veins 5, 10 and 15 cm above the medial malleolus

The common sites where the superficial veins connect with deep veins

---

[17] The varicosities should collapse when the patient lies down and the veins are at the level of the heart. If they remain engorged, you should suspect an arteriovenous fistula or a physical obstruction to the venous drainage of the leg instead of varicose veins. Are the veins pulsatile? Is there a thrill or a bruit? Is there a pelvic or abdominal mass?

[18] This does not have to be up in the groin; two thirds of the way between the knee and groin is fine as there are rarely important perforators below the saphenofemoral junction above the knee (see fig above).

I would like to perform PERTHES' TEST[19]**. Leaving the tourniquet on, could you go up and down on tiptoes please?'**
If the veins get better:
'The deep venous system appears to be functioning.'
If the veins get worse and the patient develops severe discomfort:
'There may be problems with the deep venous system.'

---

[19] **Principles of Perthes' test:** You have controlled the varicose veins by blocking off the superficial venous system with the tourniquet. The venous drainage of the leg is now carried out exclusively by the deep venous system as it would if the patient had surgical disconnection of the saphenofemoral junction. By getting the patient to go up and down on her toes you are increasing arterial blood supply and activating the calf pump – the calf muscles are squeezing the blood out of the deep veins and encouraging venous return. If the deep veins are patent this will reduce venous engorgement of the limb. If the deep system is not patent or the valves are incompetent, the effect will be the opposite. With the deep system incapable of draining the leg and the superficial system temporarily disconnected, the increased blood supply into the exercising leg has nowhere to drain, and the patient will experience a bursting pain of venous engorgement. This test illustrates why it is so important to check the patency of the deep venous system before carrying out varicose vein surgery. If the presenting complaint of venous insufficiency and engorgement of superficial veins has these problems secondary to a non functioning deep venous system (for example, after a deep vein thrombosis) then stripping the superficial system on which the patient is relying will only make it worse. To avoid this:
1. Ask about a history of DVT
2. Be suspicious of unilateral varicose veins or those in an unusual distribution
3. Confirm by ultrasound the patency and competence of the deep venous system in any patients in whom doubt exists.

Stand and say to the examiners:

'The tourniquet test can be performed at different levels. A complete examination would include an abdominal and rectal examination[20] as well as Doppler ultrasound assessment[21].'

---

[20] Especially if the varicose veins have appeared suddenly. This may be a sign of venous obstruction in the abdomen or pelvis by a space occupying lesion (e.g. ovarian or rectal carcinoma).

[21] This has now superseded the tourniquet test and Perthes' test in clinical practice and it is likely that over the next few years the examiners will increasingly ask for hand-held Doppler ultrasound examination to be performed. You must practice this before the exam – go to any vascular clinic and ask the consultant or registrar to watch you do it.

Doppler Ultrasound test:

Indications: to detect venous reflux in long saphenous, short saphenous and calf communicating veins. Valuable in detecting saphenous and deep venous reflux.

Procedure: put some ultrasound jelly on the groin and on the hand-held Doppler probe. Locate the femoral artery with the probe (it will be audible) and move the probe a centimetre medially to it over the saphenofemoral junction (this will not normally be audible). Still listening over that spot with the Doppler, squeeze the calf muscle of the same leg firmly with your other hand and let go immediately. This will squeeze some blood up the femoral vein, past the saphenofemoral junction into the common femoral vein. You will hear it WHOOSH past the junction as you listen. This will be followed by a short WOP sound as you let go the calf and the blood column falls back as far as the valve just beneath it which stops it falling any further. If the sapheno-femoral junction is incompetent, blood will not stop falling with a sharp WOP sound but will continue to leak through the incompetent valve back down into the leg, giving a long WHOOOP second sound. So WHOOSH-WOP = competent SFJ, WHOOSH-WHOOOP = incompetent SFJ. This can be repeated at any of the perforators.

In a second part to the test, you can ensure that the prolonged second sound is not due to leakage of blood back down the deep system. This would happen in the case of incompetent deep vein valves in a leg with, for example, previous DVT. Place a tourniquet round the upper thigh and repeat the test. If the long second sound WHOOOP is now shortened, it is the superficial system which has an incompetent valve, probably at the sapheno-femoral junction, so surgical disconnection of the saphenofemoral junction would probably improve the situation. If the long second sound WHOOOP is still long, the blood must be leaking back through valves in the deep system, as you have occluded the superficial system with the tourniquet. In that case, operating on the superficial veins would worsen the situation.

Other venous investigations:

Invasive ambulatory venous pressure measurement

Bipedal ascending phlebography

Injecting non-ionic contrast media into foot veins with ankle tourniquets to direct ionic contrast into the deep system – a useful method of detecting post thrombotic damage and also confirms the presence of incompetent calf communicating veins.

Varicography

Injection of surface veins with contrast (e.g. in previous surgery).

EXAMINATION OF THE ISCHAEMIC OR DIABETIC LEG

'Hello, my name is Dr Parchment Smith. Would you mind if I examined your leg? Could you lie down with your trousers and socks off please? Do you mind if I talk to the examiners as I go along?'

Stand back and LOOK.

'On general inspection I am looking for signs of cardiovascular disease[22], cigarette smoking[23] or diabetes[24]. Looking at the legs, I am looking for pallor, guttering of the veins[25], discoloration[26] and ulcers[27].'

To the patient:

'Is the leg painful[28]? Which one is worse?'

To the examiners: 'I will perform Buerger's test at the end of the examination and proceed now to PALPATION' *OR*

'As part of the inspection I would like to perform Buerger's test[29].'

To perform Buerger's test say to the patient:

'I am going to support your heel. Could you raise your leg slowly to 90° keeping your leg straight please? The foot should remain pink until 90°[30]. The second part of Buerger's test is if you sit up, swinging the legs over the edge of the bed. If the legs go engorged and purple, Buerger's test is positive.'

Crouch down and have a good, quick look at the feet while waiting for the colour change.

---

[22] Such as shortness of breath, sternotomy scars, nearby GTN spray.

[23] Such as nicotine stained teeth, hair or fingers. The huge majority of patients with peripheral vascular disease are either diabetics or smokers.

[24] **Features of diabetes** in the leg and elsewhere (see pg 297).

[25] In a severely ischaemic foot the veins are collapsed and look like pale blue gutters in the subcutaneous tissue. In a normal circulation the veins never have time to empty fully because the arteries keep refilling them, even if the leg is elevated. Venous guttering on raising the leg 10–15° above the horizontal is a sign of significant ischaemia.

[26] The ischaemic leg is typically pale but a severely ischaemic leg may be red ('sunset foot') due to acute inflammation and cellulitis secondary to tissue ischaemia. Individual toes may show the purpley-black hue of a gangrenous digit; this may be hard, well demarcated and painless ('dry gangrene') or infected, soft and moist with surrounding painful cellulitic tissue ('wet gangrene').

[27] See pg 295 and 298.

[28] Pain at rest is an indication of severe (pregangrenous) ischaemia. Painful ischaemic ulcers may be present. Absence of pain in an obviously ulcerated leg is highly suggestive of diabetes, in which ischaemia often coexists with a peripheral neuropathy.

[29] This should traditionally be done as part of 'inspection' but I advise you to omit this, proceed directly to PALPATION (pg 267) and leave the now outdated Buerger's test till the end of the examination. By telling the examiners that you plan to perform the test you give them the opportunity to tell you to skip it if they just want a quick 'spot' diagnosis.

[30] If the foot goes pale at 50° this indicates severe ischaemia. 25° indicates critical ischaemia.

'In the meantime I'll look at the pressure areas to check that there are no ulcers[31].
**As you can see by the colour, Buerger's test is positive with a Buerger's angle of
50°. Now would you lie back down again, and I'll proceed to PALPATION.'**
Feel the temperature of the foot with the back of your hand.
'The right foot is cooler than the left.'
Press the big toe with your finger and see how long the colour takes to return.
'Capillary refill time is normal on the left but slowed at 4 seconds[33] **on the right.
I am now going to palpate the PULSES**[34]**. I'm just going to feel the main artery in
your groin, sir**[35]**.'**
Palpate both femoral pulses[36]*, popliteal pulses*[37]*, dorsalis pedis*[38] *pulses and
posterior tibial*[39] *pulses. Finally palpate for an aortic aneurysm.*
**'Can I just feel the artery in your tummy, sir. Now I'm going to listen for a bruit.
Just breathe normally.'**
Get your stethoscope out to AUSCULTATE. Listen[40] *over the aorta*[41]*, renal arteries,
femoral arteries, and superficial femoral artery as it emerges from the adductor
canal about two-thirds of the way down the thigh on the antero-medial aspect*[42]*.*

---

[31] Heel, malleoli, head of fifth metatarsal, tips of toes, between the toes and the ball of the foot are typical sites
for ischaemic ulceration. In the diabetic foot neuropathic ulcers on the soles of the feet may also be seen.
[32] This is traditional because the physician's palm is warm and moist (especially in exams!) and therefore not as
sensitive to temperature differences as the cool, dry back of the hand.
[33] Two seconds is normal.
[34] In a diabetic, the pulses may be normal in a patient with ischaemic toes due to small vessel disease.
Alternatively they may be reduced, as diabetics are also predisposed to large vessel disease.
[35] Warn the patient you are going to feel his groin! Personally, I usually start with the foot pulses and work up,
but this is not traditional, and was questioned by the examiners when I did the exam, so I think it is safer to start
with the femoral pulses and work down. Whichever you choose, have a justification and be prepared to switch
rather than argue if the examiners insist.
[36] Halfway between the pubic symphysis and the anterior superior iliac spine (the mid inguinal point – the
femoral nerve lies lateral and the vein lies medial to it).
[37] The most difficult to feel reliably – try to feel it NOW on your flatmate/ brother/ mum or you will wish you
had in your exam. Letting the knee relax and flex slightly, hold it with both hands and feel in the popliteal fossa
with your fingers keeping both thumbs on the tibial tuberosity. The pulse is usually lower than you think, and
best felt against the posterior surface of the tibia below the joint line.
[38] Feel across the dorsum of the foot. The artery runs from a point midway between the malleoli to the cleft
between the first and second metatarsal bones.
[39] The posterior tibial artery lies one third of the way between the tip of the medial malleolus and the point of
the heel but can be more easily felt 2.5 cm higher where it runs just behind the medial malleolus.
[40] With the small bell of the stethoscope, not pressing too hard.
[41] The aorta bifurcates at the level of the umbilicus.
[42] This is a common place for stenosis and it is gratifying to hear a bruit here in a leg with palpable femoral
pulses but no palpable pulses distally.

'There is a bruit over the right femoral artery.'
Turn to the examiners.
'To complete the examination I would examine the rest of the vascular tree, especially the carotid arteries[43]. I would look for heart murmurs, atrial fibrillation[44] and check the blood pressure in both arms[45]. I would also perform a neurological examination on the legs[46].
Finally I would like to assess the ankle-brachial pressure index[47].'

---

[43] Listening for a carotid bruit.

[44] Both sources of emboli which can cause acute severe ischaemia. In addition arteriopathies often have a history of ischaemic heart disease which can result in murmurs or AF.

[45] To exclude subclavian or innominate artery disease.

[46] See pg 177 neurological examination of lower limb. Especially important in a diabetic, where you would expect glove and stocking anaesthesia and mononeuropathies affecting single nerves or trunks. A complete cardiovascular examination should include a full neurological examination including fundoscopy, as cerebrovascular disease in any area of the brain can result from arteriopathy.

[47] To do this you need a Doppler probe and a sphygmomanometer with a large enough cuff to encircle the patient's thigh. The patient lies supine. The brachial systolic blood pressure (i.e. the pressure at which the brachial pulse becomes inaudible when the cuff is inflated around the upper arm) is compared with the pressure at which the foot pulse becomes inaudible when the cuff is inflated around the thigh. The ankle-brachial pressure index (ABPI) is the ankle pressure expressed as a percentage of the brachial pressure. If the ankle pressure is greater than the brachial pressure the ABPI is greater than one and ischaemia is unlikely. If the ankle pressure is 70% or less of the brachial pressure, ischaemia is more likely and further investigations may be indicated. Note that ABPIs may appear to be greater than one in the presence of ischaemia if the large arteries of the legs are so calcified that inflation of the cuff fails to compress them. This is typical in diabetic large vessel arteriopathy, so diabetic patients often have misleadingly high ABPIs even if they have significant ischaemia.

EXAMINATION OF THE ISCHAEMIC ARM

'Hello, my name is Dr Parchment Smith. Would you mind if I examined your arms? Could you sit with your top off please? Do you mind if I talk to the examiners as I go along?'

Stand back and LOOK.

'On inspection of the patient I can see no obvious signs of cardiovascular disease. The patient is not short of breath, overweight or cyanosed and there are no signs of previous cardiac surgery[48].'

Take the hands.

'On inspection of the hands I am looking for cyanosis, nicotine staining[49], clubbing[50], vasculitic lesions[51], wasting of the pulp of the finger[52], skin changes, pallor or discoloration.'

FEEL the temperature of the hands with the back of your own hands.

'The hands feel warm and well perfused. I would like to check the CAPILLARY REFILL[53] – it is normal at less than 2 seconds.'

Feel the radial PULSE.

'The pulse is 70 beats per minute and regular[54].'

Raise the patients arm so the wrist is above the heart and feel the character of the pulse with the flat of the palm.

---

[48] Such as a sternotomy wound. Look also for tell-tale hints like sugar free drinks or a GTN spray on the bedside table.

[49] Heavy smokers are more prone to arterial disease and cardiac disease which can cause emboli.

[50] Causes of clubbing which relate to an apparently ischaemic arm:
    Carcinoma of the bronchus may cause thoracic outlet syndrome or hypercoagulability.
    Cyanotic congenital heart disease can be a source of emboli.
    Thyrotoxicosis is a common cause of atrial fibrillation which can be a source of emboli.
    Bacterial endocarditis can cause emboli resulting in splinter haemorrhages.

[51] In embolic disease, small vessel disease or spasm (e.g. Raynaud's phenomenon), small scars or painful ischaemic ulcers may be seen, most often in the fingertips and nailbeds. Repeated paronychia (infections around the nail) may occur and be slow to heal. Unilateral changes suggest emboli from a cardiac or subclavian source (e.g. in thoracic outlet syndrome). Bilateral changes suggest Raynaud's phenomenon.

[52] Repeated episodes of digital artery spasm or temporary blockage by emboli causes the fingers to become wasted, thin and pointed. This is most marked at the pulps. The hand becomes cold and the joints stiff. This can occur in peripheral atherosclerosis or in longstanding Raynaud's phenomenon.

[53] Do this by pressing on the patient's fingertip to blanch it, then count how long it takes for the colour to return. Normal is less than 2 seconds.

[54] Atrial fibrillation can cause emboli.

'The pulse is not collapsing[55].'
Lower the hand. Feel the other radial pulse simultaneously.
'There is no radio-radial delay[56]. I'm just going to pull on your arm while I feel the pulse … and the other side.'
While feeling the pulse, put gentle traction on the shoulder by pulling the upper arm out from the body[57].
'There is no weakening of the pulse while stretching the thoracic inlet. I will now perform ALLEN'S TEST. Could you make a fist please?'
Occlude both the patient's radial and ulnar arteries by pressing down on both pulses at the wrist with your thumbs[58].
'Now open the palm.'
It will be white. Let go of the thumb over the ulnar artery (keeping the pressure on the radial artery) and watch the palm pink up – it should take just a couple of seconds to start going pink.
'The ulnar artery looks patent. Can we do that again please? Make a fist.'
Press on both arteries again.
'Now open your palm.'
Release the thumb over the radial artery only and watch the palm pink up.
'The radial artery looks patent.'
Feel the brachial pulse.
'The brachial pulses are normal. I would like to know the blood pressure in both arms. Can I just feel for the pulse in your armpit? And now in your neck.'
Feel for the axillary, the subclavian and the carotid pulse on each side.
'The pulses feel normal and symmetrical. I am just feeling for a CERVICAL RIB[59]. Now I would like to listen for a bruit in the carotid and subclavian arteries.'

---

[55] Suggesting aortic valve incompetence.
[56] Classically suggests aortic dissection.
[57] The pulse is diminished in certain positions in thoracic outlet syndrome (see pg 319). This includes traction on the shoulder. This is not diagnostic but if the pulse is not similarly obliterated on the asymptomatic side it raises suspicions. Another test is to ask the patient to turn his head towards the affected side, take a deep breath in and hold it. In thoracic outlet syndrome the scalenus anterior is most likely to obstruct the subclavian in this position, obliterating the radial pulse. The structures that can cause thoracic outlet syndrome include abnormal first rib, scalenus anterior, clavicle, scalenus medius, heads of the median nerve, transverse processes of cervical vertebra, or pathological features such as a previous fractured clavicle or first rib, tumour or lymphadenopathy.
[58] Press on the pulses AFTER the patient has made a fist.
[59] Very rarely felt on examination. There may be a fullness at the root of the neck behind the clavicular head of the sternocleidomastoid or a prominent subclavian artery pulse but it is usually not enough to justify a diagnosis. It is diagnosed on X-ray (see pg 319).

Listen over each in turn. Finally, stand up and say to the examiners:
'A complete examination would include a cardiovascular survey of the heart[60], the lower limb[61], and a neurological examination of the arm[62].'

---

[60] See pg 276 because ischaemic heart disease (which can cause murmurs and arrhythmias which you would detect on examination) is a source of emboli.
[61] See pg 266 a commoner site than the upper limb for peripheral vascular disease, one would expect the legs to be affected in a patient with generalised arteriopathy.
[62] See pg 169 because some seemingly ischaemic symptoms may be neurological in origin. Also the two disorders can coexist (e.g. in diabetics).

EXAMINATION OF THE ABDOMINAL AORTIC ANEURYSM

'Hello, my name is Dr Parchment Smith. Would you mind if I examined you? Would you lie down flat with just one pillow under your head? Do you mind if I talk about you as I go along?'

Stand back and LOOK.

'On initial inspection this gentleman looks comfortable at rest. There is an obvious pulsatile swelling in the upper abdomen. He does not look shocked, pale or in pain, and is not breathless. I would like to start the examination by looking at the HANDS[63].'

Pick up the hands, feel the pulse.

'The pulse is 70 beats per minute, regular and equal in both wrists[64]. The palms are not cold or clammy[65], there is no pallor in the palmar creases[66] and no nicotine staining[67]. I would like to know the blood pressure in both arms[68].'

Look in the EYES.

'There is no arcus senilis or xanthomata[69]. In the NECK the character of the carotid pulse is normal and there are no bruits[70].'

Now look at the ABDOMEN.

---

[63] By declaring this you give the examiners the chance to tell you that they just want you to feel the abdomen. Don't spend too long on the preliminaries, just indicate that you are looking for signs of the predisposing factors for aneurysm (hypertension, atherosclerosis due to smoking or hyperlipidaemia) and factors suggesting a leak (shock, tachycardia, anaemia, tenderness).

[64] In any patient with an aneurysm it is important to confirm that they are cardiovascularly stable with no tachycardia. Radio-radial delay (a discrepancy between the two radial pulses) is a well-known but rarely seen sign of aortic dissection.

[65] Signs of shock.

[66] Indicating anaemia, relevant because it may indicate:
1. Fitness for surgery
2. Another, unrelated cause for an upper abdominal mass (stomach cancer lying across the aorta may present as a mass transmitting pulsations. It will not be expansile.)
3. A slow leak, e.g. in an inflammatory aneurysm

[67] Smokers are more prone to arterial disease and have a poorer prognosis in major surgery.

[68] Hypertension is a risk factor for aortic aneurysms. Discrepancy in blood pressure in both arms indicates large vessel atherosclerosis or aortic dissection.

[69] Both signs of hyperlipidaemia.

[70] A patient undergoing aortic aneurysm repair who had significant carotid stenosis would be at high risk of intraoperative stroke.

'On inspection of the ABDOMEN there is an abnormal pulsating mass above the umbilicus. I am looking for scars, especially sternotomy[71] or laparotomy scars[72]. Is your tummy tender[73]? Can I feel the lump please?'

Place your hand over the lump gently trying to feel its extent and margins.

'Is this tender? Firstly I am trying to feel the character of the lump. It is firm, non-tender and pulsatile[74].'

Put your hands either side of the lump and allow them to be visibly pushed apart by the pulsations.

'It is also expansile[75]. I estimate the transverse diameter to be about 5 cm[76]. I can feel the upper limit which suggests it is infrarenal[77]. I cannot feel a bi-lobed structure below the umbilicus which would suggest it is not extending into the iliacs. I can move it slightly from side to side but not up and down. Can I feel in the groins please?'

Palpate the femoral pulses.

'The femoral pulses are palpable – indeed the left also feels aneurysmal[78]. I'm now going to listen for a bruit.'

Auscultate over the aneurysm, either side of it just under the ribcage (for renal artery bruits) and over the femoral pulses.

Stand up and say to the examiners:

'To complete my examination I would like to examine the heart and the legs for cardiac and peripheral vascular disease[79].'

---

[71] Previous cardiac surgery has implications for any major surgery planned.

[72] Previous surgery may make aortic aneurysm repair more difficult because of adhesions.

[73] A tender abdominal aortic aneurysm raises the suspicion of a leak or sudden expansion. If it is tender, the patient should not be sitting in an MRCS exam bay!

[74] Although an aneurysm is pulsatile, this is not a specific sign as any lump near an artery is likely to be pulsatile. Rest your hand on the lump and hold it still to appreciate the pulsation.

[75] Unlike the non-specific sign of pulsatility, an expansile mass is generally an aneurysm or (rarely) an extremely vascular tumour. An expansile mass will push the hands in opposite directions, whereas both hands will move in the same direction (usually up) when resting on a pulsatile mass.

[76] You can only estimate accurately if you have felt a few aneurysms, the diameter of which had been assessed by ultrasound – so start scouring the wards and clinics for these now! The transverse diameter of a normal (non aneurysmal) aorta is 2–3 cm and can be palpated in a slim patient. Patients with aneurysms around 5 cm are usually under surveillance and very stable so ideal for exams; it is unlikely that a patient whose aneurysm had suddenly expanded to 8 cm would be put into an exam for repeated palpation!

[77] Only 1–2% are suprarenal.

[78] There is an increased incidence of other aneurysms in a patient with an abdominal aortic aneurysm. Rare in patients with aneurysms.

EXAMINATION OF AN ULCER

'Hello, my name is Dr Parchment Smith. Can I have a look at this please? Do you mind if I describe it to the examiners? Is it painful at all?[80]'

Site[81].

'There is a large painful ulcer[82] on the right medial malleolus.'

Look at and describe the size, shape, depth[83] and edges[84].

'It is about 8 cm in diameter, irregularly round in shape with sloping edges. It is about 3 mm deep.'

---

[79] Although atherosclerosis is a risk factor for aortic aneurysms, severe peripheral vascular disease is surprisingly rare in patients with aneurysms.

[80] Whether the ulcer is painful is very useful information, as neuropathic ulcers and ulcers in people with diabetic neuropathy are typically painless, whereas venous or arterial ulcers are typically painful.

[81] Different ulcers have typical sites. The commonest ulcers are a venous ulcer (pg 283 typically on the medial side of the gaiter area), a neuropathic ulcer (pg 298 typically in an area susceptible to trauma such as the sole of the foot or the heel) and an ischaemic ulcer (pg 295 typically at the periphery of the limb or pressure areas).

[82] An ulcer is a defect or excavation of the surface. It applies not only to skin and epithelium, but the surface of any tissue or organ.

[83] Note the depth in millimetres or describe it in relation to the structures (e.g. superficial, through full thickness of skin, down to bone, down to tendon).

[84] Types of edge:

Flat sloping edge: A healing ulcer. Usually shallow. Typical of venous ulcer.

Punched out/vertical edge: Follows rapid death and sloughing of a full thickness of skin without successful attempts at self-repair. Typical of neuropathic or vascular ulcers. Historically typical of syphilitic ulcer (now rare).

Undermined edge: when infection affects subcutaneous tissues more than the skin, e.g. pressure sores. Historically typical of tuberculous ulcer (now rare).

Rolled edge: develops when there is slow growth of tissue in the edge of an ulcer. Almost diagnostic of a basal cell carcinoma (see pg 47).

Everted or heaped edge: develops when tissue at the edge of the ulcer is growing quickly and spilling over the normal skin. Typical of a carcinoma.

Look at the base[85].

'The base is covered in healthy granulation tissue with one or two sloughy areas. There is no obvious discharge or visible tendons or bone[86].'

Feel the surrounding tissues, feeling for foot pulses, observing capillary refill, pointing out any signs of venous disease (see pg 283) /ischaemia (see pg 295) /diabetes (see pg 297) /neuropathy (see pg 298).

'The surrounding tissues show evidence of chronic venous disease/ischaemia/neuropathy.'

Diagnosis.

'My diagnosis is[88]...'

---

[85] The base or floor of an ulcer may look:

Healthy with pink granulation tissue (usually associated with shallow sloping edges and evidence of a margin of previously involved surrounding skin which is now healing).

Sloughy with green or yellow infected areas stuck to it. This is ally associated with a discharge and should be swabbed and treated with topical antibiotics if needed (rarely) and with a dressing which dissolves and lifts off the slough. Venous ulcers and pressure sores are commonly sloughy.

Necrotic with black or grey dead tissue – these will have to slough off, be lifted off with a suitable dressing or débrided before the ulcer can begin to heal. Vascular or neuropathic ulcers may have this appearance. Pressure sores often start off as necrotic areas.

Avascular with a pale, clean shiny base. This is usually associated with deep, punched out edges and peripheral vascular disease. These ulcers are usually slow to heal and may need the circulation improving by angioplasty or surgery. Tissue loss like this is one of the indications for a peripheral bypass if angioplasty is not suitable and bypass is possible.

[86] Apart from demonstrating the depth of the ulcer, the significance of bone or tendon at the base of an ulcer is that this is not a suitable surface to apply a split skin graft onto, as there is no underlying blood supply.

[87] The vascular and neurological status of the surrounding skin is crucial in determining the type of ulcer, especially in a foot ulcer. The exceptions are an obvious malignant ulcer in another site, e.g. trunk or face, in which case the draining lymph nodes are much more important. In a foot ulcer, the very least that should be done is to feel for the foot pulses (see examination of ischaemic limb, pg 266), look for and evidence of venous insufficiency (see examination of varicose veins, pg 261) and check sensation (see neurological examination of lower limb, pg 177).

[88] Common ulcers you will see in your exam: venous (see pg 283), ischaemic (see pg 295), diabetic/neuropathic (see pg 298) or a mixture of these. Neoplastic ulcers e.g. basal cell carcinoma (see pg 47), squamous cell carcinoma (see pg 49), malignant melanoma (see pg 51) and Marjolin's ulcer (see pg 49) should also be recognised. Less common exam cases include vasculitic ulcers (due to rheumatoid arthritis or scleroderma), syphilitic or tuberculous ulcers. Pyoderma gangrenosum, necrobiosis lipoidica and lymphangiosarcoma can also present as ulcers.

EXAMINATION OF THE HEART[89]

'Hello, my name is Dr Parchment Smith. Do you mind if I examine you? Could you sit at 45° with your shirt off please? Do you mind if I talk to the examiners as I go along?'

LOOK from the end of the bed, hands behind your back.

'On initial inspection, the patient is not breathless[90], cyanosed[91] or pale[92]. There is no malar flush[93] or obvious scars[94]. I cannot see any ankle oedema[95]. Can I look at your hands please? I am looking for clubbing[96] and splinter haemorrhages[97]. The pulse rate is 70 beats per minute and regular[98].'

Lift the hand above the patient's head and continue to feel the pulse.

'The pulse is not collapsing[99].'

Feel the other pulse at the same time.

'There is no radio-radial delay[100].'

Feel the brachial pulses.

'I would like to know the blood pressure. Can I look in your eyes? The sclera are not pale[101]. Can I look in your mouth? There is no central cyanosis[102]. Turn your head away slightly please. The JVP looks normal[103]. I'm just going to press gently on your tummy – it rises on pressing the liver as expected[104].'

---

[89] The commonest examination in the medical MRCP exam, it is rarely asked for in the MRCS. But with a vascular and thoracic bay, it seems sensible to make sure you can assess the cardiac status of a patient efficiently. Of course, as a vital part of preoperative assessment in the clinical setting, you will be familiar with the examination, but just make sure you can do it slickly and know where to listen for murmurs and what they mean.

[90] Could indicate left heart failure.

[91] Can be central or peripheral.

[92] Indicating anaemia.

[93] Red cheeks associated with mitral stenosis.

[94] Midline sternal (valve replacement) or left thoracotomy (mitral stenosis).

[95] Right heart failure.

[96] Associated with cyanotic congenital heart defects and subacute bacterial endocarditis.

[97] Caused by infective endocarditis.

[98] Regularly irregular pulse suggests heart block. Irregularly irregular is atrial fibrillation.

[99] Typical of aortic valve regurgitation or persistent ductus arteriosus.

[100] Suggests aortic dissection or coarctation.

[101] Anaemia.

[102] Congenital cyanotic heart disease.

[103] When the patient is sitting at 45° the JVP should be no more than 3 cm above the sternal angle (which is level with the base of the neck). The JVP is elevated in right heart failure, congestive cardiac failure, tricuspid incompetence, volume overload and pulmonary hypertension.

[104] If it doesn't there may be some obstruction of the vena cava.

The carotid pulse[105] **has a normal character**[106]**.'**

Look at the chest.

'On inspecting the precordium there are no visible scars or pulsations. I'm just going to feel for your heart ... first the apex beat[107]**, then over the left sternal edge**[108]**, then over the manubrium**[109]**. There are no heaves or thrills. Now I'm going to listen.'**

Take out your stethoscope for auscultation.

'Could you roll over to your left please? I'm just listening over the mitral area[110]**. Can you sit up now please and breathe in then out... now hold it – this is the tricuspid area**[111]**.'**

---

[105] Palpated just lateral to the trachea (one at a time!).

[106] A 'water-hammer' carotid pulsation is due to a rigid aorta, high cardiac output, aortic regurgitation, persistent (??patent) ductus arteriosus.

[107] **The apex beat** is the most lateral and inferior point at which the fingers are raised with each systole. The normal apex beat is in the fifth left intercostal space 1cm medial to the midclavicular line. Localise the apex beat as follows: feel for the first palpable intercostal space on the left 1cm medial to the midclavicular line. This is the second intercostal space. Count down to the fifth space and feel around here for the most lateral inferior point at which you can feel the heart beating.

Strong/lifting apex beat suggests mitral or aortic incompetence.

Double apex beat suggests hypertrophic cardiomyopathy.

Tapping apex beat (palpable first heart sound) suggests mitral or tricuspid stenosis.

Forceful sustained apex beat suggests aortic stenosis or hypertension.

Deviated apex beat displaced laterally or inferiorly suggests enlarged heart.

[108] Thrills or tapping here indicates mitral valve disease.

Sternal heave indicates right ventricular hypertrophy (pulmonary hypertension).

[109] Palpable pulmonary second sound suggests pulmonary hypertension

precordial thrill suggests aortic stenosis

[110] See fig pg 278 **Mitral area:**

Site: left fourth intercostal space 1cm medial to the mid clavicular line.

Patient's position: Rolled over towards the left.

Murmurs you will hear: Pan systolic into axilla   = mitral regurgitation

                          Mid diastolic   = mitral stenosis

[111] See fig pg 278 **Tricuspid area:**

Site: fifth intercostal space on left border of sternum.

Patient's position: sat up breathing out.

Murmurs you will hear: Early diastolic into apex   = aortic regurgitation

Less common right sided murmurs and septal defect murmurs can best be heard here also

(pan-systolic=tricuspid regurgitation/VSD, ejection systolic=pulmonary stenosis/ASD, mid diastolic= tricuspid stenosis).

Breathe normally and rest back as I listen over the pulmonary area[112] and aortic area[113]. Now let me listen to the arteries in the neck[114]. Finally, could you lean forward so I can listen to your lung bases[115] and check for sacral oedema[116].'

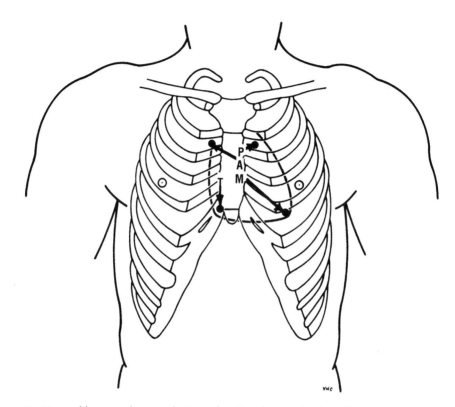

Position of heart valves and sites of optimal auscultation. P = pulmonary valve; A = aortic valve; M = mitral valve; T = tricuspid valve. Arrows indicate position where valves may be heard with the least interference.

---

[112] See fig above **Pulmonary area:**
Site: second intercostal space on left border of sternum.
Patient's position: sitting at 45°.
You will hear: increased splitting of second heart sound= right bundle branch block, pulmonary stenosis, ventricular septal defect, mitral regurgitation, atrial septal defect
[113] See fig above **Aortic area:**
Site: second intercostal space on right border of sternum.
Patient's position: sitting at 45°.
Murmurs you will hear: ejection systolic into carotid arteries = aortic stenosis
                          early diastolic = pulmonary regurgitation
[114] The ejection systolic murmur of aortic stenosis can be heard radiating into the carotids. Listen also for a carotid bruit.
[115] Crepitations suggest pulmonary oedema secondary to left heart failure.
[116] Secondary to right heart failure. Often more marked than ankle oedema in bedridden patients.

C   The Cases

Varicose Veins
Top Five Case: either varicose veins, venous skin changes or venous ulcers were seen by over half of candidates in our survey. Together accounted for over 25% of cases in this bay.

[117]Aetiology of varicose veins:

Idiopathic (primary varicose veins)

Deep vein thrombosis, pregnancy, pelvic tumours, congenital disorders (see Klippel Trenaunay syndrome, pg 327)

Factors predisposing to varicose veins:

Family history, female sex, parity, occupation.

Pathology:

Primary weakness of the wall of the vein causes dilatation just below the valve which causes valvular incompetence leading to varicosity.

Symptoms:

Unsightliness, ache on standing, night cramps, ankle swelling, skin changes, ulceration

Treatment:

Elastic support stockings

Surgery

'High tie' (Sapheno-femoral disconnection and ligation) stripping and multiple avulsions

The saphenous vein and all the tributaries which enter the saphenous vein near the sapheno-femoral junction are ligated and divided. The saphenous vein itself must be ligated flush with the femoral vein but must not narrow it. A stripper is then passed into the saphenous vein, down the thigh and out of an incision just above the knee. The vein is thus stripped from the thigh, and previously marked varicosities below the knee are avulsed through individual stab incisions. Stripping the long saphenous vein below the knee is often discouraged because of its close association with the sural nerve which supplies sensation to the medial side of the foot. The short saphenous vein can be similarly disconnected at the sapheno-popliteal junction with the patient lying prone. Bandage the whole leg firmly.

Tributaries entering near the sapheno-femoral junction:

Superficial inferior epigastric vein

Deep external pudendal vein

Superficial external pudendal vein

Posteromedial vein of the thigh

Anterolateral vein of the thigh

Superficial circumflex iliac vein

These should be ligated along with the saphenous vein to prevent recurrence.

Postoperative complications:

Tie on the sapheno-femoral/sapheno-popliteal junction slips off - always do a transfixion stitch for this important tie. If it slips off immediate re-exploration is indicated.

Wound infection (especially groin)

Haematoma or bleeding- minimised by firm bandaging

Recurrence – often because tributaries (above) have been missed. Later recurrences may reflect underlying valvular weakness in the superficial venous system.

VARICOSE VEINS[117]

Carry out examination of varicose veins (see pg 261).

'On inspection there are visible dilated varicose veins on both legs, in the distribution of the long saphenous vein. There is evidence of venous insufficiency in the gaiter area with oedema, pigmentation, lipodermatosclerosis and eczema. On the lower right leg there is a large venous ulcer (see case, pg 283). There is a palpable saphena varix in both groins with a cough impulse. There is a positive tap test. The tourniquet test reveals that the veins are controlled at the sapheno-femoral junction. Doppler examination confirms an incompetent sapheno-femoral junction and a competent deep system. The foot pulses and perfusion are good. This patient has varicose veins with signs of venous insufficiency. Indications are that a high tie and stripping would improve her symptoms.'

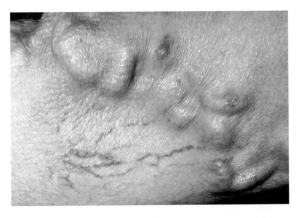

Varicose veins showing ulceration and superficial flare veins

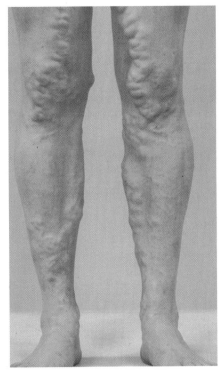

Gross bilateral varicose veins

Venous Ulcer

[118] Healthy granulation tissue in a healing ulcer.

[119] If long-standing and stationary.

[120] If infected and enlarging.

[121] **Management of a venous ulcer**

Remember this 8-point plan:

1. Exclude coexisting ischaemia and treat if present

By measuring ankle-brachial pressure index (see pg 266, examination of the ischaemic limb) the degree of ischaemia, if present, can be defined. Mixed ulcers exist where arterial and venous factors prevent healing, and they are much more difficult to treat than simple venous ulcers. In such mixed ulcers any ischaemic component must be corrected first if possible (by angioplasty or surgery) before the venous element is treated. This is because (a) an ulcer will not heal in the absence of sufficient blood supply, and (b) the methods of treating a venous ulcer will further compromise the blood supply and lead to complications.

2. Elevation

This improves venous return but it is notoriously difficult to ensure compliance and some patients are admitted to hospital just to ensure their bed is on a slope and their feet are elevated above the hips while at rest.

3. Four layer bandaging

These layers are   a) non-adherent dressing to protect the ulcer
   b) wool to cushion the dressing and protect the vulnerable surrounding skin
   c) graduated compression bandage – the functional component of the dressing which encourages venous return. It runs from foot to thigh.
   d) tubular bandage – an elastic bandage which merely keeps the whole dressing in place and stops the compression bandage from unravelling.

4. Weekly dressing and measuring

Preferably in a specialist clinic. 80–90% are healed within 12 months. Complications such as infection and Marjolin's ulcer are looked out for at these weekly assessments. Infected ulcers should be swabbed and treated with topical agents (e.g. Betadine dressing) not systemic antibiotics.

5. Plastic surgery

If healing is not progressing excision of ulcer base and skin grafting may be appropriate.

AFTER HEALING:

6. Investigate venous system

e.g. by Doppler, venous pressure measurements or phlebography to assess the sites of valve incompetence and function of the deep venous system.

7. Saphenous surgery

Successful in preventing reulceration in patients with normal deep veins but contraindicated in post thrombotic limbs.

8. Preventative measures

TED stockings, avoid minor trauma

VENOUS ULCER

Carry out examination of an ulcer (see pg 274).

'There is a large, shallow, painful, ulcer on the medial side of the gaiter area in a well-perfused foot with good pulses. The edges are gently sloping or terraced and the base is red and velvety[118]/white and fibrous[119]/yellow, sloughy and offensive[120]. Surrounding tissues show signs of long-standing venous disease including oedema, haemosiderin deposition, lipodermatosclerosis and varicose veins. This is a venous ulcer[121].'

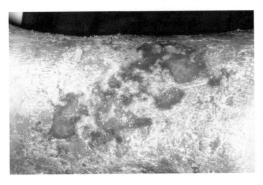

Chronic venous ulceration in a leg with signs of venous insufficiency

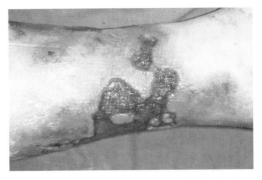

A healing venous ulcer with healthy, healing surrounding skin, red velvety granulation tissue and islands of regenerating epithelium

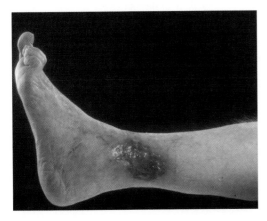

An acute venous ulcer in the gaiter area

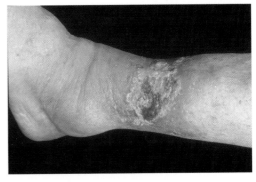

Chronic venous skin changes of the gaiter area – oedema, haemosiderin deposition and lipodermatosclerosis

Deep Vein Thrombosis
Common case: seen by over 1 in twenty of the candidates surveyed.
[122] Risk factors for DVT

Patient	Procedure	Underlying disease
Old	Type of operation (pelvic)	General injury
Female	Type of anaesthesia (GA)	Local injury
Winter	Long operation	Malignancy
Caucasian	Immobilisation	Cardiac failure
Sedentary occupation	Bedrest	Myocardial infarction
Obesity	Dehydration	Arterial ischaemia
Pregnancy		Protein C and S deficiency
Drugs		Venous disorders
Combined oral contraceptive pill		Previous DVT/PE
Intravenous saline		Varicose veins
Haemostatic treatment		Vasculitis (e.g. Buerger's, Behçet's)
Other drugs		Congenital venous abnormalities
		(e.g. Klippel Trenaunay syndrome)

Incidence
98% arise in the deep veins of legs and pelvis, 2% at other sites. If no prophylaxis were used, 30% of all patients over 40 having major surgery would develop DVTs (60% after hip surgery).

Pathogenesis of DVT
Remember Virchow's triad – a common exam question. Stasis, wall damage and hypercoagulability make up the triad, and disruption of any one of these predisposes to thrombogenesis. Aschoff's theory of thrombosis is a four-stage hypothesis.
1. Corallin thrombus plug forms (platelets adhere to endothelial surface, fibrin and red cells are deposited on top
2. Blood flow occluded
3. Rapidly propagating thrombus forms
4. Thrombus becomes organised

Differential diagnosis for DVT
Torn gastrocnemius muscle superficial thrombophlebitis
Ruptured Baker's cyst acute arteritis/haemarthrosis of the knee
Calf haematoma Achilles tendonitis
Lymphoedema and cellulitis Peripheral oedema
Acute arterial ischaemia Sarcoma
Obstruction of veins and lymphatics Myositis ossificans
Fractured femur

Prophylaxis of DVT

Preoperative:	Intraoperative	Postoperative:
Stop pill six weeks before	Care in positioning	Heparin or dextran
Keep mobile	Flowtron boots	Early mobilisation
Identify high-risk patients	Keep time on the table	Deep breathing to aid venous return
Subcutaneous heparin or iv dextran	to a minimum	Clinical vigilance for signs of DVT
	Keep well hydrated	TED stockings
		Elevate foot of bed
		Feet up when sat out
		Don't cross legs

Continues pg 286

DEEP VEIN THROMBOSIS[122]

Spot diagnosis.

'The left lower leg is swollen[123], red, hot and tender. There is pitting oedema to the knee. The calf muscle is hard and tender[124], and passive dorsiflexion of the foot causes pain in the calf (Homan's sign[125]). There are bruises on the abdomen/thigh in keeping with subcutaneous injections of low molecular weight heparin. This is a deep vein thrombosis.'

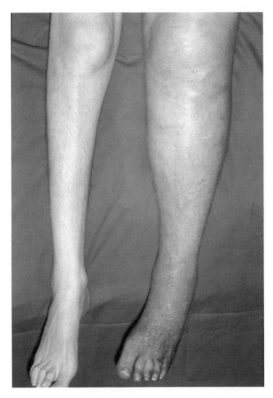

DVT of left leg which appears red and swollen

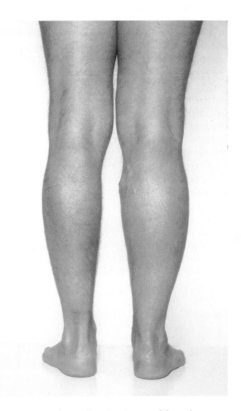

Deep vein thrombosis. Note dilated superficial veins on the right

Deep Vein Thrombosis **continued**
Complications of DVT:
<u>Pulmonary embolus</u> – most originating from femoral, iliac and pelvic veins

<u>Venous gangrene</u> – rare complication of massive ileofemoral thrombosis. Phlegmasia alba dolens (white leg) is followed by phlegmasia cerulea dolens (blue leg) and finally venous gangrene and toxaemia.

<u>Pulmonary hypertension</u> – develops after recurrent emboli

<u>Paradoxical embolus</u> – in the presence of a patent foramen ovale or ductus arteriosus, emboli from venous thrombosis can produce an arterial occlusion in the limbs or brain.

Management of DVT:
Anticoagulation (LMW heparin, warfarin)

Thrombolysis with streptokinase or TPA

Inferior vena cava filter (e.g. Mobin-Uddin umbrella, Greenfield filter)

[123] May be just around the ankle or extend to the groin depending on the extent of the thrombosis.

[124] Few conditions make the calf muscle stiff and hard, although many make it tender.

[125] Although the classic bedside test for DVT, Homan's test is unreliable. Some say that repeatedly performing the test may dislodge thrombus and cause a pulmonary embolus, but others say that most emboli come from the large veins, not the calf veins. Because of this controversy, you may find it wiser to offer to perform the test and proceed only if the examiners appear to approve of it.

Superficial thrombophlebitis:
<u>Definition:</u> venous thrombosis affecting the superficial veins.

<u>Causes:</u> Varicose veins, sclerotherapy, trauma, chemical irritation, local sepsis. Associated with carcinoma and DVT.

<u>Clinical:</u> Painful, hard, hot reddened subcutaneous cord.

<u>Treatment:</u> Analgesia and external elastic support. Condition is usually self-limiting. Surgical treatment is rarely indicated unless the upper end of the long saphenous vein is involved (superficial vein ligation described by John Hunter 1784).

<u>Complications:</u> Recurrence should suggest thrombophlebitis migrans associated with underlying carcinoma. Coexistent DVT is common; ultrasound or venography may be indicated.

SUPERIOR VENA CAVA OBSTRUCTION[126]

Spot diagnosis.

'The patient has a markedly swollen head and neck, which are suffused and cyanosed. The neck veins are distended and do not collapse on elevation or with respiration. He is short of breath at rest. The diagnosis is superior vena caval obstruction. I would like to ask the patient about associated symptoms[127], examine his neck[128] and listen to his chest[129].'

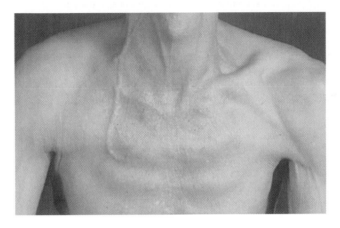

Dilated veins on the right of the neck suggesting SVC obstruction

---

Superior Vena Cava Obstruction
[126] **Causes of SVC obstruction**

Acute obstruction	Chronic obstruction	Iatrogenic
Carcinoma bronchus	Retrosternal goitre	Central TPN
Thymoma	Slow growing mediastinal tumour	
Lymphoma	Constrictive pericarditis	
Carcinoma thyroid	Mediastinal fibrosis	

Investigations:
Chest X-ray, chest CT may show lung or mediastinal tumour
Bilateral brachial vein injections of contrast to determine extent of occlusion
Management:
Exclude terminal disease
Obtain tissue diagnosis
Treat underlying cause (e.g. by radiotherapy)
Caval bypass to right atrium
[127] Tinnitus, epistaxis, a non-productive cough and dysphagia are all related symptoms that can be attributed to the underlying cause, the effects of venous congestion, and direct pressure effects of a mass in the neck or mediastinum.
[128] For goitre, central line scars or lymphadenopathy.
[129] For pulmonary effusion due to carcinoma bronchus.

Axillary Vein Thrombosis
Accounts for 1–2% of all venous thromboses.
[130] **Causes:**
Idiopathic
Cervical rib
Thoracic outlet obstruction (see pg 319)
History:
Affects right hand most commonly and develops after excessive or unusual exercise e.g. painting a room (nick-named 'effort thrombosis').
Patients are often young (35–45 years)
Presents with discomfort and weakness
Investigations:
Chest X-ray and CT thorax to exclude Pancoast's tumour or lymphoma; cervical spine X-ray to exclude cervical rib. Brachial venography is required to confirm diagnosis and extent of thrombosis.
Management:
Conservative – especially if patient presents late. Most untreated patients develop good collateral pathways and become symptom free after a few months.
Anticoagulants – usually given for 3 months to prevent propagation of thrombus or the faint possibility of pulmonary embolus.
Thrombolysis – Streptokinase or TPA may reduce late sequelae of chronic venous insufficiency.
Surgical decompression – combined with thrombectomy.
Surgical bypass – utilising internal jugular vein.
Course of axillary vein
- Brachial artery venae comitantes join basilic vein at the lower border of teres major axillary vein
- Runs upwards on the medial side of the axillary artery
- Ends at the lateral border of the first rib by becoming the subclavian vein
- Tributaries include
  cephalic vein
  highest thoracic vein
  thoraco acromial vein
  lateral thoracic vein
  subscapular vein
  anterior circumflex humeral vein
  posterior circumflex humeral vein
The last six correspond with the branches of the axillary artery.

AXILLARY VEIN THROMBOSIS[130]

Spot diagnosis or examination of upper limb (see pg 169).

'The right arm is painful and weak. The fingers, hand and forearm feel cool and are swollen and blue. There is pitting oedema on the dorsum of the hand and the subcutaneous veins appear distended with enlarged collateral veins over the shoulder and chest. The upper limb pulses are present and undiminished. The finger movements are diminished, but sensation is intact and movement of the rest of the arm is limited only by pain and swelling. A tender cord can be felt along the course of the axillary vein (see opposite). There is no palpable cervical rib or cervical lymphadenopathy. The diagnosis is axillary vein thrombosis.'

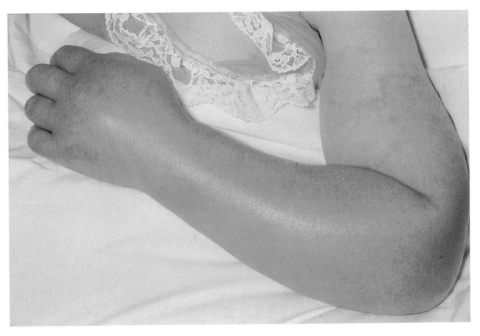

Patient with axillary vein thrombosis showing a swollen oedematous arm

Ischaemic Leg

Top Five Case: excluding diabetic legs, ischaemic legs were seen by more than half of the candidates surveyed. Accounted for over 20% of the cases in this bay.

[131] Peripheral vascular disease of lower limbs

Aetiology

The main cause of arterial disease in the lower limb is <u>atherosclerosis</u>, either thrombosis or embolic.

Other causes include

> <u>Thromboembolism from other source</u> (cardiac, aortic or other aneurysms)
>
> <u>Anatomic or developmental anomalies</u> (popliteal entrapment syndrome, persistent sciatic artery, adventitial cystic disease, fibromuscular dysplasia)
>
> <u>Inflammatory conditions</u> (Buerger's disease, Vasculitis, repetitive trauma)
>
> <u>Vasospastic conditions</u> (Raynaud's phenomenon, ergotism, iv drug use)
>
> <u>Hypercoagulable states</u> (anticoagulant deficiency e.g. protein C or S, polycythaemia, malignancy, thrombocytosis)

Symptoms:

Intermittent claudication involving the calf in SFA disease, the thigh and buttock in iliac disease.

Rest pain and night pain indicates more severe insufficiency.

Ulceration from small ulcers to major tissue loss.

If told to ask some questions in the exam:

<u>To confirm the pain is claudication</u>

How far can you walk before you get the pain?

Is it worse going uphill or in the cold weather?

Is it just in the calf or in the buttock and thigh as well?

Does it go away within seconds when you stop (e.g. to look in a shop window)?

<u>To assess severity and progression</u>

How long have you been suffering from this pain on walking?

Do you get pain that wakes you in the night? Do you swing your leg out of bed to help it go away?

Do you get pain at rest? (indicates onset of critical ischaemia)

Have you ever had ulcers or sores on your leg? (tissue loss is an indication for intervention)

<u>To assess risk factors and treatment options</u>

Are you diabetic?

Do you smoke?

Are you on aspirin?

Have you ever had your cholesterol checked?

Have you ever had any angiograms or ballooning to stretch your arteries?

Have you ever had a heart attack, angina or a stroke?

Do you get symptoms in your other leg?

Investigations:

Ankle brachial pressure index (see pg 268).

Contrast angiography (generally only needed if intervention is planned).

Magnetic Resonance Angiography (MRA).

Assess risk factors such as blood sugar, cholesterol, blood pressure, lipids.

Assess comorbidity such as cardiac, renal and lung function.

Continues pg 292

ISCHAEMIC LEG[131]

Carry out examination of ischaemic/diabetic leg (pg 266).

'This (male, middle-aged to elderly) patient has nicotine stained fingers. His legs are pale, with venous guttering, cyanosis and rubor around the feet. The left foot is painful at rest with two painful ulcers, one on the heel and one on the middle toe. Buerger's test is positive with an angle of 50° on the right and 30° on the left suggesting ischaemia. The feet are cool and capillary refill is delayed at four seconds. The femoral pulses are present, but on the left the popliteal pulses are diminished and the foot pulses are absent. On the right the pulses are present. There is a bruit over the left superficial femoral artery two-thirds of the way down the medial thigh. This patient has significant bilateral peripheral vascular disease worse on the left with a likely atherosclerotic stricture at the left adductor hiatus complicated by rest pain and tissue loss. I would like to have a hand held Doppler and sphygmomanometer to check the ankle brachial pressure indices.'

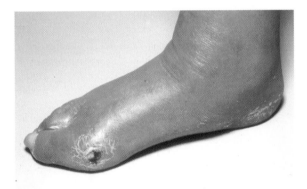

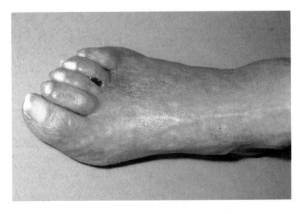

Chronically ischaemic right foot with dependent rubor and ulceration

Ischaemic leg continued
Management of peripheral vascular disease
<u>Claudication is managed conservatively if possible</u>
Stop smoking
Treat hypertension, diabetes, hypercholesterolaemia
Lose weight
Take 75–325 mg aspirin daily
Avoid diuretics and beta blockers
Follow a graded exercise programme to increase collateral circulation
Do not get an angiogram unless you are planning intervention
80% of claudicants remain stable or improve when treated as above over 1 year, 50% over 5 years
10% develop indications for intervention and 5% die of cardiovascular disease each year
Indications for intervention
Worsening life-limiting claudication despite the above measures
Rest pain
Tissue loss (ulcers)
Sudden deterioration (e.g. acutely ischaemic limb)
Options for intervention
<u>Percutaneous endovascular revascularisation</u>
Balloon angioplasty
Stenting
Best in focal SFA stenosis or isolated iliac lesions. Extensive disease may require surgery
<u>Surgery</u>
Endarterectomy
Patch angioplasty
Saphenous vein bypass (in situ valvotomed or reversed).

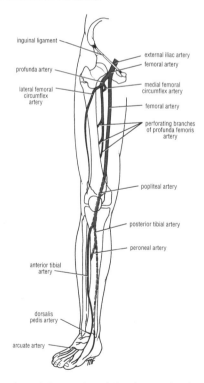

Arterial supply of the lower limb

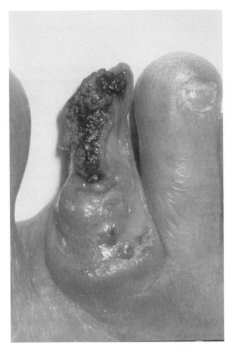

Wet gangrene of toe due to Buerger's
disease

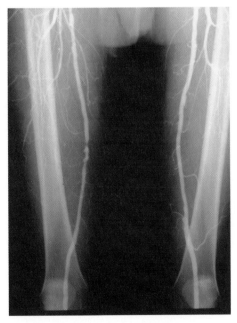

Arteriogram of lower limbs showing
stenosis of the superficial femoral artery

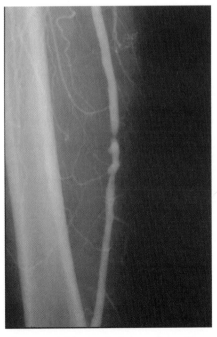

Close up of stenosis in previous figure

Ischaemic Ulcer

[132] Heel, malleoli, head of fifth metatarsal, tips of toes, between the toes and the ball of the foot are typical sites for ischaemic ulceration.

[133] See pg 266.

[134] Even if the ulcer is painful, examination of the ischaemic leg (especially in a diabetic) will often show loss of superficial and deep sensation, weakness of movement and loss of reflexes.

Management of an ischaemic ulcer

An ulcer will not heal in the absence of sufficient blood supply, so the main aim of management is to restore circulation to the affected limb.

1. Angioplasty: in more fortunate patients, an angioplastiable lesion will be detected and the situation can be improved by angioplasty.

2. Bypass: in those without an angioplastiable lesion, surgical reconstruction may be possible. Critical ischaemia (rest pain) and tissue loss (ulceration) are said by some vascular surgeons to be the only indications for bypass surgery (which is not now routinely offered to patients with simple claudication due to high rates of restenosis).

3. Amputation: in some unfortunate patients (e.g. those with extensive atherosclerosis or small vessel disease) bypass is not possible and amputation is the only option to relieve pain and prevent progressive tissue loss, infection and gangrene.

4. Local care: in the meantime, nursing care includes avoiding ill-fitting footwear, applying non-adherent dressings, avoiding compression bandages, and prescribing topical antiseptics if necessary.

5. Conservative measures: the usual advice to improve circulation (see pg 292, ischaemic leg) such as give up smoking, improve walking distances, take regular aspirin (or anticoagulants if indicated) and reduce cholesterol should be given as appropriate.

Other causes of ischaemic ulceration

By far the most common causes of ischaemic ulceration is atherosclerosis (usually of the large arteries) and diabetic arteriopathy (affecting both large and small arteries).

Other causes include:

Large artery: embolism.

Small artery: Raynaud's disease (see pg 321), Scleroderma (see pg 323) Buerger's disease (see pgs 290, 293) embolism.

Physical agents: pressure, radiation, trauma, electric burns.

ISCHAEMIC ULCER

Carry out examination of an ulcer (pg 274).

'There is a small, painful ulcer over heel of the left foot[132]. It is punched out in appearance, with steep edges and a pale, bloodless/sloughy infected base. The underlying tendon/joint/bone can/cannot be seen in the base. The leg itself is pale and cool with absent foot pulses and no obvious signs of venous disease. This is an ischaemic ulcer. I would like to formally examine the leg for ischaemia[133] and neuropathy[134].'

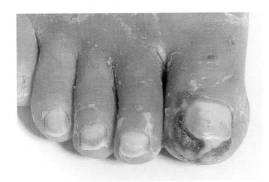

Ulceration between the toes in an ischaemic foot

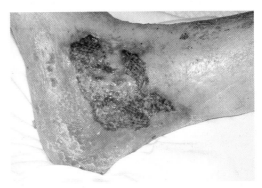

Ischaemic ulceration of the heel

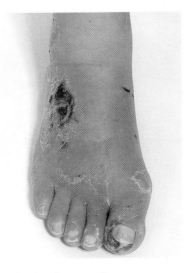

Multiple ulcers and wet gangrene on a critically ischaemic left leg

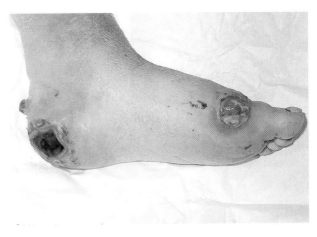

Ischaemic foot with patches of ulceration on typical pressure areas: heel and head of first metatarsal

Diabetic Leg

Top Five Case: diabetic legs or feet were seen by more than one in six of the candidates surveyed. Accounted for over 7% of the cases in this bay.

Features of diabetes in the leg and elsewhere

[135] <u>Neuropathic ulcers</u>: or signs of trauma secondary to insensate foot (e.g. may stand on a tack and not notice it for days).

<u>Charcot's joint</u>: painless disorganised joint due to decreased sensation (see pg 229).

<u>Loss of foot arches</u>: due to peripheral neuropathy.

<u>Shiny hairless leg</u>: is said to be typical but is non-specific.

<u>Amputated toes</u>: small vessel disease often leads to loss of digits either by surgery or autoamputation of a gangrenous digit.

<u>Necrobiosis lipoidica diabeticorum</u>: erythematous plaques over shins with a waxy appearance and brown pigmentation. Can scar, become scaly or ulcerate.

<u>Infections</u>: such as paronychia due to poor circulation and being immunocompromised.

<u>Xanthomata</u>: grey-yellow plaques of lipid in the skin often in the skin of the eyelid.

<u>Acanthosis nigricans</u>: brown pigmentation of the skin, typically in skin folds such as the axilla.

<u>Granuloma annulare</u>: groups of flesh coloured papules on extensor surfaces of hands and fingers.

Note that ABPIs may appear to be greater than one in the presence of ischaemia if the large arteries of the legs are so calcified that inflation of the cuff fails to compress them. This is typical in diabetic large vessel arteriopathy, so diabetic patients often have misleadingly high ABPIs even if they have significant ischaemia. (See footnotes on pg 268).

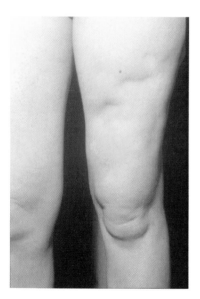

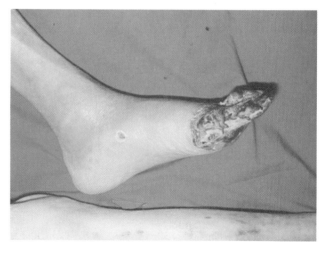

Demarcated gangrenous great toe in a diabetic

Lipoatrophy in a diabetic

DIABETIC LEG

Carry out examination of an ischaemic/diabetic leg (see pg 266).

'There is, in this patient, evidence of previous digital amputation of the right great toe. The sole of the left foot has a painless neuropathic ulcer (see pg 298) and there is a Charcot's joint (see pg 229) at the left ankle. There is loss of the foot arches, lipoatrophy and necrobiosis lipoidica diabeticorum (see opposite). There is loss of sensation in a stocking distribution bilaterally. The femoral and popliteal pulses are present bilaterally, as are the foot pulses on the left and the ankle-brachial pressure index is more than one[135], but the feet are cold, ulcerated and discoloured with poor capillary refill. This patient is diabetic with significant neuropathy and small vessel arteriopathy of both legs.'

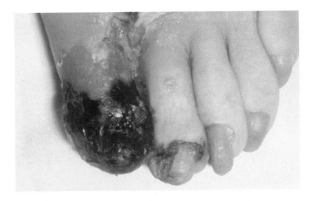

Wet gangrene in the toe of a diabetic

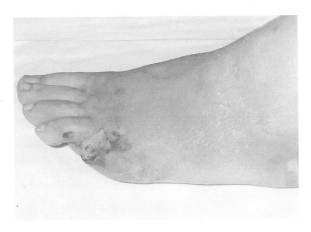

Autoamputation of a digit in the foot of a diabetic

NEUROPATHIC ULCER

Carry out examination of an ulcer (see pg 274).

'This is a small, painless ulcer on the sole of the foot (of a diabetic?). The ulcer is deep, with punched out edges and pink granulation tissue in the base. The surrounding skin is insensate and has good capillary refill[136]. There are good foot pulses and no evidence of venous insufficiency. This is a neuropathic ulcer. I would like to ask if the patient is diabetic and carry out a neurological examination of the lower limb.'

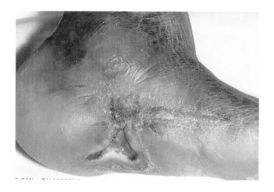

Neuropathic ulcer in a diabetic foot

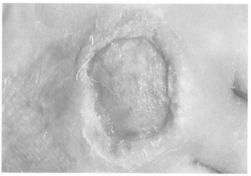

Punched out neuropathic ulcer on sole of foot

Neuropathic ulcer

[136] It is common to have dual pathology, for example in diabetics with neuropathy where coexisting peripheral vascular disease produces a mixed ulcer which delays healing. This may occur even in the presence of good foot pulses, as small vessel disease is more common in diabetics. Checking the capillary refill around the ulcer gives a good indication of whether there is a reasonable blood supply, but beware infected ulcers when superficial cellulitis may mask underlying ischaemia.

Causes of neuropathic ulcer:

Peripheral neuropathy: Diabetes mellitus, nerve injury, leprosy.

Spinal cord lesions: Spina bifida, tabes dorsalis, syringomyelia.

AMPUTEE[137]

'There is (in this male, middle-aged smoker) a left below knee amputation. It appears to have been performed by a Burgess-Romano trans-tibial technique with a long posterior flap. It is well shaped, an appropriate length and well healed. There is/is no evidence of previous vascular surgery on that leg[138]. The opposite leg shows evidence of peripheral vascular disease (see examination, pg 266).'

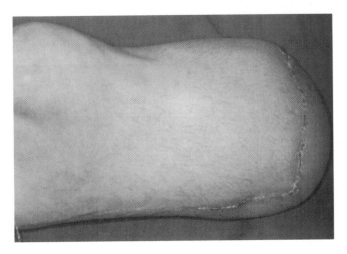

Below knee (trans-tibial) amputation

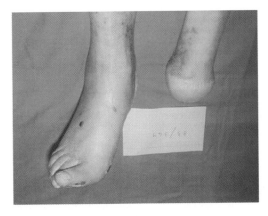
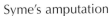

Syme's amputation

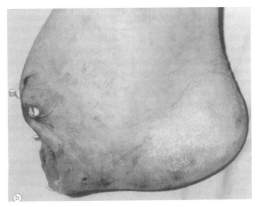

Chopart's amputation

---

[138] Look for scars in the groin and medial thigh and knee.

Amputee

Very common case: seen by over 1 in 10 of the candidates surveyed.

[137] **Amputations**

Commonest cause in developed countries:	end stage peripheral vascular disease; diabetes
Commonest cause in developing countries:	trauma; infection

Pre-operative care

Counselling.

Optimise nutrition, hydration and cardiac and respiratory status.

DVT prophylaxis.

Be sure vascular salvage bypass is inappropriate.

Selection of amputation levels

Should not rely solely on clinical assessment.

Digital or part foot amputations only suitable for those with small vessel disease and no large vessel compromise (e.g. some diabetics, vasculitides) or in those undergoing revascularisation procedures (bypass or angioplasty).

Transtibial (below knee amputation – BKA) should always be attempted if feasible.

Usually feasible if thigh systolic pressure is >70 mmHg or if angiography show good inflow to the profunda artery.

Transfemoral (above knee amputations – AKA) cannot always be avoided but have many disadvantages.

Types of amputation

Digital

Ray (includes most of metatarsal bone).

Part foot transmetatarsal (e.g. in revascularised limb or selected diabetics).

Lisfranc's (midfoot amputation – rare in vascular disease).

Chopart's (leaves behind calcaneous and talus – rarely used).

Syme's (distal 1cm of tibia and fibula excised and heel flap sutured under to form stump. Useful in trauma especially of young patients, but limited use in peripheral vascular disease).

Below knee Gold standard for end stage peripheral vascular disease (see below).

Above knee Most common for end stage peripheral vascular disease (see below).

Advantages of BKA

Maximises chances of patient mobility

Preserves limb length

Reduced energy and oxygen requirements compared with AKA

Much higher chance of rehabilitation than AKA

Much less likely to be wheelchair bound than AKA

Live longer and have better quality of life than AKA

Principles involved in performing a BKA

10 cm distal to tibial tuberosity is ideal transection level.

Burgess-Romano technique involves long posterior flap (see fig on opposite pg).

Fascia overlying soleus and gastrocnemius must be preserved with posterior skin flap, muscles may be excised.

Posterior tibial nerve should be pulled down then excised to allow it to retract.

Fibula must be divided proximal to tibia.

Tibial transection should be bevelled and filed to leave no sharp points.

Deep fascia of posterior flap is sutured to deep fascia or periosteum anteriorly.

Principles involved in performing an AKA
Performed too often in this country for peripheral vascular disease.
Use anterior-posterior flaps as shown below.
Keep stump as long as possible without compromising healing.
Transect nerves 5cm proximal to bone transection level.
Ideally residual adductor muscles should be fixed to the lateral femur to prevent it lying abducted.
Quadriceps should be fixed to the posterior femur to cover stump and prevent it lying flexed.
These last two are rarely done, usually because the AKA is often left to junior team members.
Postoperative management
Pain control (spinal, epidural PCA, epidural catheter placed alongside sciatic nerve intraoperatively).
Wound care (antibiotics, reduce oedema, avoid trauma e.g. plaster of paris dressing).
Nutrition.
Treatment of concurrent medical illness (e.g. diabetes, cardiac disease).
Management of contralateral limb (may also have vascular disease).
Early mobilisation and fitting of prosthesis.
Attention to psychological problems.

Long-term prognosis
Limited life expectancy (far less 5 yr survival rate than Dukes B colon cancer patients).
50% develop critical ischaemia in other leg.
Many continue to smoke and so are at risk of cancer, respiratory and cardiovascular disease.
Diabetes, cardiac and cerebrovascular disease increase morbidity and mortality.

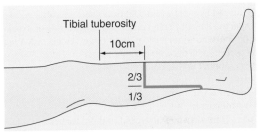

Skin incisions for transtibial amputation

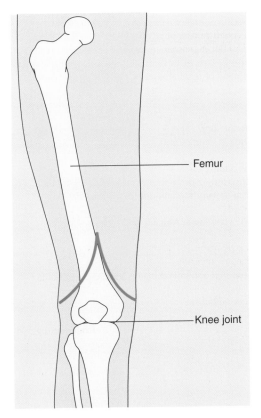

Skin incisions for transfemoral amputation

Abdominal Aortic Aneurysm

Top Five Case: aneurysms (including femoral and popliteal) were seen by over a quarter of the candidates surveyed. Accounted for 12% of cases in this bay.

[139] **Abdominal aortic aneurysm (AAA)**

Definition: Localised region of abnormal dilatation of the abdominal aorta defined as >3 cm diameter or at least 50% greater than the normal artery above it.

Epidemiology: Rupture is the 13th leading cause of death in the USA. Incidence increases with age. More common in men, smokers, hypertensives and Caucasians.

Complications

Aneurysmal rupture:

The major complication of AAA. Thrombosis and embolisation are rare in comparison. Caused by increasing wall tension and decreasing wall thickness as the aneurysm enlarges in line with La Place's law:

Wall stress = blood pressure × radius/wall thickness.

Thrombosis

Usually accompanied by acute bilateral lower limb ischaemia, AAA thrombosis is associated with a poor outcome.

Embolisation

Investigations

Clinical examination is only 50% diagnostic due to obesity, unco-operative patient, lumbar lordosis, adjacent tumour, aortic tortuosity. An aneurysm under 4 cm can rarely be felt except in thin individuals.

Plain X-ray: in < 50% of patients calcium in the aneurysm wall allow visualisation on plain abdominal (preferably lateral) X-ray.

Ultrasonography: good for initial diagnosis and screening, relationship with renal arteries but not good for imaging suprarenal aorta, iliacs, retroperitoneal leak, obese patients.

CT: useful in cases where USS is limited (see above), to plan elective surgery and in stable patients with suspected leak but time consuming, high doses of irradiation, contrast material given.

MRI: More accurate evaluation of other vessels, MRA very useful but expensive, not widely available and can't be used in patients with pacemakers.

Angiography: only used in selected cases such as where assessment of renal arteries or iliac artery disease is needed.

Cause of AAA:

Atherosclerosis.

Ehlers-Danlos syndrome types I and IV (abnormal collagen production).

Marfan syndrome (Autosomal dominant condition often affecting the aortic root).

Tuberous sclerosis (rare autosomal dominant syndrome).

Takayasu's disease (inflammatory aortitis of children and young adults).

Syphilitic aneurysm (thoracic aortic endarteritis obliterans of the vaso vasorum in untreated tertiary syphilis).

Mycotic aneurysm (due to bacterial infection commonly in drug users or the immunocompromised).

Polyarteritis nodosa (a vasculitis affecting the vasa vasorum).

Intima-media mucoid degenerative aneurysms (in middle-aged hypertensive Africans and Indians – aetiology unknown).

Symptoms

75% asymptomatic.

Leaking aneurysms present with the characteristic triad of diffuse mid-abdominal pain, shock and a pulsatile abdominal mass.

Other presentations include back pain, flank pain, thrombosis or embolism.

Continues pg 304

ABDOMINAL AORTIC ANEURYSM[139]

Carry out examination of abdominal aortic aneurysm (pg 272).

'There is an expansile abdominal mass consistent with an abdominal aortic aneurysm of about 5 cm in diameter apparently extending from below the renal arteries to just above the bifurcation. It is non-tender and the patient is cardiovascularly stable.'

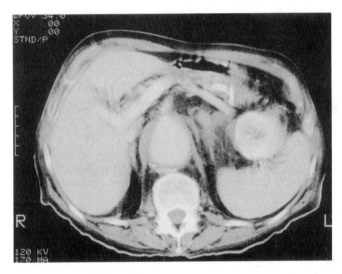

CT showing abdominal aortic aneurysm

Abdominal Aortic Aneurysm

Indications for surgery

It is important to operate on an aneurysm before it ruptures. Elective AAA repair caries a mortality of 3.5–5%, whereas for the small proportion of patients with ruptured AAA who live long enough to make it to surgery, the mortality is 30–80%. The most important predictive factor of aneurysm rupture is size.

In aneurysms >6 cm 3 year survival is <50% if untreated, so these clearly need replacement if possible. Small aneurysms (less than 4 cm) tend not to rupture and enlarge very slowly, so these clearly are best left alone. Controversy surrounds intermediate sized aneurysms (4–6 cm). The rate of rupture of aneurysms 4–6 cm is 6% per year over 3 years. The UK small aneurysm trial confirms a low rate of rupture of aortic aneurysms less than 5.5 cm in diameter. The risk of surgery varies also depending on the age and fitness of the patient. Many surgeons would agree that, where the risk of surgery is less than 5% mortality, elective repair should be considered for patients with aneurysms over 5.5 cm. Smaller aneurysms should be scanned regularly.

Surgery of AAA

The transperitoneal endoaneurysmorrhaphy is the most common, where a synthetic graft is sewn into the opened aneurysm sac via an abdominal incision. Variations of this include a retroperitoneal approach (used for inflammatory aneurysms, battle-scarred abdomens, horseshoe kidney or suprarenal aneurysm), exclusion bypass technique and endoluminal stenting (for infrarenal aneurysms).

Complications of surgery

Intra-operative

Bleeding (especially with ruptured aneurysms).

Limb ischaemia due to a large dislodged embolus needing embolectomy, or microemboli causing 'trash foot', or thrombosis secondary to prolonged clamping.

Early post-operative

Cardiac: over 50% of postoperative deaths including MI, arrhythmias, CCF.

Pulmonary: including atelectasis, pneumonia.

Renal failure: especially in those with pre-existing renal impairment or perioperative hypotension.

Gastrointestinal: infarction of the GI tract is surprisingly rare considering how often the inferior mesenteric artery is sacrificed. Acute gastritis is common.

Cerebrovascular: Stroke can be avoided by preoperative carotid endarterectomy in patients at risk.

Late post-operative

Graft infection (1%) may occur years after the surgery and is increased in the presence of malnutrition, immunosuppression, chronic disease, skin infections, groin incisions, ischaemic feet.

Aortoenteric fistulas are rare but catastrophic. Enclosing the graft in the old aneurysm sac reduces this risk.

Anastomotic aneurysms most commonly occur in aortic bi-femoral grafts.

Lymph leaks can cause seromas.

Sexual dysfunction is a result of damage to the autonomic plexus.

Recurrence of aneurysm proximal to the graft occurs in 3–8% of patients.

Graft thrombosis: rates are 3% at 10 years.

SUBCLAVIAN STEAL SYNDROME[140]

Carry out examination of ischaemic upper limb (pg 269).

'This patient describes claudication symptoms and dizziness on exercising the right arm. There are decreased pulses in the right arm and the blood pressure is reduced compared with the left. There is a supraclavicular bruit. The diagnosis is subclavian steal syndrome.'

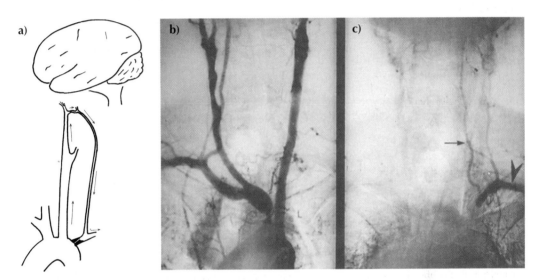

a) Diagramatic representation of flow b) arteriogram showing no flow up the right vertebral or subclavian arteries c) later film shows retrograde flow down the vertebral artery (arrow), filling the subclavian artery (arrowhead)

---

[140] **Pathogenesis of the subclavian steal syndrome:**
Atherosclerosis rarely causes upper limb ischaemia because of good collaterals and the decreased frequency of atheroma in these vessels. When it does, it is usually subclavian artery stenosis. If the occlusion is in the proximal part of the subclavian artery, patients may experience vertebrobasilar symptoms when they exercise the affected limb. This is because the vertebral artery on the side of the stenosis acts as a collateral – blood flow actually reverses – 'stealing' blood from the circle of Willis and cerebral vessels.

Causes of subclavian obstruction:
Atherosclerosis, arteritis, embolism, thoracic outlet syndrome (see pg 319).

Diagnosis: arteriography

Treatment: Reconstruction of subclavian artery by:
    subclavian bypass
    carotid-to-subclavian bypass
    subclavian to carotid anastomosis

If axillary or brachial artery is occluded, a long vein bypass must be taken from a healthy artery above the occlusion to an unaffected segment beyond, tunnelling the bypass through the thoracic outlet. These bypasses are often difficult to perform and tend to occlude early.

Femoral Artery Aneurysm

[141] Aetiology:

True femoral artery aneurysms (rare).

Atherosclerosis: commonest cause of true femoral artery aneurysm. A third are asymptomatic. Risk of rupture is low (5–15%) due to the muscular fascial surrounding compartment but pressure of expansion can cause occlusion or acute thrombosis resulting in an acutely ischaemic limb.

Infection: used to be a common cause of true femoral artery aneurysms due to septic emboli from endocarditis, but now that antibiotics are in use they are much less common.

False femoral artery aneurysms (common)

Puncture aneurysms following cannulation of or aspiration from the femoral artery.

Para-anastomotic false aneurysm should raise the suspicion of an infected graft. Other predisposing factors include synthetic graft, silk sutures, small arterial wall tissue bites, haematoma.

Mycotic false aneurysms: common in intravenous drug addicts.

Symptoms: 29% asymptomatic, 30% local symptoms (groin swelling, hyperaesthesia, local pain). Other presentations include: peripheral ischaemia from aneurysm thrombosis or emboli, groin pain radiating into leg, distal neuropathy, or, in mycotic false aneurysms, red hot tender swelling +/- necrosis of overlying skin.

Investigations:

Angiography or MRA visualises the aorta and iliacs as well as the distal circulation to identify other aneurysms in true aneurysms, and the run off and other anastomotic sites in para-anastomotic aneurysms.

Colour flow duplex scanning: used to identify iatrogenic puncture aneurysms and show effectiveness of direct pressure on stopping the leak. Quick and effective way of confirming mycotic aneurysm which may need immediate surgery.

Management:

True atherosclerotic femoral artery aneurysms over 3 cm: elective interposition graft with Dacron or PTFE (veins are too small).

Infected false aneurysms: ligation of healthy arteries proximal and distal, wide débridement of infected tissues, and bypass, (maybe extra anatomic). Alternatively, arterial ligation may be possible without reconstruction if there is good collateral circulation.

Iatrogenic false aneurysm following percutaneous catheterisation: ultrasound guided compression treatment (10 minute sessions) or surgery if symptomatic, rupturing or thrombosed.

[142] Such as dusky toes or purpuric skin lesions.

[143] 85% of patients with true atherosclerotic femoral artery aneurysms have an aortic, iliac or popliteal aneurysm, and 70% are bilateral. Aortic and iliac aneurysms take precedence over femoral aneurysms as far as treatment goes, as they cause more complications.

FEMORAL ARTERY ANEURYSM[141]

'There is (in this middle-aged smoker) a 4 cm pulsatile swelling in the right groin midway between the pubic tubercle and the anterior superior iliac spine. The mass is expansile, and there is an audible bruit. There are no overlying scars or bruises indicating previous surgery or intervention, and the swelling is not red, hot or tender which would indicate infection. The distal circulation, sensation and power of the limb are normal, and there is no evidence of embolic disease[142]. This is a femoral artery aneurysm, and the presence of nicotine stained fingers and absence of evidence of iatrogenic injury or infection point to a true atherosclerotic aneurysm. I would like to examine the other groin and the abdomen and popliteal fossae[143].'

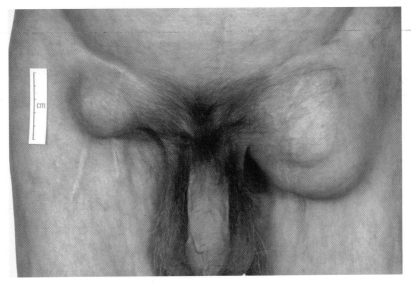

Bilateral femoral artery aneurysms

Popliteal Artery Aneurysm
Common case: seen by more than 1 in 20 of candidates surveyed.
[144] Popliteal artery aneurysm.
Definition: External diameter >2 cm or >one and a half times the normal proximal popliteal artery diameter.
Epidemiology: Commonest over the age of 50. More common in men than women.
Aetiology: Atherosclerosis is by far the most common. Also popliteal entrapment syndrome, collagen disorders (such as Behçet's disease), fibromuscular dysplasia, infection and blunt or penetrating trauma.
Symptoms: One third asymptomatic. Distal embolisation may cause claudication, rest pain, gangrene or acute ischaemic event. Acute occlusion of the aneurysm causes acute lower limb ischaemia. Tibial nerve compression results in pain in the distribution of that nerve. Popliteal vein occlusion or thrombosis may occur resulting in deep vein thrombosis. Acute ischaemic emergencies (due to aneurysmal thrombosis or embolisation) are the presenting complaint in 52–77% of cases resulting in amputation of 16–20% of patients.
Investigations: Aim to determine extent and shape of aneurysm, presence of intraluminal thrombus and the condition of inflow and outflow vessels. Methods include duplex scanning, angiography or MRA, CT or MRI. Colour flow duplex examination is best for monitoring aneurysms which are not operated on.
Management: Acute ischaemia with sensory and motor impairment: urgent bypass surgery +/- distal vessel thrombectomy or intra-arterial injection of thrombolytic agent.
Occluded aneurysm without critical ischaemia: thrombolysis retains more of the limb run-off vessels.
Asymptomatic: elective surgery – conservative management is associated with poor outcome.
Surgery: Interposition saphenous vein bypass graft with aneurysm exclusion usually by medial approach (although posterior or supragenicular approaches can also be used). Vein grafts in patients with good run-off perform better than synthetic grafts and results are good with 75–100% 5 year patency.
[145] The tibial nerve supplies sensation to the sole of the foot and power to the great toe flexors. The peroneal nerve supplies sensation to the anterior and lateral surface of the lower leg and foot, and power to the ankle and foot extensors. Both may be compressed by a large popliteal aneurysm.
[146] 38–58% bilateral. 32% associated with more proximal aneurysms.

POPLITEAL ARTERY ANEURYSM[144]

Spot diagnosis or examination of a lump (pg 29).

'There is (in this middle-aged to elderly man) a 3 cm pulsatile swelling in the popliteal fossa. The mass is expansile and has an audible bruit on auscultation. The distal limb shows no sign of ischaemia or embolic disease (see examination of ischaemic limb, pg 266), and sensation and power are intact[145]. This is a popliteal artery aneurysm. I would like to examine the opposite popliteal fossa, the groins and the abdominal aorta[146].'

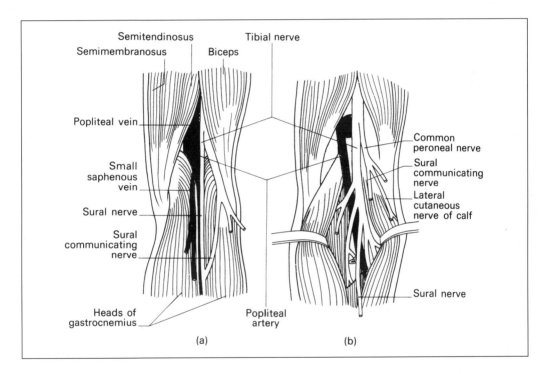

Popliteal fossa anatomy

Surgical Arteriovenous Fistulae

Top Five Case: surgical or congenital a-v fistulae were seen by over one in five of the candidates surveyed. Accounted for nearly 10% of the cases in this bay.

[147] **Surgical arteriovenous fistulas**

These cause grossly dilated veins and are created primarily for ease of vascular access in patients with renal failure who need regular haemodialysis. It avoids the need for long-term percutaneous central venous catheter which carries risks of infection, venous stenosis and thrombosis.

Types of arteriovenous fistulae

<u>Autogenous</u>: direct joining of a vein with a neighbouring artery usually end vein to side artery using the Brescia-Cimino technique.

<u>Autogenous bridge</u>: a vein and artery are joined using a separate vein graft (e.g. saphenous vein).

<u>Synthetic straight bridge grafts</u>: PTFE or other synthetic graft material is used to bridge between an artery and a vein. Other graft materials include bovine carotid arteries, human umbilical vein or cryopreserved cadaveric vein grafts.

<u>Loop grafts</u>: usually synthetic. An artery and vein are joined by a loop of graft tunnelled subcutaneously.

Sites of arteriovenous fistulae

In order of preference: radiocephalic, brachiocephalic, forearm loop, upper arm straight. The non-dominant hand and more distal sites are usually considered first.

Pre-operative questions you should know to ask

Dominant hand.

Previous attempts at access and reasons for failure.

Examine forearm veins, if necessary using a proximal tourniquet (40 mmHg).

Aim for autogenous but warn of risks of synthetic bridges in case veins aren't good enough.

Perform Allen's test (see pg 270) to evaluate potential arterial inflow sites. Non-palpable pulses should not be used.

Exclude local or systemic infection.

Post-operative complications

<u>Nerve injury</u>: especially radial and median.

<u>Thrombosis</u>: usually due to poor flow, kinking or compression by haematoma.

<u>Steal phenomenon</u>: claudication symptoms due to inadequate perfusion – treated by ligating artery just distal to graft except in proximal fistulae which require bypass.

<u>Infection</u>: especially in synthetic grafts.

False aneurysm.

[148] Palpate the fistula trying to determine two things:

1. Is there any synthetic material present? This is probably a PTFE bridge graft.

2. Is there a long U-shaped loop of distended vessel? This is probably a loop graft as opposed to a straight bridge graft or a direct Brescia-Cimino end-to-side graft.

SURGICAL ARTERIOVENOUS FISTULAE[147]

Spot diagnosis.

'There is (in this young or middle-aged patient) a grossly dilated pulsatile vessel in the forearm of the non-dominant arm with an overlying scar. There is an audible bruit. The distal limb is well perfused with good pulses and no signs of venous insufficiency. There are/are no signs of previous, more distal surgery or surgery on the opposite arm. There is a scar on the neck compatible with a previous central venous line. The patient is not uraemic and looks well nourished and in good health. This is a surgical arteriovenous fistula[148] created for ease of venous access, probably for haemodialysis in a patient with renal failure.'

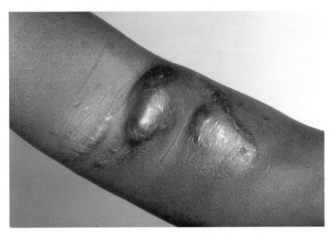

Surgical arteriovenous fistula at the antecubital fossa of a renal dialysis patient

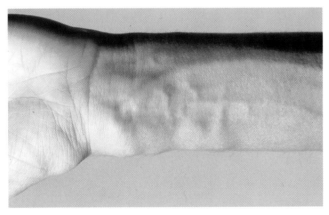

Surgical arteriovenous fistula at the wrist of a renal dialysis patient

311

Congenital Arteriovenous Fistulae

[149] **Definition:** a pathological connection between arteries and veins. May be localised, diffuse, large or small. May form aneurysms. Rare (<1 per million).

Localised fistula (cirsoid aneurysms)

Investigations: selective arteriography and CT scanning.

Differential diagnoses:

Metastatic deposits of a typically vascular tumour such as thyroid carcinoma (important to exclude this).

Traumatic arteriovenous fistulae.

Treatment:

Expectant if asymptomatic or develops during pregnancy.

Therapeutic embolisation using clot, Gelfoam, lead shot, superglue, wire.

Surgical excision. Simple ligation of feeding vessels is ineffective. Sclerosants and laser have been tried.

[150] Common in the head, neck and limbs.

[151] It has been described as looking like a bag of pulsating worms.

[152] **Parkes-Weber syndrome**

Complications:

Lipodermatosclerosis and ulceration as a result of chronic venous insufficiency.

High output cardiac failure and cardiomegaly.

Severe thrombocytopenia.

Differential diagnoses:

Klippel-Trenaunay syndrome (see pg 327).

Lymphoedema (see pg 325).

Diagnosis:

Venography, arteriography, thermography.

Treatment:

Expectant, embolisation, excision, microsphere injection, surgical 'skeletalisation' under tourniquet control.

Complications of treatment:

Embolisation, infarction, recurrence. May need amputation.

Branham's bradycardic response: Occluding the circulation of the enlarged limb with a sphygmomanometer cuff causes a bradycardia because it increases the peripheral resistance.

CONGENITAL ARTERIOVENOUS FISTULAE[149]

Case 1 Cirsoid aneurysm

Carry out examination of a lump (see pg 29).

'There is a soft, warm, pulsatile swelling on the left arm[150] covered by dilated cutaneous channels in the overlying skin[151]. It is hemispherical, about 4 cm in diameter with a smooth edge. It is fluctuant, compressible and has a palpable thrill and audible bruit. This is a localised arteriovenous fistula, or cirsoid aneurysm.'

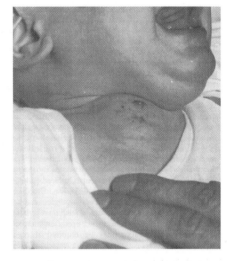

Cirsoid aneurysm

Case 2 Parkes-Weber syndrome[152]

Spot diagnosis or carry out examination of varicose veins (see pg 261).

'This patient has an enlarged left leg, which is covered in dilated veins and shows features of lipodermatosclerosis and ulceration. The leg is warm and pink and increased in both length and width. There is bony as well as soft tissue enlargement. The dilated veins are pulsatile with palpable thrills and audible bruits on auscultation. The veins do not collapse on elevation. These are multiple arteriovenous fistulae. The condition is called Parkes-Weber syndrome, also known as Robertson's giant limb.'

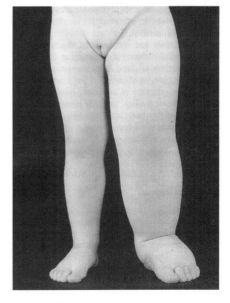

Parkes-Weber syndrome

313

Carotid Artery Disease

Common case: seen by over 1 in 20 of candidates surveyed.

[153] **Definitions:**

Transient ischaemic attack (TIA) is a focal neurologic deficit completely resolving within 24 hours.

Amaurosis fugax or transient monocular blindness (TMB) is a monocular visual disturbance or loss, commonly described as a descending curtain or mist completely resolving within 24 hours.

Reversible ischaemic neurological deficit (RIND) lasts longer than 24 hours but resolves completely within 30 days. Despite this recovery, CT scans may show residual lesions in up to 30% of TIAs and up to 60% of RINDs.

Stroke leaves a permanent neurologic deficit ranging from a mild weakness to a coma with permanent paralysis.

Epidemiology:

One-third of ischaemic strokes originate from atherosclerosis of the great vessels supplying the brain, one-third from the heart and one quarter from small vessel occlusions (lacunar strokes) now also known to be due to great vessel atherosclerosis.

Risk factors for atherosclerosis of the carotid artery

Smoking, obesity, family history, male, hypertension, diabetes, hypercholesterolaemia, hyperlipidaemia.

Investigations:

Carotid artery duplex scan determines vessel diameters and flow velocities with accuracy in good hands of up to 95%.

Carotid angiograms are used where duplex accuracy is uncertain, or if disease is suspected outside the cervical region. Aortic arch injections allow visualisation of the aortic arch branches and the vertebral arteries, but overlapping vessels and insensitivity for ulcerated carotid lesions are drawbacks. Selective carotid artery catheterisation shows the carotid bifurcation and intracranial vessels more clearly and identifies areas of irregularity or ulceration. Complications of angiography include haematoma, pseudoaneurysm, adverse dye reactions and neurological events caused by emboli, hypotension or vascular spasm. TIAs occur in 0.8–4% and permanent deficits in 0.1–1.3% of carotid angiograms.

MRA (Magnetic Resonance Angiography) is replacing invasive angiography.

Medical management of carotid artery disease

Control of hypertension, cholesterol, lipids and diabetes.

Stop smoking.

Aspirin (dose controversial).

Antiplatelet drugs such as Ticlopidine.

Warfarin is used to prevent stroke from cardiac or hypercoagulable cause, but not for carotid atherosclerosis.

Indications for carotid endarterectomy

Symptomatic stenoses >70%.

Some asymptomatic stenoses (see pg 316).

Crescendo TIAs with severe stenosis.

Fluctuating neurological defect post CVA with severe stenosis.

Acute stroke with severe stenosis (after patient is neurologically stable).

Continues on pg 316

CAROTID ARTERY DISEASE[153]

'There is, in this patient with a history of a TIA affecting his right side, a bruit over the left carotid artery. The patient denies previous strokes or TIAs and has never had amaurosis fugax of the left eye. He has no residual neurology. The diagnosis is symptomatic left carotid artery disease[154], and evaluation of the extent of his carotid artery stenosis would be needed before offering him a carotid endarterectomy[155].'

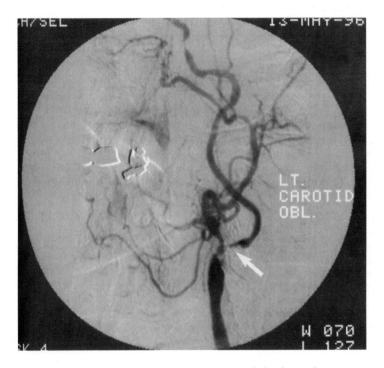

Digital subtraction carotid arteriogram with high grade internal carotid stenosis and ulceration. Arrow shows stenosis at the origin of the internal carotid artery.

Carotid Artery Disease continued
How important trials have determined treatment regimes
Patients with neurologic symptoms in the previous four months in the territory of a carotid artery with 70–99% stenosis (European Carotid Surgery Trial 1998 and North American Symptomatic Carotid Endarterectomy Trial (NASCENT) 1991 showed benefit in these patients when compared with optimal medical treatment alone).
Management of asymptomatic patients is more controversial. Asymptomatic patients with a carotid artery stenosis of more than 60% were shown to benefit from carotid endarterectomy in the Asymptomatic Carotid Atherosclerosis Study (ACAS) in 1987, so much so that the trial was stopped by the National Institute of Health in 1994. However, statistically significant differences were not seen for three years, so general surgery in asymptomatic patients tends to be reserved for
> Patients with low operative risk and good life expectancy
> High grade stenosis (e.g. over 80%)
> Progressive or ulcerated lesions

Carotid artery surgery
Internal carotid endarterectomy involves removing the plaque of atheroma and the media leaving the adventitia of the artery. It can be done under general or regional block anaesthetic. Incision along anterior border of sternocleidomastoid. Some surgeons routinely use a shunt, some do so selectively. Some use intra-operative transcranial Doppler to monitor the flow, some do not. Some surgeons routinely use a vein or prosthetic patch to enlarge the diameter, some do so selectively.

Complications of carotid endarterectomy
Perioperative stroke due to
cerebral ischaemia during clamping
embolisation of debris during or after the operation
thrombosis at the endarterectomy site
Cervical haematoma
Cranial nerve neuropraxia especially
recurrent laryngeal
hypoglossal
marginal mandibular
glossopharyngeal
superior laryngeal
Recurrent stenosis (5–15% of patients) due to hyperplasia or recurrent atherosclerosis. If symptomatic, reoperation is indicated.

Carotid artery angioplasty and stenting
New treatment modality which may become more popular.

[154] Although neck bruits are neither sensitive nor specific for carotid bifurcation stenosis, their presence in association with neurologic symptoms is an important clinical finding.

[155] He will be eligible only if he has >70% stenosis in the artery supplying the affected area.

OSLER-WEBER-RENDU SYNDROME[156]

Spot diagnosis.

'This patient has multiple telangiectasia[157] on the face and on the mucosa of the mouth[158] and nose. She has pale sclera and looks anaemic. There are also telangiectasia on the hands. The skin is not tight, shiny and smooth as in patients with scleroderma, and although there are telangiectasia on the hands there are none of the features of scleroderma (see pg 323). This patient has Osler-Weber-Rendu syndrome. I would like to ask the patient if she has ever had problems with nose bleeds, rectal bleeding, melaena, haemoptysis or chronic anaemia needing iron treatment.'

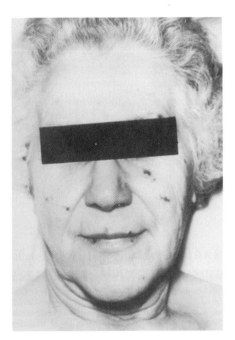 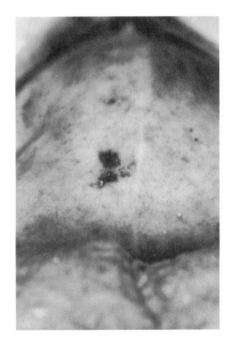

Osler-Weber-Rendu syndrome

Osler-Weber-Rendu syndrome (see also pgs 66, 67)

[156] Also known as **Hereditary Haemorrhagic Telangiectasia**, this is a rare autosomal dominant genetic condition. The telangiectasia are found throughout the gastrointestinal and genitourinary systems. The main clinical implications are repeated bleeding from these sites which increase in frequency with age and can result in anaemia. Coagulation screening tests are normal.

Treatment:
Cautery of bleeding points (e.g. endoscopically).
Oral oestrogen: converts columnar to stratified squamous epithelium and may reduce bleeding.
Long term iron therapy if necessary.
[157] Small groups of dilated venules that blanch on pressure and bleed easily after minor trauma.
[158] Look in mouth and under tongue

Cervical Rib/Thoracic Outlet Syndrome

[159] **Cervical rib** occurs in 0.4% of the population, usually C7. 60% are symptomatic.

Clinical signs as outlined opposite are almost always unilateral, can progress to areas of necrosis or patchy gangrene. Acute thrombosis may cause massive ischaemia of the upper limb but this is unusual due to a good collateral circulation.

Mechanism: The rib can compress the artery against any of the following:

Scalenus anterior

2 heads of scalenus medius

Heads of the median nerve

Hypertrophied neck muscles (e.g. in swimmers)

Clavicle (previous fracture increases risk)

Congenital band between rib and clavicle

Transverse processes of cervical vertebrae

Abnormal first rib (eg. fracture, tumour etc)

Differential diagnosis:

Thoracic outlet syndrome is over-diagnosed. You must exclude:

Cervical spondylosis

Spinal cord tumours

Pancoast's tumour

Supraspinatus tendonitis

Buerger's disease

Cervical disc protrusions

Syringomyelia

Osteoarthritis of shoulder

Ulnar neuritis

Carpal tunnel syndrome

Axillary vein thrombosis

Atherosclerosis

Takayasu's disease

Investigations:

X-ray of cervical spine, shoulder and thoracic inlet. Axillary arteriograms with arms in different positions may show thrombosis, kink, emboli of small vessels, aneurysm.

Treatment:

Conservative: posture, physiotherapy.

Surgical decompression: most commonly excision of cervical rib or first rib.

[160] **Thoracic outlet syndrome** is compression, occlusion or damage of the subclavian artery in the neck most often by a cervical rib. It may be associated with signs of compression of the somatic and sympathetic nerves and the main veins draining the upper limb. Compression by other structures at the thoracic inlet has been reported and includes:

a congenital fibrous band where a cervical rib would be found

muscular hypertrophy (e.g. in swimmers of the scalenus muscles)

previous fractures of the first rib or clavicle

tumours or lymphadenopathy in the neck

[161] Cervical rib is rarely visible or palpable unless it is large or the patient is very thin.

[162] 70% of cervical ribs are bilateral but the symptoms are usually unilateral.

[163] Often the only clinical clue to an underlying cervical rib.

[164] Ipsilateral contracted pupil, enophthalamos (eyeball not as protruberant as the other side), slight ptosis (eyelid drooping) due to damage to the sympathetic nervous system, in this case by compression as the nerves run out of the spinal cord at C8/T1/T2 to the sympathetic chain, stellate ganglion and carotid sympathetic plexus.

[165] See axillary vein thrombosis, pg 289.

[166] If axillary vein thrombosis occurs, collateral veins develop on skin over shoulder and scapula.

[167] Like a soldier standing to attention.

[168] This nerve root loops over the cervical rib.

CERVICAL RIB[159]/THORACIC OUTLET SYNDROME[160]

Carry out examination of the ischaemic upper limb (pg 269).

'There is a bony swelling[161] in the left side[162] of the root of the neck. The subclavian artery pulsation is more prominent[163] on this side and has a bruit. There is no sign of Horner's syndrome[164]. There are signs of venous obstruction of the left upper limb[165], including distended arm veins[166] which do not collapse even on elevating the arm, cyanosis of the hand and arm and pitting oedema. There are signs of arterial spasm or ischaemia affecting the fingers and the hands. The radial pulse is decreased on the left on traction of the shoulder, and when the shoulders are braced back[167] and the patient turns his head away. There are also signs of T1 root compression[168] in the wasted small muscles of the hands and loss of sensation on the medial side of the arm. The diagnosis is thoracic outlet syndrome secondary to a cervical rib.'

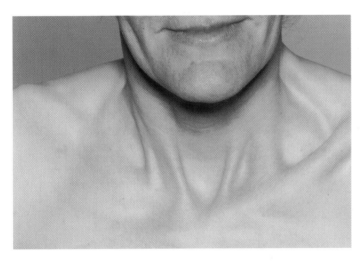

Bilateral cervical ribs, the left more obvious as a swelling above the clavicle

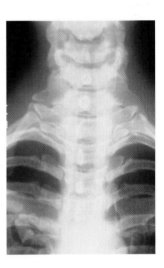

A plain X-ray showing cervical ribs

Raynaud's Disease/Phenomenon
Common case: seen by over 1 in 20 of candidates surveyed.
[169] **Raynaud's phenomenon:** a series of colour changes in the skin of the hands or feet following exposure to the cold in the order 'WBC'(white, blue, crimson).

Raynaud's disease: Primary idiopathic Raynaud's phenomenon which cannot be ascribed to a known cause.

Pathology: <u>White phase</u>: severe arterial spasm.

<u>Blue phase</u>: a very slow trickle of deoxygenated blood through dilated capillaries and venous congestion caused by persistent venous spasm.

<u>Red phase</u>: reactive hyperaemia following relaxation of arteriolar spasm making the skin red, hot and painful.

Causes of Raynaud's phenomenon:

<u>Idiopathic</u>: (primary idiopathic Raynaud's disease). Usually in young girls. May be hereditary.

<u>Irritation of nerves</u>: cervical spondylosis, cervical disc protrusion, cervical rib, thoracic outlet syndrome, spinal cord diseases, old poliomyelitis.

<u>Emboli from</u>: subclavian artery aneurysm, stenotic subclavian artery, damaged subclavian crossing cervical rib.

<u>Scleroderma</u>: as part of the CREST syndrome of Calcinosis, Raynaud's, oEsophageal (American spelling) dysmotility, Sclerodactyly and Telangiectasia (see next case).

<u>Systemic disease</u>: diabetes, hypothyroidism, Systemic Lupus Erythematosus, malnutrition.

<u>Occupational</u>: vibrating tools, refrigeration units, repeated cold water.

<u>Drugs</u>: combined Oral Contraceptive Pill, beta blockers.

<u>Blood abnormalities</u>: cold agglutinins, cryoglobulins.

Investigations:

Aim to exclude the above causes. Full blood count, U&Es, ESR, cryoglobulins, antinuclear factor, thyroid function tests, antithyroid antibodies, antimitochondrial antibodies. If suspicious of CREST syndrome, barium swallow. If suspicious of subclavian artery or large vessel disease, angiography may be indicated.

Treatment:

If Raynaud's phenomenon, treat underlying cause (see above).

For primary Raynaud's disease:

<u>Conservative</u>: reduce exposure to the cold (warm or even heated gloves, avoid cold water), stop smoking.

<u>Medical</u>: nifedipine, prostacyclins, thamoxamine, stanazolol have all been used.

<u>Surgical</u>: cervical sympathectomy (cervical or transaxillary approach, or laparoscopic).

[170] You may be asked (as I was in my MRCS exam) to 'ask a few questions and look at the hands of this girl whose hands are painful in the cold.' It is immediately obvious what the diagnosis is, but what you get marks for are the questions you ask and the way in which you examine what is, essentially a normal upper limb. The scheme on the pg opposite shows how to get maximum mileage out of eliciting important and relevant negative findings.

RAYNAUD'S DISEASE/PHENOMENON[169]

Carry out examination of ischaemic upper limb (see pg 269).

Case 1[170]

'The (young female) patient gives a history of hands which become extremely painful in the cold and show characteristic colour changes of turning white, blue and crimson in turn. She has no family history of this, and has no history of working with vibrating tools, refrigeration units or cold water. She denies diabetes or scleroderma, and is not on the contraceptive pill or beta-blockers. On examination of the upper limb, the hands show no discolouration at present, there are no splinter haemorrhages, wasting of the pulps of the fingers or ulcers. The peripheral pulses and capillary refill are normal, there is no diminution of the radial pulse with traction, and there is no audible subclavian bruit. Palpation of the neck reveals no signs of cervical rib or previous clavicle fractures. There is no obvious focal neurology, although I would like to perform a full neurological examination of the upper limb (see pg 169). My diagnosis is primary idiopathic Raynaud's disease.'

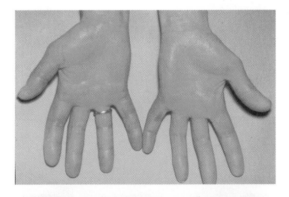

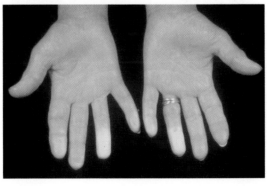

Raynaud's disease

Raynaud's Disease/Phenomenon

[171] Other related disorders (NOT Raynaud's phenomenon).

Acrocyanosis – persistently blue, cold hands and feet. Susceptible to chilblains.

Erythrocyanosis frigida/Bazin's disease

This is a form of cold sensitivity on a part of the leg frequently exposed to the wind, rain and cold. It affects healthy girls aged 15–25 years of stout build with fat, often hairless legs. The lower posterior and medial aspect of the lower leg becomes red-blue and swollen. The swollen area is tender, susceptible to chilblains and superficial ulceration. Often the swelling is more noticeable than the discolouration and can be mistaken for lymphoedema. For those of you old enough to remember the popular 'Viz' magazine, it is highly likely that the blotchy-legged characters in the 'Fat Slags' comic strip suffered from this condition!

[172] The severity of the signs and the calcinosis should alert you to the fact that systemic sclerosis (also known as scleroderma) is the cause of the symptoms rather than Raynaud's disease. This should point you towards looking for the other signs of scleroderma or CREST syndrome (oesophageal involvement, telangiectasia).

[173] The mouth often looks small and pinched.

[174] CREST syndrome – (see pg 320)

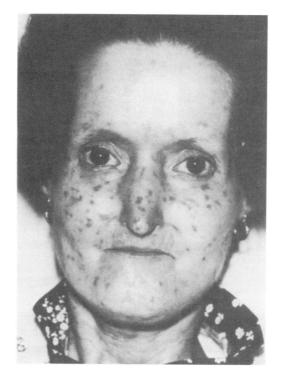

CREST syndrome. Note multiple telangiectasia and small mouth with tight skin due to scleroderma

Case 2[171]

'The (middle-aged female) patient gives a history of hands which become extremely painful in the cold and show characteristic colour changes of turning white, blue and crimson in turn. On examination of the hands, they are reddish-blue in colour with dry, smooth, shiny, tight skin and brittle nails. Several trophic changes can be seen which include vasculitic lesions, tiny scars and ulceration of the fingertips, finger pulp atrophy and paronychia. There are nodules of calcinosis[172] palpable in some of the fingers. The wrist pulses are normal, as are the other pulses in the upper limb. On inspection of the patient's face the skin is smooth, shiny and tight especially around the mouth[173] and there is telangiectasia of the face and pigmentation. The diagnosis is Raynaud's phenomenon secondary to scleroderma/CREST[174] syndrome.'

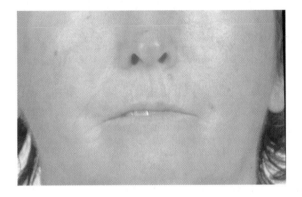

Scleroderma – note the small mouth with smooth shiny tight skin

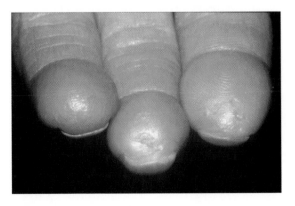

Scleroderma – note fingertip atrophy and ulceration due to vasculitic lesions

Lymphoedema
Common Case: seen by over 1 in 20 of candidates surveyed.
[175] **Definition:**
Lymphoedema is an accumulation of tissue fluid as the result of a fault in the lymphatic system, primarily affecting the legs (80%).
In contrast, oedema is an accumulation of tissue fluid in patients in whom a lymphatic abnormality has not been confirmed.
Classification:
There are three main categories into which the oedematous lower limb can be classified: Oedema which is not real lymphoedema, secondary lymphoedema and primary lymphoedema.
1. Oedema which is not real lymphoedema (i.e. not a result of a fault in the lymphatic system)

Systemic	Venous	Others
Cardiac failure	Post thrombotic syndrome	AV malformations
Renal failure	Iliac venous obstruction	Lipoedema
Hepatic failure	Klippel Trenaunay syndrome	Lipodystrophy
Hypoproteinamia	Extrinsic pressure -tumour	Disuse (e.g. if wheelchair bound)
Allergic disorders	-retroperitoneal	Fat
Hereditary angioedema	fibrosis	Factitious
Idiopathic cyclical oedema	-pregnancy	Gigantism

2. Secondary lymphoedema (i.e. known cause of lymphatic system failure)
Surgical excision: after block dissection. Occurs in <10% of cases. Worse after radiotherapy.
Radiotherapy: Produces block of fibrous tissue which cannot be transgressed by new lymphatic pathway.
Filariasis: infestation by *Wuchereria bancrofti* leading to tropical disease elephantitis. Also TB and other chronic infections.
Silica: this ore in soil can enter the lymphatic system through bare feet and blocks the inguinal nodes.
Cancer: e.g. breast.
3. Primary lymphoedema (lymphatic system failure of unknown cause)
Usually unilateral. Initially pitting then progresses to non-pitting.
Milroy's disease is congenital hereditary primary lymphoedema due to aplasia of lymph trunks. It is rare (accounts for 3% of primary lymphoedema). Most other cases of primary lymphoedema are due to abnormal or occluded vessels. 20% have a family history of swollen legs.
Investigations: Renium and antimony labelled technetium colloid injection. Ilioinguinal colloid uptake of < 0.3% at 30 minutes is diagnostic. Rapid clearance occurs in venous oedema.
Treatment:
Exclude other causes of oedema
Compression stockings
Compression device e.g. Flowtron boots
NOT diuretics
Occasionally debulking surgery or bypass surgery (indicated in <10% of patients)
Methods include enteromesenteric bridge (pelvic plexus joined to iliac nodes to bypass blocked pelvic nodes. Must be done before distal lymphatics obliterate. Poor outcome.
[176] Due to shoes.

LYMPHOEDEMA[175]

Spot diagnosis.

'There is a grossly enlarged left leg with non-pitting swelling extending from the foot to the groin. The skin of the lower leg is thick and pigmented, with warty skin excrescences. The toes are squared off[176]and there is a moist ulcer secreting clear watery fluid. In the groins there are grossly enlarged inguinal lymph nodes but no sign of previous surgery or radiotherapy. This is chronic lymphoedema.'

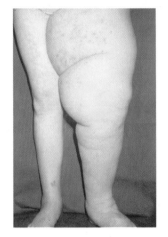

Unilateral secondary
lymphoedema

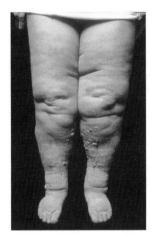

Chronic idiopathic
(primary) lymphoedema

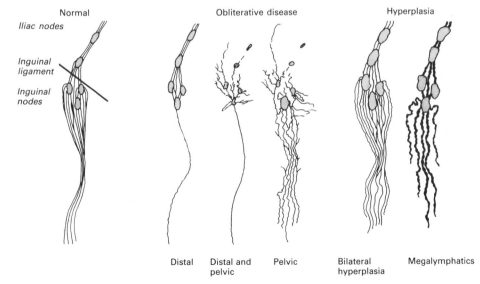

Classification of primary lymphoedema

Klippel-Trenaunay Syndrome

[177] Diffuse mesodermal abnormality associated with lymphatic and other congenital abnormalities. Usually detected soon after birth when the naevus, limb hypertrophy and varicose veins become apparent.

Complications and associations:

Pelvic venous anomalies in 25% which may cause rectal bleeding or haematuria.

Lymphoedema, spina bifida, syndactyly, coxa vara, digital agenesis, atresia of ear canal, clinodactyly, increased incidence of DVT.

Investigations:

Arteriography, bipedal ascending venography (to confirm deep vein function). Exclude Parkes-Weber syndrome where multiple av fistulae results in limb hypertrophy (see pg 313).

Treatment:

Conservative:

Elastic stockings

Camouflage creams

Cover with DVT prophylaxis during surgery.

Surgery:

Only if deep veins are normal, no history of DVT, symptoms not relieved by conservative measures.

Ligation of deep to superficial communication. Varices stripped out or avulsed. Recurrence common.

Limb debulking (result usually unsightly).

Epiphyseal stapling (to arrest growth of bone).

Amputation of giant digit/s.

[178] There may also be bone hypertrophy and limb lengthening leading to abnormal gait, joint problems and lumbar backache.

[179] The aberrant lateral varicose vein connects with persistent primitive lateral limb vein which has failed to regress.

KLIPPEL-TRENAUNAY SYNDROME[177]

Spot diagnosis.

It may be appropriate to carry out examination of varicose veins (see pg 261).

'There is an enlarged left leg with soft tissue hypertrophy[178]. There are extensive varicose veins unusually situated on the lateral side of the limb[179] with none of the normal signs of venous insufficiency. These veins are not pulsatile, and there does not appear to be an arteriovenous shunt. There is an extensive pale purple naevus on the same limb. The combination of a cutaneous naevus, varicose veins bone and soft tissue abnormalities suggest the Klippel-Trenaunay syndrome.'

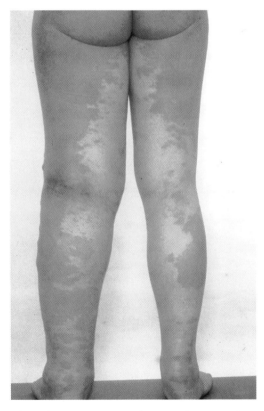 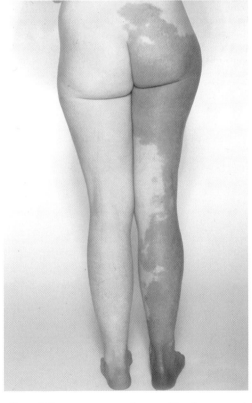

Klippel-Trenaunay syndrome. The extensive pale purple naevus is obvious, as is the soft tissue hypertrophy. The dilated lateral varicose veins are just visible

Klippel-Trenaunay syndrome. The bony and soft tissue overgrowth can be seen by the fact that the affected right leg is longer than the left, causing pelvic tilting when standing

Hyperhidrosis

Common Case: seen by over 1 in 20 of candidates surveyed.

[180] Hyperhidrosis is not an infection (see hidradenitis suppurativa, pg 77) but an increase in sweat production from sweat glands usually of the hands, axilla or feet. The majority are idiopathic, but secondary hyperhidrosis includes:

Hyperhidrosis erythematosus traumatica: a rare occupational form of the condition in which sweating occurs in skin in contact with a vibrating tool.

Syringomyelia can cause facial hyperhydrosis.

Frey's syndrome post parotidectomy (see pg 120) where 'gustatory sweating' is caused by disturbance of sympathetic and parasympathetic nerve fibres.

Treatment of hyperhidrosis:

1. Painting with aluminium hexachloride
2. Excision of hair bearing axillary skin
3. Cervical sympathectomy for palms   )   cervical, transaxillary, laparoscopic
5. Lumbar sympathectomy for feet   )   routes

Avoid total sympathectomy -> postural hypertension

Cervical sympathectomy

This is a misnomer – it is an upper thoracic sympathectomy carried out through a cervical incision. The sympathetic chain is divided below the third thoracic ganglion and the grey and white rami to the second and third ganglia are also cut. In this way the vasoconstrictor pathways to the head and upper limb (from segments T2, 3 and 4) are divided, preserving the stellate ganglion, which are sympathetic connections to the eyelid and pupil.

Transthoracic transpleural sympathectomy

The upper thoracic chain can also be removed via the second intercostal space, the incision being placed on the medial wall of the axilla. The lung is allowed to collapse and the chain identified as it lies on the heads of the upper ribs. Resection of the T2–4 segment results in a warm dry hand.

HYPERHIDROSIS[180]

Spot diagnosis.

'This patient complains of profuse sweating of the hands, axilla and feet. The hands are moist and warm. This patient has hyperhidrosis.'

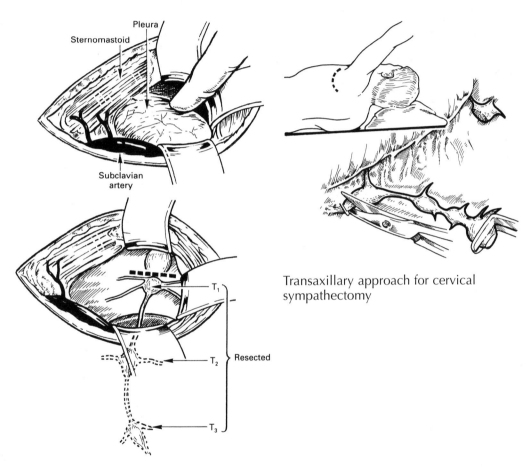

Transaxillary approach for cervical sympathectomy

Cervical approach for cervical sympathectomy

Temporal Arteritis[181]

Also known as giant cell arteritis, this is a vasculitis closely related to polymyalgia rheumatica.

Diagnosis: 2 cm biopsy of superficial temporal artery under local anaesthetic through an incision directly over the vessel (always palpate and mark the course of the vessel before infiltration of the lignocaine and adrenaline). 60% of biopsies show the characteristic histological features:

> florid intimal thickening
> a round cell infiltration through all layers of the arterial wall
> destruction of the internal elastic lamina
> giant cells

Treatment: is high dose systemic steroids, gradually reducing as symptoms abate. Since steroids reduce the incidence of blindness and only 60% of biopsies are diagnostic, treatment should be started on grounds of clinical suspicion only. Some say this negates the need for a biopsy.

[182] Twice as common in women as in men.

[183] Including blurred vision, amaurosis fugax, diplopia, visual hallucinations. Visual loss occurs in between one third and one half of patients and becomes permanent if left untreated. It is caused by ischaemic changes in the ciliary arteries causing optic neuritis or infarction. Initially fundoscopy is normal but ischaemic papillopathy and thrombosis of the central retinal artery may occur. Ophthalmoplegia may also be a feature.

[184] This is variable – pulsation is often still felt.

[185] If you are confident at doing these – if not don't volunteer! You could say 'send them for full visual acuity testing, fundoscopy and visual field mapping' and leave it to the ophthalmologist! Testing visual fields is simple if practised – get the patient to cover one eye with their hand and look straight ahead, preferably at a fixed point. You then steady their forehead with one hand and ask them to tell you when they can see your other hand. With index finger wiggling, bring your hand into the patient's line of vision from behind her head at 2, 4, 7 and 11 o'clock. Repeat on the other side. Visual acuity can be done using a Snellen chart with the patient covering one eye at a time.

TEMPORAL ARTERITIS[181]

Spot diagnosis.

'There is (in this woman[182] over 60) a history of malaise, fever, myalgia, frontoparietal headache and visual disturbance[183]. The left temporal artery is thickened and prominent, tender to touch, with absent pulsation[184] and reddened overlying skin. This patient has temporal arteritis. I would like to examine/arrange for assessment of the visual acuity, visual fields and retina[185].'

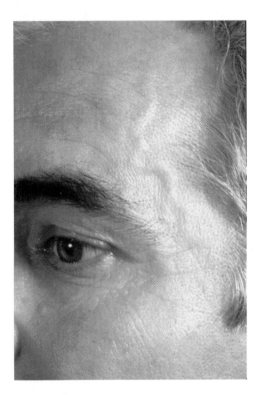

Temporal arteritis

D   Detailed Results of Survey

CIRCULATORY SYSTEM

Total of 122 cases reported in the survey

TOP 5 CASES (accounted for 79.5% of all Circulatory System cases)

Type of case	Number seen in survey	Breakdown and details of cases
Venous disease of legs	32	17 Varicose veins (3 with saphena varix) 9 Chronic venous skin changes (5 lipodermatosclerosis) 6 Venous ulcer Questions included examine, do Trendelenburg's test, use Doppler probe, aetiology, treatment, anatomy.
Ischaemic leg (excluding diabetic leg)	29	13 Examine leg with peripheral vascular disease (PVD) 7 Examine leg post bypass surgery or stenting 3 Look at this angiogram 6 Amputations due to PVD Questions included history, examination, measuring of ankle-brachial pressure indices, anatomy of pulses, treatment of PVD, Beurger's test, sources of emboli, how is angiography performed, complications of amputation.
Aneurysm	15	7 Abdominal aortic 4 Popliteal 1 Femoral 2 False (1 groin post femoral-distal vein graft, 1 radial) 1 Brachial artery post surgical AV fistula formation Questions included risk factors, management, indications for surgery, angiograms, other sites for aneurysms, look at CT scan.
Arteriovenous fistula	12	9 on forearm for renal transplant patients 1 In groin for renal transplant 1 Multiple Cimino fistulae and false aneurysm 1 Congenital AV malformation 1 in Superficial Lesions bay, 2 in Abdomen and Respiratory bay. Questions included indications, complications, what is a Brescia fistula, what is a Cimino fistula.
Diabetic feet	9	3 Ischaemic toe 2 Ulcer 2 Amputation 2 Peripheral vascular disease Questions included examine feet, examine legs, why are the pedal pulses present?

OTHER CASES

Type of case	Number seen in survey	Breakdown and details of cases
Venous disease of upper body	5	2 IVC obstruction 2 Axillary vein thrombosis 1 ?cervical varicose veins (examiners did not know either!) Questions included examine, investigations, management, anticoagulation
Upper limb ischaemia	4	I Subclavian artery thrombosis 1 Axillary artery thrombosis 1 Critical ischaemia 1 Thoracic outlet syndrome Questions included Allen's test.
Carotid disease	3	1 Bruit and history of transient ischaemic attack 1 Carotid artery stenosis – signs not specified 1 Carotid aneurysm (in Superficial Lesions bay)
Lymphoedema	3	Including congenital and gross bilateral lymphoedema
Raynaud's	3	Examine hands and take history
Hyperhidrosis	3	Questions included anatomy of sympathetic chain, typical history
Deep vein thrombosis	3	Questions included history, examination, aetiology, diagnosis, investigations, management, use a Doppler, interpret venogram
Osler-Weber-Rendu syndrome	12	1 in Superficial Lesions bay.
Ankylosing spondylitis	2	Questions included cervical spine examination, hip and knee examination, X-ray features.
Paget's disease	2	Both tibia. Questions included complications and X-ray features.
Gout	1	Tophi on finger, asked differential diagnosis. In Superficial Lesions bay.
Winged scapula	1	In Superficial Lesions bay.
Ankle	1	Arthritis after tibial fracture (with X-ray)
Ingrowing toenail	1	In Superficial Lesions bay
Lower limb neurology	1	
Bone graft	1	
Exostosis	1	
Osteochondrosarcoma of chest wall	1	In Superficial Lesions bay

CHAPTER FIVE

CLINICAL BAY 4
THE TRUNK

CONTENTS

THE TRUNK

A   The Bay

In the MRCS (Eng) examination the Trunk or Abdomen and Respiratory bay incorporates the abdomen, cardiorespiratory system, groins and genitalia. The bay lasts 10 minutes during which time the candidates are expected to see 3–4 patients. This will be extended to 15 minutes after December 2002 (see pg 5 for details of the changes). There are five marks available, three for clinical approach and two for discussion.

The aim of the bay is to determine the candidate's ability to examine the chest or abdomen, describe physical findings and demonstrate a sound knowledge of the process of investigation which is likely to produce a differential diagnosis. Results of relevant investigations may be shown and discussed.

Generally there are two examiners; (a general surgeon examiner will be present) one giving instructions and asking questions and one recording the marks.

EXAMINATION OF THE ABDOMEN

Introduce yourself and get the patient into position[1].
'Hello, I'm Dr Parchment Smith. Would you mind if I examined your tummy? Can you lie flat? Are you comfortable? Do you mind if I talk about you as I go along?'
Stand back, hands behind your back, and look at the patient and their surroundings.
'On initial INSPECTION Mrs. X looks well/ill/thin[2]. She is comfortable/in pain and her colour is good/pale/jaundiced. Around her I can see an intravenous drip/sick bowl.
Mention anything else which is immediately obvious and relevant. Pick up both hands.
'Can I just have a look at your HANDS first? I'm looking at the nails for clubbing[3], leukonychia[4], koilonychia[5]. In the palm I'm looking for Dupuytren's contractures[6], palmar erythema[7], pale palmar creases. On the skin of the hands I'm looking for jaundice, scratch marks[8], purpura[9], tattoos[10].
To the patient:
'Could you hold both arms straight out please? And cock your palms back like this please? I'm looking for a LIVER FLAP[11].

---

[1] Lying flat with one pillow at the most, head and legs relaxed (legs not crossed) and arms relaxed by the side.
[2] Weight loss not only occurs in carcinoma, but in many other abdominal disorders such as inflammatory bowel disease, malabsorption and coeliac disease.
[3] The two gastrointestinal causes of clubbing are chronic liver disease and inflammatory bowel disease (ie Crohn's disease and ulcerative colitis).
[4] White nails caused by hypoalbuminaemia in chronic liver disease.
[5] Spoon-shaped nails caused by iron deficiency anaemia.
[6] Feel the palms. This thickening of the palmar fascia is better felt than seen. It is commonly associated with chronic liver disease but is also familial or idiopathic.
[7] Compare the patient's palm colour with your own. This redness of the palms sparing the centre, caused by increased circulating oestrogen in liver failure. Is also seen in pregnancy and rheumatoid disease and may be idiopathic.
[8] Jaundiced patients are itchy (icteric).
[9] People with chronic liver failure bruise more easily due to loss of clotting factors.
[10] Hepatitis B may be contracted through tattoo needles.
[11] You will never see this sign of advanced liver disease and encephalopathy in an examination setting, but it may be seen on the wards.

Can I just look into your EYES? Look up please.'
Gently draw the skin below the eye down to look at the conjunctiva .
'The conjunctiva is pale[12]/not pale and the sclera is jaundiced[13]/not jaundiced. Now I'm looking at the MOUTH for angular stomatitis[14] and telangiectasia[15]. Could you open your mouth and stick out your tongue please? I'm looking for a smooth, red beefy tongue[16], a pale tongue[17] or a blue tongue[18]. I'm going to shine a pen torch in the mouth to look for ulcers[19], Peutz-Jeghers spots[20], telangiectasia and the general state of dentition.'
To the patient:
'Now I'm going to feel your NECK for any lumps or bumps.'
Feel in the left supraclavicular fossa for Virchow's node[21].
'Could I take off your top/pull down your night-dress so I can see your CHEST AND SHOULDERS?'
To the examiners
'I am looking for spider naevi[22], gynaecomastia[23], scratch marks and axillary hair loss.'
'Now I would like to have a look at the ABDOMEN. Normally I would like the patient exposed from nipples to knees[24].'

---

[12] Pale conjunctiva is a clinical sign of anaemia (it does not prove that the patient is anaemic, only the haemoglobin measurement can do that).

[13] The sclera is the best place to see early or mild jaundice, or jaundice in Asian or black patients.

[14] Cracks at the corners of the mouth may indicate iron deficiency (but beware dribbly old ladies who also have cracked corners of their mouths!).

[15] A localised collection of non-contractile capillaries forms a red spot or telangiectasis. Telangiectasia may be found in and around the mouth and tongue, and may occur elsewhere in the gastrointestinal causing bleeding and anaemia. It may be part of a hereditary syndrome (Osler-Weber-Rendu hereditary haemmorrhagic telangiectasia) or as part of the auto immune syndrome CREST.

[16] Vitamin B12 deficiency.

[17] Clinical sign of anaemia.

[18] Cyanosis in liver disease.

[19] Seen in Crohn's disease.

[20] Small brownish black macules on the lips and buccal mucosa (not tongue) may be associated with intestinal polyps in Peutz-Jeghers disease. The polyps may cause obstruction, intussusception or GI TRACT bleeding.

[21] The left supraclavicular node is classically one of the first palpable nodes to enlarge in gastric cancer.

[22] A bright red spot on the skin with branching spider-like rays caused by dilatation of superficial cutaneous arteries. Up to six may be normal, but more than that in the area drained by the superior vena cava (face, arms, upper trunk) may indicate liver disease.

[23] Abnormal breast tissue (in males only) may indicate an increase in circulating oestrogen in liver failure. Loss of axillary and chest hair and microgonadism may occur for the same reason.

[24] Always say this although the examiners never require it to be done. The underpants should be pulled down to the pubis to spare the patient's modesty and expose most of the abdomen.

Stand back and take a look. To the patient:
'Take a deep breath in and out please? Now cough[25].'
To the examiners:
'On INSPECTION there is no obvious distension[26], swelling[27], visible peristalsis or pulsation[28] of the abdomen. Looking at the skin, there are no scars (see pg 344) or fistulae. There are no distended abdominal veins[29]. I would now like to PALPATE the abdomen for masses and organomegaly (see pg 395).'
Kneel down. Ask the patient:
'Are you tender anywhere[30]? Just relax, arms by your sides'
Light palpation in the nine areas, then deeper in the four quadrants resting over the epigastrium to feel for an aortic aneurysm. Then, starting in the right iliac fossa, palpate for the liver:
'Take deep breaths please in and out.'
Then, starting again in the right iliac fossa, palpate for the spleen:
'And again, deep breaths. I'm just going to pull you towards me.'
Deep palpation for spleen with patient rolled towards you. Then ballot for the kidneys[31].
'I'm now going to PERCUSS the abdomen.'
Percuss from the right nipple down for the liver, left nipple down for the spleen, and pubic bone up for the bladder. Then tap from one flank to the other for flank dullness. If there is flank dullness, or there is a liver edge, or jaundice, you should demonstrate shifting dullness[32].
'I'm going to LISTEN FOR BOWEL SOUNDS.'

---

[25] This should reveal any abdominal herniae. If you suspect any, ask the patient to lift both legs off the bed, keeping the knees straight. Divarication of the recti and incisional hernia (see pg 369) should be palpated to feel the extent and nature of the margins of the defect in the aponeurosis.

[26] e.g. in ascites.

[27] Asymmetrical swelling may be seen due to constipation, organomegaly or a mass in the abdomen.

[28] e.g. aortic aneurysm.

[29] e.g. in portal hypertension. Abnormal veins should be stroked slowly in both directions to determine the direction of flow. In IVC obstruction the flow is upwards, in SVC obstruction it is downwards and in portal hypertension a caput medusae of veins flowing ray-like away from the umbilicus may be seen.

[30] If they are, touch that bit last.

[31] A common exam. question: differences between a kidney and a spleen: A spleen is not ballotable, moves diagonally with respiration not vertically, is dull to percussion not resonant and you can't get above it.

[32] For shifting dullness: tap from the resonant centre to the right side until you hear the note turn dull towards the flanks. LEAVE YOUR FINGER ON THE SPOT that was dull while the patient rolls away from you onto her left side. Wait for the fluid to settle, then tap on the same spot which now, being uppermost, should have gas beneath it and be resonant.

Auscultate over all four quadrants[33], the epigastrium[34], and over the liver[35]
Finally stand back and say
'To complete my examination I would like to examine the GROINS, EXTERNAL
GENITALIA and do a pr. I would also check for ANKLE OEDEMA.'

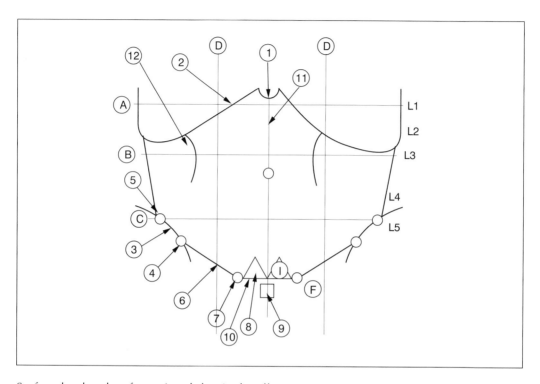

Surface landmarks of anterior abdominal wall

---

[33] There should always be bowel sounds. A silent abdomen may indicate peritonitis. Loud bowel sounds are called borborygmi. High pitched 'tinkling' bowel sounds may indicate obstruction.
[34] You may hear an aortic bruit. If you do, renal artery bruits may be heard either side of the umbilicus and femoral bruits over the femoral arteries.
[35] A liver bruit may be heard in active hepatitis, tumour or arteriovenous malformation.

(A) **Transpyloric line:** halfway between jugular notch and pubic symphysis at L1 (pancreas lies here)

(B) **Subcostal line:** under lowest rib (rib 10 at L3)

(C) **Intertubercular line:** between the two tubercles of the iliac crest (L5)

(D) **Mid-clavicular line:** through mid-inguinal point, halfway between anterior superior iliac spine and symphysis pubis

(1) **Xiphoid process:** Xiphisternal junction is at T9

(2) **Costal margins:** ribs 7–10 in front and 11 and 12 behind. Tenth costal cartilage is the lowest at L3

(3) **Iliac crest:** anterior superior iliac spine (ASIS) to posterior superior iliac spine (PSIS). Highest point L4

(4) **ASIS**

(5) **Tubercle of iliac crest:** 5 cm behind ASIS at L5

(6) **Inguinal ligament:** running from ASIS to pubic tubercle

(7) **Pubic tubercle:** tubercle on superior surface of pubis. Inguinal ligament attaches to it, as the lateral end of the superficial inguinal ring

(8) **Superficial inguinal ring:** inguinal hernia comes out above and medial to the pubic tubercle at point marked (I). Femoral hernia below and lateral to the pubic tubercle at point marked (F)

(9) **Symphysis pubis**: midline cartilaginous joint between pubic bones

(10) **Pubic crest**: ridge on suerior surface of pubic bone medial to pubic tubercle

(11) **Linea alba**: symphysis pubis to xiphoid process midline

(12) **Linea semilunaris**: lateral edge of rectus. Crosses costal margin at ninth costal cartilage (tip of the gall bladder palpable here)

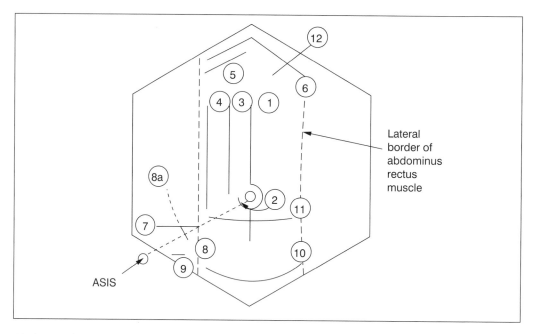

Abdominal incisions

(1) Midline incision through the linea alba: this provides good access, can be extended easily and is quick to make and close. It is relatively avascular. Is more painful than transverse incisions. Incision crosses Langer's lines. Poor cosmetic appearance. Narrow linea alba below umbilicus. Some vessels cross the midline. May cause bladder damage.

(2) Subumbilical incision: used for repair of paraumbilical hernias and laparoscopic port.

(3) Paramedian incision: 1.5 cm from midline through rectus abdominus rectus. Was the only effective vertical incision in the days when the only available suture material was catgut. Takes longer to make than midline incision. Does not lend itself to closure by 'Jenkins rule' (use four times the length of the suture as the length of the wound). Poor cosmetic result. Can lead to infection in the rectus sheath. Other hazards include: the tendinous intersections must be dissected off; need to divide falciform ligament above umbilicus on the right; if rectus is split more than 1 cm from medial border, the intercostal nerves are disrupted leading to denervation of the medial rectus (the rectus can be retracted without splitting to avoid this).

(4) Pararectal: now abandoned due to damage of nerves entering rectus sheath.

(5) Kocher's incision: 3 cm below and parallel to the costal margin from the midline to the rectus border. Good incision for cholecystectomy on the right and splenectomy on the left, **but** beware superior epigastric vessels. If wound is extended laterally, too many intercostal nerves are severed. Cannot be extended caudally.

(6) **Double Kocher's (rooftop) incision**: good access to liver and spleen. Useful for intrahepatic surgery. Used for radical pancreatic and gastric surgery and bilateral adrenalectomy.

(7) **Transverse muscle cutting incision**: can be across all muscles. Beware intercostal nerves.

(8) **McBurney's/Gridiron:** classic approach to appendix 'through the junction of the outer and middle third of a line from the ASIS to the umbilicus at right angles to that line'. It may be modified into a skin crease horizontal cut. The external oblique aponeurosis is cut in the line of the fibres and the internal oblique and transversus abdominus are split transversally in the line of the fibres. Beware – scarring if not horizontal – the iliohypogastric and ilioinguinal nerve – the deep circumflex artery.

(8a) **Rutherford Morrison incision**: the gridiron can be extended cephalad and laterally, obliquely splitting the external oblique to afford good access to the caecum, appendix and right colon.

(9) **Lanz**: this is a lower incision than the McBurney's and closer to the ASIS. It has a better cosmetic result (covered by bikini in ladies) but tends to divide the iliohypogastric and ilioinguinal nerves, leading to denervation of the inguinal canal mechanism which can result in increased risk of inguinal hernia.

(10) **Pfannenstiel incision**: most frequently used transverse incision in adults. Excellent access to female genitalia for Caesarian section and for bladder and prostate operations. Also used for bilateral hernia repair. The skin is incised in a downwardly convex arc into the suprapubic skin crease 2 cm above the pubis. The upper flap is raised and the rectus sheath incised 1 cm cephalic to the skin incision (not extending lateral to the rectus). The rectus is then divided longitudinally in the midline.

(11) **Transverse incision**: particularly useful in neonates and children who do not have the subdiaphragmatic and pelvic recesses of the adult. It heals securely and cosmetically with less pain and fewer respiratory problems than the longitudinal midline incision, but division of red muscle involves more blood loss and less secure closure than a longitudinal incision. It cannot be extended easily. It takes longer to make and to close. Limited access in adults to pelvic or subdiaphragmatic structure.

(12) **Thoraco abdominal incision**: access to lower thorax and upper abdomen. Used for liver and biliary surgery on the right. Used for oesophageal, gastric and aortic surgery on the left.

NB. **The ideal abdominal incision**: should allow easy and rapid access to the relevant structures; should allow easy extension, if necessary; should favour secure healing for the short-term (dehiscence) and long-term (herniation); should be relatively pain free post-operatively; should have a satisfactory cosmetic appearance.

RESPIRATORY EXAMINATION

Introduce yourself and get the patient into position[36].
'Hello, I'm Dr Parchment Smith. Would you mind if I examined your chest? Can you sit up? Are you comfortable? Do you mind if I talk about you as I go along?'
Stand back, hands behind your back, and look at the patient and their surroundings.
'On INITIAL INSPECTION Mrs. X looks well/ill/thin[37]. She is comfortable/ breathless at rest is/isn't using her accessory muscles of respiration, and her colour is good/pale/cyanosed. Around her I can see antibiotic drip/peak flow meter/oxygen/nebulisers.'
Mention anything else which is immediately obvious and relevant. Pick up both hands.
'Can I just have a look at your HANDS first? I'm looking at the nails for clubbing[38], nicotine staining[39], cyanosis[40] or pallor. I'm also looking at the hands for signs of rheumatoid disease[41] or long term steroid use[42]. I'm looking at the palms for pallor in the palmar creases and coal dust tattoos[43].'
To the patient:
'Could you hold both arms straight out please? I'm looking for a tremor[44]. And cock your palms back like this please? I'm looking for a CO_2 retention flap[45]. Can I feel your pulse?'

---

[36] Sitting in bed at 45 degrees to the horizontal.

[37] Weight loss not only occurs in carcinoma, but in emphysema and bronchiectasis.

[38] Thickening of the nailbed, loss of obtuse angle between the nail and nailbed, increased curvature of the nail side to side and lengthways, increased fluctuation of the nail bed and drumstick appearance. Respiratory causes: carcinoma of the bronchus, suppurative lung diseases (empyema, bronchiectasis, lung abscess, cystic fibrosis), mesothelioma, fibrosing alveolitis.

[39] Smoking increases risk of carcinoma, bronchitis and emphysema.

[40] Peripheral cyanosis is not reliable – it may be significant or the patient may just be cold.

[41] Linked with fibrosing alveolitis.

[42] Thin skin, bruising.

[43] Coal workers are at greater risk of lung disease, including pneumoconiosis.

[44] Caused by beta-agonists (e.g. salbutamol) commonly used for asthma or chronic obstructive airway disease.

[45] This will never occur in an exam. because it is a sign of severe CO_2 retention which would only be seen in a very ill patient whose respiratory function was severely compromised. If the examiner asks, tell him this, and say politely that you include it as part of a complete respiratory examination.

While feeling the pulse count the respiratory rate instead of the pulse[46].
'The pulse is neither bounding[47] **nor racing**[48]**. The respiratory rate is 14. Can I just look into your EYES please? Look up please.'**
Gently draw the skin below the eye down to look at the conjunctiva.
'The conjunctiva is pale[49]**/not pale/suffused**[50]**. Can you stick your TONGUE out and lift it up please? There is no central cyanosis. Now I'm going to look at your NECK. Turn to one side and relax the head. The JVP is not raised**[51]**. I'm just going to feel your windpipe, sorry if it's a bit uncomfortable. The trachea is central**[52]**.'**
Stand back again.
'I want to have a look at your CHEST now. Could you take off your top please? Put your hands on your hips[53]**. Now take two deep breaths. Lovely. On INSPECTION of the chest there are no obvious scars**[54]**, radiation burns, abnormal shape or deformity. The chest moves normally**[55]** and symmetrically with respiration. There is/is no use of accessory muscles of respiration**[56]**. There is/is no audible wheeze or stridor**[57]**. I'll now test for EXPANSION.'**
Spread the fingers and grasp the sides (not front) of the ribcage firmly under the nipples until the thumbs meet.

---

[46] The respiratory rate is slow and tedious to count. To make a quick guess, assess whether it is fast or not. If it's fast, say 24, if normal, say 14!

[47] In CO_2 retention.

[48] Tachycardia may occur if the patient is febrile e.g. in pneumonia, or acutely breathless e.g. in acute asthma.

[49] Pale conjunctiva is a clinical sign of anaemia (it does not prove that the patient is anaemic, only the haemoglobin measurement can do that).

[50] If there is superior vena caval obstruction, for example in bronchial carcinoma with enlarged lymph nodes, the venous drainage of the head will be congested and the sclera may look red and suffused.

[51] The JVP is raised in congestive cardiac failure, when the heart has failed. This is a common cause of breathlessness due to pulmonary oedema. The JVP can also be raised in SVC obstruction (see above), but in this case it will be fixed and have no hepatojugular reflex.

[52] The trachea may be PUSHED away from the affected side (pleural effusion, tension pneumothorax, space occupying mass) or PULLED towards it (collapse due to obstruction or infection, fibrosis, old TB). You may feel a tracheal tug if the chest is hyperinflated.

[53] Leave them with their hands on their hips throughout the examination for access and comfort.

[54] From thoracotomy, thoracoplasty, pneumonectomy.

[55] The movement becomes more up-and-down instead of in-and-out in conditions like emphysema.

[56] The patient braces his arms, uses his shoulder and neck muscles to help increase his chest volume. You may see the intercostal and supraclavicular spaces indrawing.

[57] Wheezy expiration is common in asthma, bronchitis, emphysema. Noisy inspiration (stridor) is due to obstruction such as mediastinal masses or secretions in the upper airway.

'Take the biggest breath you can and breathe out. Expansion is normal/reduced on the right/left/both sides[58].'

Repeat this above the nipples.

'I'm just going to tap on your chest.'

PERCUSS[59] from clavicles down, comparing sides. Don't forget the axillae.

'Percussion note is normal/dull/hyper-resonant/stony dull (say where)'

'Say '99' when I touch you.'

Assess TACTILE FREMITUS[60] with the ulnar border of the hand from the clavicles down, comparing sides.

'Tactile fremitus is normal/increased/decreased (say where)'

'Okay, now I'm going to have a listen. Breathe in and out through your mouth when I touch you with the stethoscope.'

AUSCULTATE[61] from clavicles down, comparing sides. Don't forget the axillae.

'Now say '99' when I touch you with the stethoscope.'

Assess VOCAL FREMITUS from clavicles down, including axillae.

'Now can you lean forward so I can do all that again on your back! First let me FEEL YOUR NECK for any lumps or bumps.'

Repeat expansion, percussion, tactile fremitus, auscultation and vocal fremitus on the BACK OF THE CHEST.

'Let me press on your lower back. There is/is no SACRAL OEDEMA[62].'

Finally stand back and say

'To complete my examination I would like to examine for ANKLE OEDEMA, see the PEAK FLOW READING, TEMPERATURE and SPUTUM POT for this patient. I would also like to see the X-RAYS.'

---

[58] This is a useful sign. Just remember that expansion is usually decreased on the diseased side.

[59] **Percussion:** Hyperesonant = pneumothorax or hyperinflation
Dull = Collapse, consolidation or fibrosis.
Stony dull = fluid ie pleural effusion.

[60] **Tactile and vocal fremitus:** Increased if it's solid or pus-filled (Consolidation, collapse, fibrosis)
Decreased if it's air or water (Pneumothorax, pleural effusion)
Normal in uncomplicated COAD or asthma

[61] **Breath sounds:** Vesicular is normal. Bronchial (just like if you listen over the trachea) in consolidation, collapse and fibrosis. Absent in collapse, pneumothorax, effusion. Added sounds: Crackles/crepitations are early in inspiration in COAD and asthma, late in inspiration fibrosing alveolitis and LVF, and change on coughing in bronchiectasis. A polyphonic wheeze is heard in asthma, but may be present in COAD also. Asthma and COAD have prolonged expiration.

[62] This may be a sign of congestive cardiac failure (like ankle oedema) in patients who have been sitting rather than standing.

EXAMINATION OF THE GROIN

Introduce yourself and get the patient into position.
'Hello, my name is Dr Parchment Smith. Would you mind if I examined your groin? Can you stand in front of me, on this step[63], trousers off please? Do you mind if I speak to the examiners as I go on? I'm just going to have a look first of all.'
Look at the position of the lump.
'My impression on inspection is of a large/small swelling in the right scrotum[64]/groin crease[65]/groin[66].'
If you can't see anything ask the patient.
'Is it aching or sore anywhere? Show me where[67]. OK I'll be gentle. Does the lump ever pass into the sac? I'm going to gently feel the scrotum now.'
Palpate the scrotum.

---

[63] There is usually a step by the bed. If there is, get the patient to stand on it. It looks more elegant to crouch in front of the patient looking up or straight ahead at the lump rather than being hunched over double, furtling in the low-down groin buried under the tum of a small, fat person! It will also be easier for the examiners to see the signs you are demonstrating. If there is not a step by the bed, don't bother – making an issue of it will just irritate the examiners.

[64] This could be an inguinal hernia, hydrocoele, testicular mass or epididymal cyst.

[65] An inguinal hernia usually lies above the groin crease. A lump filling the groin crease and extending down towards the upper thigh is more likely to be a femoral hernia.

[66] **Differential diagnosis of a lump in the groin**:
- Hernia – direct inguinal
           – indirect inguinal
           – femoral
- Lymph nodes
- Saphena varix
- Ectopic testis
- Femoral aneurysm
- Hydrocoele of – spermatic cord
                 – Canal of Nuck
- Lipoma of the cord
- Psoas bursa
- Psoas abscess

[67] On the one hand this might be construed as cheating, but on the other hand it is important to ascertain whether or not a lump is tender before you start, and if being so considerate has the added benefit of getting the patient to point out an otherwise invisible lump, so much the better!

'I can feel a mass in the scrotum[68]. I would like to determine three things. Firstly, can I get above it[69]? If not it is probably a hernia[70]. Secondly, can I feel the testis separate from the mass[71]? If not then the lump is either in the testis, such as a neoplasm or an orchitis, or around the testis, such as a haematocoele or a hydrocoele[72]. Thirdly does it transilluminate? Can I have the shades down please?'

Shading the front of the groin further with your hand, shine your pen torch from the back of the scrotum to see if the swelling lights up as a brilliantly illuminated pinky-red.

'If it does, it is fluid filled; either an epididymal cyst or a hydrocoele.'

If you think the swelling is a hernia:

'I think this is an inguinoscrotal hernia as I cannot get above it, it is separate from the testicle, and it does not transilluminate. I'm now going to palpate it from the side.'

Stand next to the patient[73], one hand in the small of the patient's back and the palpating hand flat on the groin parallel to the inguinal ligament. Feel the temperature, tension and composition of the lump.

---

[68] Even if you can see an obvious lump in the groin, it is important to start with examination of the testicle because
a) the hernia may extend into the scrotum
b) you need to make sure there is one, as ectopic testis is a differential of a groin lump, and
c) people with dual pathology are commonly called upon to be exam. cases.
The differential diagnosis of a lump in the scrotum is

Can't get above it	Can't feel testicle separately	Transilluminable	Can get above it, can feel
Indirect inguinal hernia	Seminoma/Teratoma	Hydrocoele	testicle separately and not
Infantile hydrocoele (rare)	Haematocoele	Epididymal cyst	transilluminable
Varicocoele	Hydrocoele		Epididymitis (incl. TB)
	Syphilitic Gumma		Spermatocoele
	Orchitis		
	Torsion		

[69] Palpate the testicle. Above it should be only the narrow leash of cord structures and the thin scrotal skin. You should be able to feel the top of the testicle.
[70] If you can't get above the lump the swelling is an inguinoscrotal hernia, a varicocoele (which looks and feels characteristic see pg 381) or (rarely in exams.) an infantile hydrocoele.
[71] Trace the cord down until you feel the testicle. Work your fingers gently around it, trying to determine if the mass is separate from the testicle or not. The epididymis arises from the posterior aspect of the testicle. Is it the epididymis that is swollen? You might find it useful at this stage to feel the opposite testicle so you can feel what is normal for this patient (assuming he does not have dual pathology)
[72] If you can feel the testis separately it is probably an epididymal swelling such as an epididymal cyst or epididymitis.
[73] The reason for standing next to the patient is to be able to place your hand in exactly the same position as the patient's hand would be when supporting or reducing the hernia – i.e. putting a hand on the hernia and lifting it upwards and backwards.

'The swelling is not hot or tense, is non tender and has fluid and gaseous components in its composition. I would just like to test for a cough impulse.'
Compress the lump gently but firmly, applying counter pressure with your hand on the back[74].
'Can you cough please? It expands[75] on coughing, so has a positive cough impulse. Now I'd like to check for reducibility. Does the lump go back in sir? Can you get it back in yourself? Will you do that please, I don't want to hurt you[76]. That's great, thank you. Now I'll take it.'
Let the patient reduce it, then you take over and hold it reduced with gentle pressure.
'I'm now applying pressure over the external ring[77]. Could you cough please? The hernia is controlled at the external ring[78].'
Slide your hand back to rest over the internal ring, keeping a steady pressure so you are still controlling the hernia.
'I am now pressing over the deep or internal ring[79].

---

[74] This stops you pushing the patient backwards

[75] It must expand, not just move, to be a positive cough impulse

[76] Often the lump has not been reduced for years, or the patient has a special knack for getting the hernia back in. In any case, hurting the patient is an automatic fail, and nothing hurts more than the tenth SHO for the day leaning on your large inguinoscrotal hernia. The examiners, familiar with this scenario from clinic, will usually let you get away with this unless they are real sadists. If the patient refuses, or says that he's never tried to put it back, you have no option but to gently try to reduce it with your flat hand from underneath the lump (not poking it in with your fingers!) lifting it upwards and backwards. Press firmly to reduce the tension in the lump. Then gently squeeze the lower part of the swelling. As the lump gets softer, lift it up towards the external ring until the hernia has all passed in through this point.

[77] Remember that the inguinal hernia reduces into or through a point above and medial to the pubic tubercle (the external or superficial ring). A femoral hernia will (if reducible) reduce into or through a point below and lateral to the pubic tubercle. The upper crease of the mons (ie where the pot belly hangs over) indicates the crest of the pubis and the level of the pubic tubercle. These, you will remember, form the inferior and lateral margins respectively of the superficial inguinal ring, just lateral the midline (see pg 361 and fig on pg 342). Once you have located this and feel the hernia is controlled by your hand, try to control it with a couple of fingers so the point at which the hernia is controlled is demonstrated more clearly. Having reduced the hernia and inspected the patient, you will have a reasonable idea whether the hernia is direct or indirect, so concentrate on demonstrating this.

[78] Both direct and indirect hernias are controlled at the external ring (but a femoral hernia will not be).

[79] The deep ring is situated 1.3 cm above the inguinal ligament, midway between the anterior superior iliac spine and the pubic tubercle. This is the 'midpoint of the inguinal ligament' just lateral to the femoral artery pulsation at the so-called 'mid-inguinal point'.

'Cough again please. The hernia is controlled at the deep ring[80]**. I'm now going to let go and observe the movement of the hernia through the canal.'**

Let go and watch the hernia reappear[81]. *If it does not reappear spontaneously, ask the patient to cough again. Stand back and say to the examiners:*

'To complete my examination[82] **I would like to examine the other groin with the patient standing and perform an abdominal and groin examination with the patient lying down**[83]**. My diagnosis is...'**

---

[80] If the hernia can only be held reduced at the external ring it is a direct inguinal hernia. If it can be controlled by pressure over the internal ring it is an indirect inguinal hernia. Bear in mind that some larger indirect inguinal hernias have an element of a direct hernia (posterior inguinal canal wall weakness) associated with it.

[81] An indirect hernia will seem to slide obliquely along the line of the canal whereas a direct hernia will project directly forward.

[82] Percussing and auscultating the lump, if it is very large and you suspect it contains bowel, may be appropriate. Bowel sounds confirm the presence of loops of bowel within the sac, which increases the risk of obstruction or strangulation.

[83] Looking for things that might have increased the intra-abdominal pressure such as a large bladder, enlarged prostate, ascites, chronic intestinal obstruction and pregnancy.

EXAMINATION OF A STOMA[84]

When asked to comment on a stoma, be methodical and state the obvious in an intelligent way. Even if you have no idea what type of stoma it is or what operation has occurred, there are ten things you should look for and comment on to get you through this case.

1. **Site**. Ileostomies are typically in the right iliac fossa, colostomies on the left. Midline loop colostomies are rarely done for relief of obstruction usually in emergency cases. Sites may vary due to exceptional circumstances, so use it as a guide rather than relying on it absolutely.

2. **Calibre**. Colostomies are the largest, followed by ileostomies then urostomies. Retraction or stenosis may make the lumen look smaller, prolapse may make a stoma look bigger.

3. **Number of lumens**. Is the stoma and end stoma or a loop or double barrelled stoma? The non-productive lumen may look tiny and retracted, you have to look for it. There may be more than one stoma, for example a colostomy and mucus fistula after a modified Hartmann's, or a colostomy and urinary diversion after a pelvic clearance.

---

[84] **Top Five Case: seen by over a quarter of candidates in our survey. Accounted for 12.5% of the cases in this bay.**

Types of stoma

Gastrostomy	Caecostomy
Jejunostomy	Colostomy
Ileostomy	Urostomy

Indications for stomata

- **Feeding** e.g. gastrostomy following GI surgery, in CNS disease, in coma
- **Decompression** e.g. gastrostomy (usually temporary), caecostomy
- **Lavage** e.g. caecostomy on table before resecting distal colonic disease with primary anastomosis
- **Diversion** e.g. ileostomy to protect at risk distal anastomosis, or to achieve bowel rest for Crohn's. Loop colostomies and double-barrelled colostomies facilitate closure later but are more difficult to manage.
- **Exteriorisation** e.g. double-barrelled colostomy (not used for malignancy), resection with end colostomy and rectal stump (Hartmann's) when primary anastomosis is impossible (e.g. perforation, ischaemia, obstruction). Resection with end colostomy and mucous fistula (like Hartmann's but easier to rejoin). Permanent colostomy (e.g. after abdomino-perineal resections in low rectal tumours). Permanent ileostomy (e.g. after panproctocolectomy for ulcerative colitis or familial polyposis coli).

Selecting a stoma site

Assess	Avoid	Problem Patients
Before operation	Wound site	Wheelchair-bound
With clothes	Bony prominences	Amputees
Lying and standing	Existing scars	Obese
Good visibility	Umbilicus	Allergies
	Groin crease/skin fold	Psychological problems

4. **Spout**. Ileostomies have a spout to keep the irritating alkaline effluent away from the skin, colostomies do not unless they are prolapsing.

5. **Bag contents**. Often the most instantly informative. Green fluid ileal contents, faeces or urine? Even if the bag has been taken off, it will be lying somewhere around, and inspection of the contents (eg any mucus, blood) is a useful part of the examination.

6. **Scars**. What previous surgery has the patient had? Look particularly for evidence of previous closures of other stomata or mucus fistulae. The absence of a midline incision in the presence of a stoma indicates a trephine (usually defunctioning) colostomy or a laparoscopic procedure. The maturity of the scars also give a clue as to how recently the surgery was performed.

7. **Complications of the stoma**. Mention the state of the stoma. Does it look healthy and well-constructed? Is it ischaemic, prolapsing, retracted, stenosed? Does it have a parastomal hernia (ask the patient to cough or raise his legs). Is the mucosa inflamed, are there polyps?

Complications of stomata

Technical Problems

- **Ischaemia/gangrene:** abdominal wall defect too tight; injury to mesenteric vessels; re-siting is necessary
- **Prolapse or intussusception:** when bowel is not anchored to abdominal wall internally; reduction is easy but re-siting is needed if prolapse is recurrent
- **Parastomal hernias:** may cause difficulties with appliances; may contain bowel at risk of obstruction/strangulation; re-siting may be needed
- **Stenosis:** poor initial siting; ischaemia; underlying disease process (carcinoma, inflammatory bowel disease); re-siting may be necessary if there is obstruction
- **Bowel contents spill over into efferent loop:** especially in loop colostomy; distal bowel is not adequately defunctioned if this occurs; split or double-barrelled stomata solve this; the efferent loop should always be sited cephalic to (above) the afferent loop
- **Reservoir ileostomies** have specific problems: valve failure; incontinence; obstruction; impaired blood supply

General Problems

- **Stoma diarrhoea:** due to underlying disease; due to inappropriate diet; can lead to water and electrolyte imbalance especially after ileostomy
- **Nutritional disorders:** vitamin B deficiency (megaloblastic anaemia); chronic microcytic normochromic anaemia
- **Kidney stones and gallstones:** caused by loss of terminal ileum; failure of bile salt absorption; excessive water loss
- **Short gut syndrome:** profuse fluid and electrolyte loss
- **Underlying disease:** may cause recurrent symptoms; Crohn's may cause peristomal fistulae or proximal obstruction
- **Psychological and sexual problems**

8. **Perineum**. Ask if the patient has a patent anal canal or a closed perineum to ascertain whether this is a temporary or permanent stoma. It will also give you a clue as to the operation: the commonest reasons for an abdominoperineal resection are a low rectal cancer, familial polyposis coli, or severe ulcerative colitis.

9. **General condition of the patient**. Is this a terminally ill patient who has been given a palliative defunctioning colostomy? Or a very thin young woman whose Crohn's disease necessitated a temporary ileostomy? Or a healthy looking middle-aged man long recovered from the low rectal tumour that needed an APR and end colostomy? Do they look malnourished or dehydrated (e.g. due to high output stoma)

10. **Type of appliance**. A one-piece is where the whole appliance is connected to the skin by adhesive and the whole appliance has to be changed. A two-piece (more common for long-standing stomata) has a base-plate with a flange. The pouch only is changed regularly. Drainable, transparent pouches with a tap on the end are used in the post-operative period when the output is large and must be monitored. Closed, opaque bags are more common in the long term and may have charcoal filters to release flatus without odour.

Practical Problems
- **Odour:** advice can be given on hygiene, diet and deodorant sprays.
- **Flatus:** can be improved by diet and special filters.
- **Skin problems:** usually due to an ill-fitting device. The problem is worsened as the stoma shrinks post-operatively. The problem can be counteracted by a barrier cream or two-piece appliance. Ileostomies with their irritant, copious output, can be particularly troublesome. The patient may need a supporting belt if spout is not big enough.
- **Leakage:** transverse loop colostomies are especially prone to leakage. A poor site may be responsible. Methyl cellulose bland paste around the appliance can help.
- **Parastomal hernia:** A flexible pouch, supporting belt and filler paste can all help with this problem. Re-siting may be necessary.
- **Stoma prolapse:** may need surgical correction.

Post operative advice
- Patient warned of problems: oedematous stoma; copious offensive early output; transparent pouch to monitor stoma.
- Self-care programme: patients observe, help them manage their own stomata

Counselling and support: from stoma care nurse.

355

C   The Cases

[85]Indirect inguinal hernia

Top Five Case: seen by 48% of the candidates in our survey. Accounted for 19.5% of cases in this bay. Inguinal hernias were a very common case seen by over a third of the candidates surveyed.

The most common type of groin hernia in children. It is thought to be caused by a congenital failure of processus vaginalis to close (saccular theory of Russell). The indirect inguinal hernia sac is the remains of the processus vaginalis. The sac extends through the deep ring, canal and superficial ring. The inferior epigastric artery lies medial to the neck. In a complete sac the testis is found in the fundus. In an incomplete sac, the sac is limited to the canal or is inguinoscrotal or inguinolabial. The indirect hernia commonly descends into the scrotum.

Predisposing factors for indirect inguinal hernias

Male (bigger processus vaginalis)

Premature twins/low birth weight (processus vaginalis not closed)

Young (compared with direct hernias which become more common with age)

Africans (lower arch in more oblique African pelvis)

On the right (right testis descends later than left)

Testicular feminisation syndrome (genotypic male but androgen insensitive so phenotypic female)

Increased intraperitoneal fluid (eg cardiac, cirrhotic, carcinomatosis, dialysis opens up processus vaginalis)

[86] Advantages of groin hernia repair under local anaesthetic (LA)

Early mobilisation

Decreased urinary retention, DVT/PE

Safer in high risk patients

Decreased cost, increased patient turnover

No reduction in complications or increase in recurrence

If not fit for general anaesthetic

The Royal College of Surgeons suggest aiming to do 30% of elective hernias as a day case (easier if LA).

INDIRECT INGUINAL HERNIA[85]

Carry out examination of groin (pg 349).

Case 1

'There is (in this young/middle-aged patient) a visible lump in the right groin extending towards the scrotum. On examination the lump has an expansile cough impulse, is not tender and the overlying skin is normal. It is reducible through a point above and medial to the pubic tubercle, and is controlled both at the superficial and deep inguinal ring. This is a reducible indirect inguinal hernia and could be repaired electively, preferably under local anaesthetic[86] if the patient is fit. I would like to examine the other side, and would normally do a cardiorespiratory assessment and examine the abdomen.'

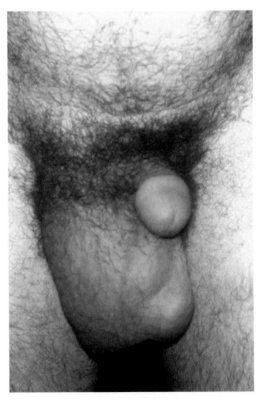

Indirect inguinal hernia on the right

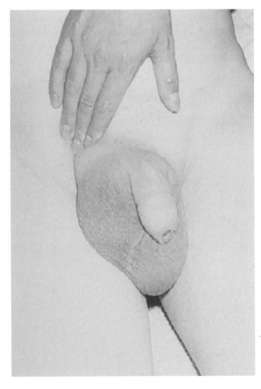

Indirect inguinal hernia controlled with pressure applied at the superficial ring

Anatomy of the inguinal canal

The inguinal ligament is the rolled-under inferior margin of the aponeurosis of the external oblique muscle and runs between the anterior superior iliac spine (ASIS) and the pubic tubercle.

The inguinal canal lies above the medial half of the inguinal ligament between the deep and superficial rings.

The deep inguinal ring is an opening in the transversalis fascia 1.3 cm above the inguinal ligament midway between the ASIS and the pubic tubercle (the midpoint of the inguinal ligament). It lies lateral to the inferior epigastric vessels.

The superficial inguinal ring is a triangular opening in the external oblique aponeurosis. The lateral crus attaches to the pubic tubercle. The medial crus attaches to the pubic crest near the symphysis. The base of the superficial ring is the pubic crest.

The floor of the inguinal canal is formed by the inguinal canal and the lacunar ligament medially.

The ceiling of the inguinal canal is formed by, lateral to medial, the transverse abdominis, internal oblique and the conjoint tendon.

The anterior wall of the inguinal ligament is formed by the external oblique strengthened laterally by the internal oblique.

The posterior wall of the inguinal canal is formed by the transversalis fascia strengthened medially by the conjoint tendon.

Contents of the inguinal canal in the male

Vas

Arteries: testicular, artery to vas, cremasteric

Veins: The pampiniform plexus

Lymphatic vessels: The testis drains to the paraaortic lymph nodes; the coverings of the testis drain to the external iliac nodes

Nerves: Genital branch of the genitofemoral (supplies cremaster muscle)

        Sympathetic nerves accompanying arteries

        Ilioinguinal nerve (enters via the anterior wall of the canal) supplying the skin of the inguinal region, upper part of thigh and anterior one-third of scrotum or labia

Processus vaginalis: The obliterated remains of the peritoneal connection to the tunica vaginalis

        All of the above are in the spermatic cord except the ilioinguinal nerve.

Case 2

'There is a large swelling in the right groin and scrotum. On examination the lump has an expansile cough impulse, is not tender and the overlying skin is normal. It is not reducible but appears to emerge from a point above and medial to the pubic tubercle. The contents of the lump have liquid and gaseous components and there is evidence of bowel sounds indicating bowel loops within it. This is an irreducible or incarcerated inguinal hernia, and should be repaired promptly if the patient is fit. I would like to examine the other side, and would normally do a cardiorespiratory assessment and examine the abdomen.'

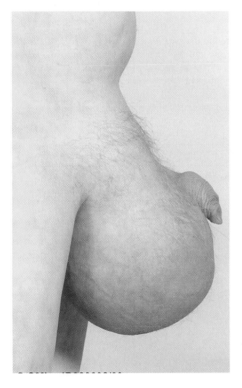

Irreducible inguinoscrotal hernia

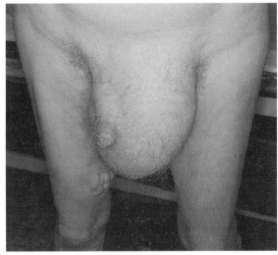

Large inguinoscrotal hernia

[87] Direct inguinal hernia

This is an acquired weakness in the abdominal wall so tends to develop in adulthood as compared with indirect hernias which are common in children. 35% of adult male inguinal hernias are direct, 5% are a combination of direct and indirect. The direct inguinal hernia sac lies behind the cord. The inferior epigastric artery lies lateral to the neck. The hernia passes directly forward through the defect in the posterior wall (fascia transversalis) of the inguinal canal. The hernia does not typically run down alongside the cord to the scrotum but may do so.

Predisposing factors for direct inguinal hernias

- Males
- Old age
- Increased intra-abdominal pressure (eg chronic cough, obesity, constipation, prostatism)
- Smoking
- Aortic aneurysm (associated with collagen defect)
- Anatomical variant of the conjoint tendon (in 10% of adult white males)

Complications of hernias

- Incarceration
- Obstruction
- Strangulation
- Reduction en masse
- Richter's hernia (only antimesenteric margin of gut is strangulated in the sac)
- Maydl's hernia (a W-shaped loop of small gut lies in the hernia sac and the intervening loop is strangulated within the main abdominal cavity)
- Littre's hernia (hernia sac containing strangulated Meckel's diverticulum)
- Spontaneous or traumatic rupture of hernia sac
- Involvement in peritoneal disease process (e.g. metastatic disease, mesothelial hyperplasia, peritonitis, endometriosis, etc)

Indications for groin hernia repair

Non-mandatory	Small, easily reducible, direct	Follow-up in one year (same for recurrent hernias)
Elective to be prioritised by job	Indirect, symptomatic direct	Because rate of strangulation of inguinal hernia is 0.3–2.9% per year - risk if irreducible or indirect
Prompt	Irreducible inguinal hernia History of <4 weeks	More risk of strangulation in first three months after appearing
Urgent	All femoral hernias	Within a month 50% strangulate
Emergency	Painful irreducible hernias	

Royal College of Surgeons Guidelines of Management of Groin Hernias

- Appropriately trained surgeon performs/supervises operation
- Special hernia centres and special interest consultants recommended
- Suggest aiming to do 30% of elective hernias as a day case (8% at present)
- Criteria for surgery should be assessed:
  - type of hernia (inguinal, femoral, reducible, partially reducible, primary, recurrent, complex)
  - type of patient (social circumstances for discharge, ASA grade) and matched to surgeon, operative technique, day case or inpatient, GA or LA
- Recommends aiming for a recurrence rate of 0.5% at five years

DIRECT INGUINAL HERNIA[87]

Carry out examination of the groin (pg 349).

'There is a small swelling in the right groin. On examination the lump has an expansile cough impulse, is not tender and the overlying skin is normal. It is easily reducible and emerges from a point above and medial to the pubic tubercle. It is controlled by pressure over the superficial ring but not by pressure over the deep ring. This is a direct inguinal hernia and could be repaired electively, preferably under local anaesthetic if the patient is fit. Alternatively, if the lump is small, asymptomatic and the patient is elderly, an easily reducible direct inguinal hernia can safely be managed expectantly. I would like to examine the other side, and would normally do a cardiorespiratory assessment and examine the abdomen.'

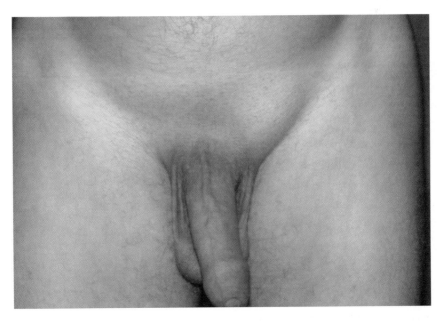

Small left inguinal hernia

Types of inguinal hernia repair

The Royal College of Surgeons Guidelines on Hernia Management suggest the Shouldice technique or mesh repair for primary uncomplicated inguinal hernias.

Shouldice repair is recommended for strangulated hernia to avoid insertion of mesh in a potentially infected wound.

Laparoscopic repair is indicated in bilateral inguinal hernias and in recurrent hernias. The mesh is most commonly stapled between the peritoneum and the fascia transversalis.

Advantages and disadvantages of prosthetic mesh repair

Advantages	Disadvantages
Easier to learn and perform by trainees	Main disadvantage is the risk of infection; incidence
Lower recurrence rate (1:1000)	may be reduced by avoiding haematomas and use of
Tension free repair	prophylactic antibiotics
Reduced analgesic requirement	

Advantages and disadvantages of Shouldice repair

Advantages	Disadvantages
Low risk of infection	More technically difficult than the mesh repair
Indicated in the presence of strangulated	High standard of training needed
bowel where mesh is not recommended	Longer operative time than mesh repair
Low recurrence rate in the right hands*	Difficult to perform tension-free repair
	Higher post-op analgesic requirement than mesh repair

* This technique was popularised by the Shouldice Clinic. Recurrence rate is <1% there, but approaches 3.5% elsewhere. At the Shouldice Clinic, the trainee surgeon is required to assist in 50 hernia repairs then perform 100 hernia repairs under supervision before being allowed to repair inguinal hernias independently.

Postoperative complications of groin hernia repair

Wound: haematoma, sepsis, sinus.

Scrotal: ischaemic orchitis, testicular atrophy, hydrocoele, genital oedema, damage to vas and vessels.

Special complications: nerve injuries, persistent post-operative pain, compression of femoral vessels, urinary retention, impotence, mesh infection.

General complications: chest infection, DVT, PE, cardiovascular problems, visceral injury.

Operation failure: recurrence, missed hernia, dehiscence.

Mortality

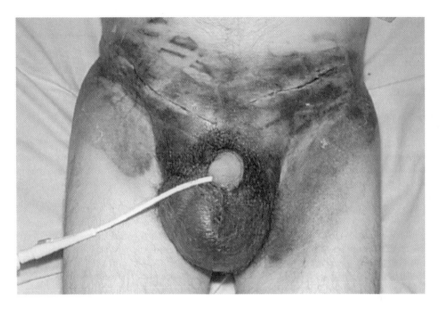

Haematoma and urinary retention, two complications of hernia repair

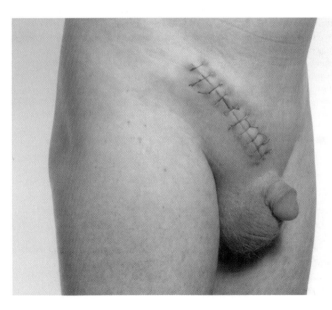

Infected hernia repair

[88] **Femoral hernia**

Epidemiology

In females, femoral hernias are as common as indirect inguinal hernias. They are found 2.5 times more commonly in females because:

- Inguinal ligament makes a wider angle with the pubis in the female.
- Enlargement of the fat in the femoral canal in fat middle-aged ladies stretches the femoral canal; this fat then disappears in old age leaving a bigger canal.
- Pregnancy increases intra-abdominal pressure and stretches the fascia transversalis.

Mechanics of femoral hernia

Femoral hernia enters femoral canal through the femoral ring. The hernia arrives in the thigh next to the saphenous opening of the femoral sheath. The cribriform fascia over the saphenous opening becomes stretched over the hernia. The hernia enlarges upwards and medially into the superficial fascia of the inguinal ligament. Typically it lies between the superficial external pudendal and superficial epigastric veins compressing the saphenous vein as it emerges through the saphenous opening.

Anatomy of the femoral sheath

The femoral sheath is a downward protrusion into the thigh of the fascial envelope lining the abdominal wall. It surrounds the femoral vessels and lymphatics for about 1 inch below the inguinal ligament. The sheath ends by fusing with the tunica adventitia of the femoral vessels. This occurs close to the saphenous opening in the deep fascia of the thigh.

The anterior wall is continuous above with the fascia transversalis, the posterior wall is continuous above with the fascia iliacus/psoas fascia. It does not protrude below the inguinal ligament in the foetal position.

The femoral sheath exists to provide freedom for vessel movement beneath inguinal ligament during movement of the hip.

Contents of the femoral sheath

- Femoral artery in lateral compartment
- Femoral veins in intermediate compartment
- Lymphatics in medial compartment or femoral canal
- The femoral branch (L1) of the genitofemoral nerve pierces the anterior wall of the femoral sheath running on the anterior surface of the external iliac artery.

NB. The femoral nerve lies in the iliac fossa between psoas and iliacus behind the fascia. Therefore it enters the thigh outside the femoral sheath.

Anatomy of the femoral canal

The femoral canal is the medial compartment of the femoral sheath, containing lymphatics. It is about 1.3 cm long with an upper opening called the femoral ring. The femoral canal allows lymph vessels to be transmitted from the lower limbs to the abdomen and is also a dead space into which the femoral vein can expand when venous return increases. The femoral canal is the path taken by femoral herniae.

Contents of the femoral canal

- Fatty connective tissue
- Efferent lymph vessels from deep inguinal nodes
- The deep inguinal node of Cloquet draining the penis/clitoris

Relations of the femoral ring

- Anteriorly the inguinal ligament
- Posteriorly the superior ramus of the pubis and the pectineal ligament
- Medially the lacunar ligament or ileopubic tract
- Laterally the femoral vein

These are also the margins of the neck of a femoral hernia. Note that three of the four are rigid making the femoral hernia prone to strangulation.

FEMORAL HERNIA[88]

Carry out examination of the groin (pg 349).

'There is (in this elderly woman) a small non-tender lump bulging into the right groin crease. On examination the lump has an expansile cough impulse[89], is not tender and the overlying skin is normal. It is reducible[90] through a point below and lateral to the pubic tubercle. This is a femoral hernia and requires repair within four weeks. I would like to examine the other side, and would normally do a cardiorespiratory assessment and examine the abdomen.'

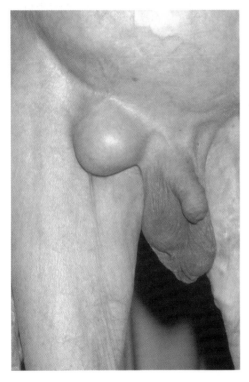

Large right femoral hernia

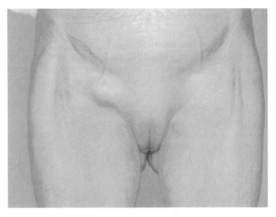

Right femoral hernia in an elderly woman

Characteristics of a typical femoral hernia

- Small (hard to find in an obese patient)
- Not reducible
- No cough impulse
- Often contains only omentum
- May contain a knuckle of bowel (most common site for a Richter's hernia)
- More common on the right
- 35–50% of all strangulated groin hernias in adults are femoral hernias

Differential diagnosis of femoral hernia

Inguinal hernia	Femoral artery aneurysm
Enlarged lymph gland	Sarcoma
Sapheno-varix	Ectopic testis
Ectopic testis	Obturator hernia
Psoas abscess	Psoas bursa
Lipoma	

Repair of femoral hernia

The main aims are to remove the peritoneal sac and repair the defects. Methods include:

The crural/low/Lockwood approach is the simplest – used for elective repair but not recommended for strangulated hernia

High/inguinal/Lothiessen approach reveals the femoral canal through the inguinal canal

High/extraperitoneal/McEvedy approach- safest for strangulated hernia.

Royal College of Surgeons Guidelines on Repair of Femoral Hernias

The Royal College of Surgeons recommends the high inguinal approach, except in thin females when a low crural approach is acceptable.

In complex, recurrent or obstructed hernias the high extraperitoneal approach is advised.

[89] A narrow neck and adherence of the contents to the peritoneal sac mean that many femoral hernias do not have a cough impulse.

[90] The size of most femoral hernias can be reduced by firm pressure, but often cannot be completely reduced because the contents are often adherent to the peritoneal sac.

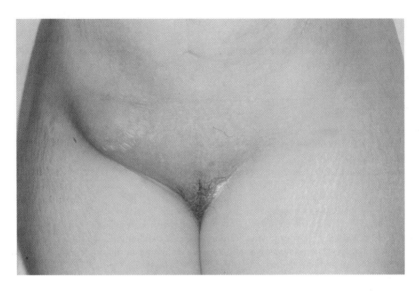

Red hot tender strangulated right inguinal hernia

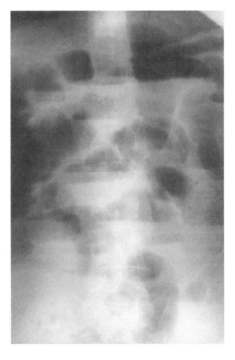

Dilated small bowel loops with fluid
levels on the plain abdominal X-ray
of patient above picture

[91] **Incisional hernia**

Incisional hernia was a very common case seen by over 1 in 10 of the candidates in our survey.

Definition: Diffuse extension of peritoneum and abdominal contents through a weak scar

Incidence: 6% of abdominal wounds at 5 years, 12% at 10 years. More common in Caesarean section and gynaecological wounds.

Causes of incisional hernia:

Technical failure by surgeon: haematoma, necrosis, sepsis, inept closure, poor incision, drains or stomata

Tissue factors: age, immunosuppression, obesity, malignancy, malnutrition, infection

High risk incisions: lower/upper midline, lateral muscle splitting, subcostal, parastomal, transverse

Preoperative conditions: cardiopulmonary disease, obesity, local skin/tissue sepsis

Surgical repair of incisional hernia

Layer to layer anatomical repair (if there is no tissue loss)

Mesh repair

Keel repair (Sac invaginated by successive lines of sutures)

Recurrence rates vary from 1–46% – lower (10%) with mesh repairs.

Divarication of the recti can be mistaken for an incisional hernia, as it can occur after multiple midline incisions. Other causes include multiple pregnancies and prolonged abdominal distension. The linea alba stretches and fails to hold together the two longitudinal rectus abdominus muscles. The resulting gap may be as much as several inches, and allows a diffuse bulge to appear between the recti, more pronounced superiorly where the origin of the rectus muscles is further apart (on the lower ribs) than their insertion at the pubis. Surgery is unnecessary unless there is a local defect within the divarication as they rarely strangulate.

INCISIONAL HERNIA[91]

Spot diagnosis, or may be found during examination of abdomen (see pg 339).

'There is a non-tender reducible lump with an expansile cough impulse under an old scar. The lump is about 10 cm by 6 cm and a defect in the abdominal wall can be felt which is about 4 cm by 2 cm. The extent of the hernia can be seen more clearly when the patient, lying flat, raises both straight legs just off the bed. This is an incisional hernia. The wide neck and easy reducibility points to a low risk of strangulation.'

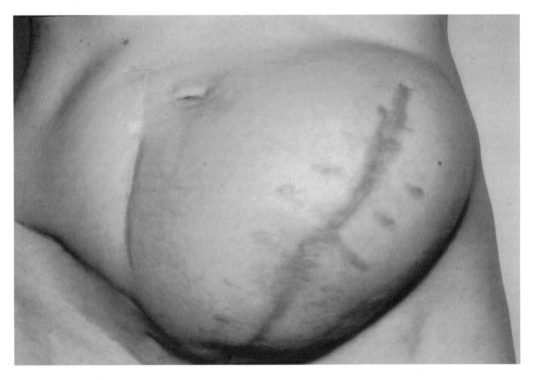

Abdominal incisional hernia

[92] **Paraumbilical hernia**
Common case: seen by nearly 1 in 10 of the candidates in our survey
More common with increasing age, M = F.

Causes
Increased intra-abdominal pressure, e.g. ascites, multiple pregnancy, malignancy, chronic obstructive pulmonary disease or obesity.

Anatomy
The sac protrudes through a defect in the linea alba near the umbilical cicatrix but, unlike the true umbilical hernia, not through the cicatrix itself. Progressively increases in size. Usually contains just omentum but may contain transverse colon and sometimes small intestine. The neck of the sac is often very narrow compared with the sac contents and very fibrous. Contents adhere to one another, the coverings and the omentum.

Coverings
Skin, superficial fascia, rectus sheath, transversalis fascia and sac. These stretch and fuse into a thin membrane, through which peristalsis may be seen.

Complications
Redness, excoriation, ulceration, gangrene, becoming pendulous, infection, faecal fistula, strangulation, incarceration and obstruction.

Clinical features
Usually irreducible. May present with pain due to incarceration and subacute obstruction. Strangulation is common due to narrow neck.

Difficulties with surgical repair
This may have significant mortality in old patients with large hernias. Problems include:
- Patients tend to be old with co-morbidity
- High risk of strangulation
- Difficult anatomy and reduction
- May have increased intra-abdominal pressure after reduction, which exacerbates respiratory problems. Pre-operative weight loss and chest physiotherapy may help.

Techniques of surgical repair
Mayo's operation 'vest over pants' – lower edge of rectus (pants) is brought up and fixed by non-absorbable sutures to behind the upper flap.
Mesh repair – especially useful if there is tissue loss.

Umbilical hernias
Incidence
- 3% neonates have umbilical hernias, most resolve spontaneously
- 3:1000 live births need further surgery
- More common in negro children

Anatomy
Peritoneal sac penetrates through linea alba at umbilical cicatrix to lie in subcutaneous tissues between skin cicatrix. There is a narrow rigid neck at the aponeurosis.

Prognosis
- All decrease in size as child grows
- Few persist after puberty
- Some cause disfigurement or incarcerate
- Only a minority need an operation
- Must preserve the umbilicus to avoid stigmatising child
- Similar Mayo 'vest over pants' repair to adult repair (see above); Absorbable polymer used.

PARAUMBILICAL HERNIA[92]

Spot diagnosis or may be found during examination of the abdomen (see pg 339).

'There is (in this obese, middle-aged woman) a non-tender reducible lump with an expansile cough impulse adjacent to the umbilicus. The umbilicus is pushed to one side and is stretched into a characteristic crescent shape. The lump is about 3cm in diameter and there is a fingertip-sized defect felt in the linea alba after it is reduced. This is a paraumbilical hernia. As strangulation is relatively common in these small-necked hernias, I would suggest surgical repair if the patient is fit. If the hernia is symptomatic, irreducible or has appeared recently, repair should be prompt.'

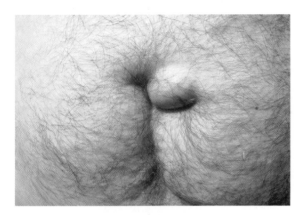

Paraumbilical hernia

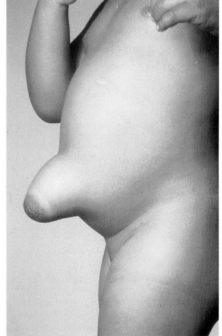

Congenital 'true' umbilical hernia in an infant

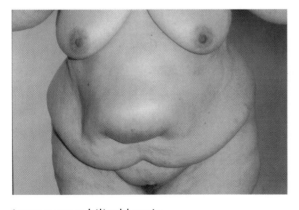

Large paraumbilical hernia

EPIGASTRIC HERNIA[93]

Examination of a lump (see pg 29) or may be found during examination of abdomen (see pg 339).

'There is (in this young male patient) a small firm non-tender lump in the epigastrium[94]. It is irreducible, with no cough impulse. This is a likely epigastric hernia but the differential diagnosis is a lipoma.'

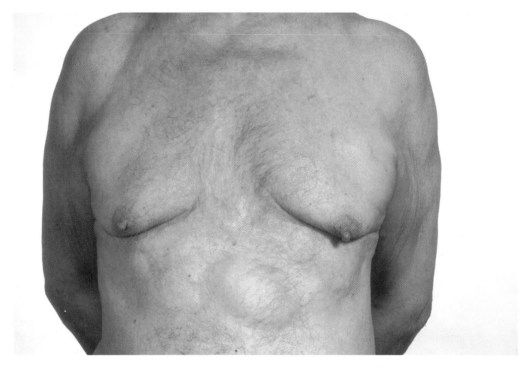

Epigastric hernia

---

[93] This is a protrusion of extra-peritoneal fat or peritoneum through one of the lozenge-shaped fissures commonly found between the latticed fibres of the linea alba. Epigastric hernias can occur in children or adults and may cause disproportionate epigastric pain and upper gastro-intestinal symptoms. They are cured by excision of sac and repair of linea alba. 30% have co-existing intra-abdominal disease causing symptoms and so should be fully investigated.

Stop here if you are pretty sure this is what it is or if you have been given any hints e.g. 'This man has been complaining of pain after eating'. However, in the absence of hints it is often impossible to differentiate an epigastric hernia from a lipoma, as they are often irreducible and have no cough impulse due to their small neck. An ultrasound scan would differentiate the two.

[94] Or in the line of the linea alba anywhere from umbilicus to xiphisternum.

SPIGELIAN HERNIA[95]

Carry out examination of a lump (see pg 29).

'There is a diffuse swelling at the lateral border of the left rectus muscle. Although not acutely tender, the patient reports it as an aching lump. It is/is not reducible, arises from the deep tissues and the skin moves over it freely. There is no superficial bruising overlying the lump. This is likely to be a Spigelian hernia, but the differential diagnosis is a rectus sheath haematoma.'

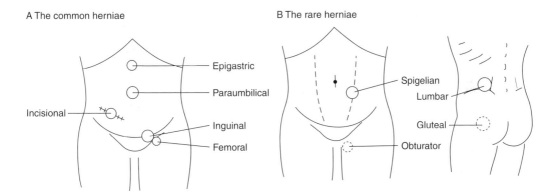

A The common herniae — Epigastric, Paraumbilical, Incisional, Inguinal, Femoral

B The rare herniae — Spigelian, Lumbar, Gluteal, Obturator

Sites of hernias (A) Common (B) Rare

---

[95] **Spigelian hernia**
These are also known as **semilunar line hernias** and account for 1% of abdominal hernias. The hernia protrudes through bands of internal oblique muscle as it enters the semilunar line. Most occur below the umbilicus adjacent to line of Douglas. It is usually deflected laterally by the external oblique and can be found near the iliac crest. The sac may enter rectus sheath and be confused with rectus muscle haematoma. They are more common in women than men. They present as an aching lump and are diagnosed by ultrasound scan. They may strangulate. Repair is by excision of peritoneal sac and closure of the aponeurotic defect.
Other rare hernias
Lumbar hernia
These tend to occur after renal operations, lumbar abscesses or paralysis of lateral lumbar muscles by poliomyelitis or spina bifida. Spontaneous lumbar hernias occur through the lumbar triangle of Petit (formed by the iliac crest, posterior external oblique and anterior latissimus dorsi) or the quadrilateral lumbar space (formed by the 12th rib, lower border of serratus posterior inferior, anterior border of erector spinae and internal oblique).
Gluteal hernia emerges through greater sciatic notch.
Obturator hernia emerges through obturator foramen.
Sciatic hernia emerges through lesser sciatic notch.

[96] **Hydrocoele**

Scrotum was a Top Five Case: seen by nearly a third of candidates in our survey. Accounted for 13% of cases in this bay. In particular the hydrocoele was a very common case and was seen by a quarter of the candidates in our survey.

Definition

A hydrocoele is an abnormal quantity of serous fluid within the tunica vaginalis.

The most common type is the vaginal hydrocoele which the processus vaginalis is obliterated and the fluid collects only around the testicle. Thus the cord structures can be felt above the swelling, and the testicle cannot be felt separately.

Also common (but not seen so often in exams) is the congenital hydrocoele, seen in infants, where the hydrocoele communicates with the peritoneal cavity due to a patent processus vaginalis. They usually resolve within the first 6–12 months of life, but need surgery if they persist after a year.

An infantile hydrocoele is rare and involves the processus vaginalis being obliterated at or near the deep inguinal ring, but remaining patent in the cord and the scrotum. Thus fluid collects around the cord as well as around the testicle. In an infantile hydrocoele the cord cannot be palpated above the testicle, and it may therefore be confused with an inguinoscrotal hernia.

A hydrocoele of the cord is also rare and is a type of infantile hydrocoele where the fluid collection is restricted to the cord. Thus unlike all the other types of hydrocoele, the testicle can be felt separately (hydrocoele of the cord is known as the 'third testis' as is an epididimal cyst). This can also be mistaken for a hernia.

Causes

Primary hydrocoele: (Appears gradually and becomes large and tense; occur in children or elderly.)
Idiopathic

Secondary hydrocoele: (Appears rapidly in the presence of other symptoms, are not tense and often contain some altered blood. Occur most commonly between age 20 and 40.)
Trauma
Epididymo-orchitis
Tumour
Lymphatic obstruction

Management

Exclude tumour: Testicular tumours can present as hydrocoeles, so initially investigations are geared towards excluding tumour as an underlying cause. In the past aspirating the hydrocoele in order to palpate the testicle was considered reasonable; now this is absolutely contraindicated as it may seed the tumour to the scrotal skin. Ultrasound imaging is the minimum investigation. Hydrocoeles which arise suddenly in young men are particularly suspicious.

Jaboulay's procedure: Sac incised longitudinally, everted and approximated behind the cord.

Lord's operation: Small incision through the scrotum and tunica allowing the testicle to be lifted from the sac and the scrotum. The sac is then plicated to the junction of the testis and epididymis.

Postoperative complications

Recurrence
Haematoma
Infection

HYDROCOELE[96]

Carry out examination of the groin (see pg 349).

'There is (in this middle-aged/elderly man) a large non-tender swelling filling the left scrotum. I can feel the cord above the swelling, but I cannot feel the testicle separate from the lump. It is brilliantly transilluminable, fluctuant and dull to percussion. The surface is smooth and well-defined and the consistency is tense/lax. The skin of the scrotum is freely mobile over the swelling. This is a vaginal hydrocoele. An abdominal examination and scrotal ultrasound are important to exclude an underlying cause.'

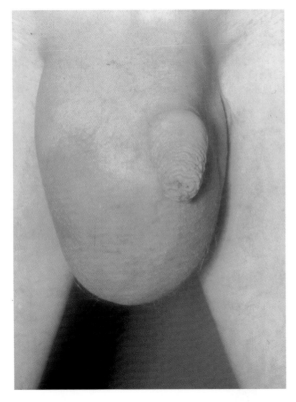

Right hydrocoele

Other causes of intrascrotal swelling:

<u>Acute epididymitis</u>
Chlamydia the commonest cause, followed by gonorrhoea, presenting between 18 and 35 years of age.
Adults over 35 are most commonly affected by *E. coli* secondary to urinary outflow obstruction.
Other causes include smallpox, chickenpox, *E. coli* in children.
In the early stages a swollen tender epididymis lies behind a normal testis. Later, generalised tenderness, oedema, congestion and reactive hydrocoele can make it impossible to differentiate from torsion.
Treatment is by antibiotics.

<u>Chronic epididymitis</u>
Usually due to tuberculosis, but can be caused by sarcoidosis, coccidioidomycosis and unresolved acute epididymitis (see above). Tuberculous epididymitis usually presents as a painless hard nodule separate from the testicle, but if it caseates it can envelop the testicle and cause a secondary hydrocoele. Ulceration through the scrotum may occur. Antituberculous medical therapy may resolve this, if not, an epididectomy may be necessary.

<u>Torsion of the testicle</u>
Unlikely to feature in an exam. Acutely tender, high riding testicle with thickened cord +/– a secondary hydrocoele.

<u>Haematocoele</u>
Collection of blood within the tunica vaginalis, usually caused by trauma or underlying malignant disease. The swelling has the same clinical features as a hydrocoele, except it is not transilluminable and may be tender.
Chronic haematocoeles become hard and non tender and may be mistaken for a testicular tumour (see pg XX)

<u>Gumma of the testis</u>
This is due to syphilis is rare and causes a hard, insensate, enlarged 'billiard ball' testis.

<u>Orchitis</u>
Acute orchitis in the absence of epididymitis is invariably due to a viral infection, usually mumps.

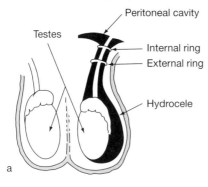
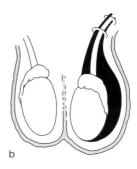
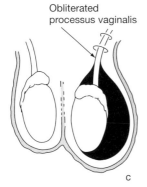
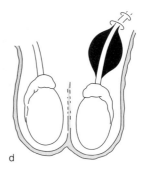

Hydrocoele: 4 types
    a) Congenital hydrocoele   b) Infantile hydrocoele
    c) Vaginal hydrocoele   d) Hydrocoele of the cord (see pg 374)

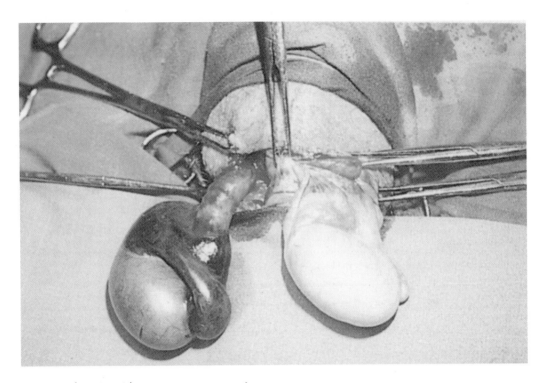

Torsion of testis with gangrene at operation

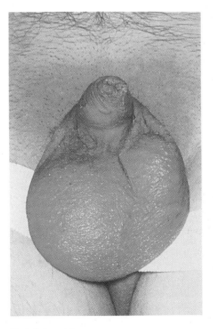

Epididymitis

[97] **Epididymal cyst**

Definition: Fluid filled swellings connected with the epididymis. May be a <u>true epididymal cyst</u> containing clear fluid or a <u>spermatocoele</u> containing grey, opaque fluid with spermatozoa. Since these are difficult to distinguish, they tend to both be called epididymal cysts.

Symptoms: Commonly occur in men over 40. Usually an asymptomatic swelling which appears like a 'third testicle'. They enlarge slowly, over years are often multiple and may be bilateral. May develop pain or discomfort.

Treatment: Conservative especially in young men as surgery can disrupt sperm transport and reduce fertility. Cyst enucleation can be done in older patients, and epididectomy is necessary occasionally to avoid operating on frequent recurrences.

[98] Varies from a few millimetres to over 10 cm in diameter.

EPIDIDYMAL CYST[97]

Carry out examination of groin, (see pg 349).

'There is a non-tender swelling in the right scrotum. It is 4 cm in diameter[98], ovoid in shape with a well-defined, smooth but bosselated surface. It is firm, fluctuant, dull to percussion and brilliantly transilluminable. It is separate to the testicle and lies above it and behind the cord structures. The cord structures can be felt above the mass, and it is not reducible. This is an epididymal cyst. I would like to examine the other side.'

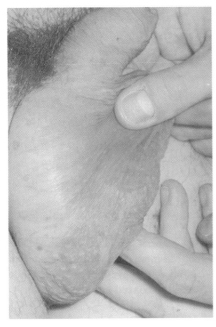

Epididymal cyst. A mass is felt in the scrotum above and separate to the normal sized testicle

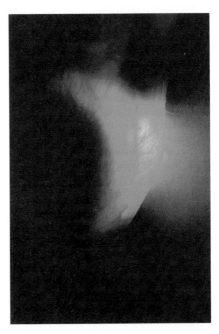

Epididymal cyst. The mass but not the whole scrotum transilluminates

[99] **Varicocoele**

Definition: A bunch of dilated and tortuous veins in the pampiniform plexus (ie varicose veins of the spermatic cord)

Symptoms: Occur in 25% of normal young men, usually unnoticed. Can if large, cause a vague dragging sensation and aching pain in the scrotum or groin, and will cause that scrotum to hang lower than the other side. The testis below a large varicocoele may be a little smaller and softer than the testis on the other side, and bilateral varicocoeles may be associated with subfertility.

The sudden appearance of a varicocoele in a middle-aged or old man raises the suspicion of retroperitoneal disease.

Varicocoele repair:

Scrotal approach: rarely used because you can't be sure you've ligated all the veins.

Retroperitoneal approach: incision above the anterior superior iliac spine, testicular artery and veins identified, veins divided and ligated.

Inguinal approach: more difficult to identify testicular artery.

Embolisation: by sclerosing solutions or balloon catheter (risk of PE).

Post-operative complications:

Recurrence (via obturator collaterals).

Harder, more prominent varices until thrombus organises.

Hydrocoele formation.

[100] 98% of varicocoeles occur on the left because:

1. The left spermatic vein forms a more vertical angle with the left renal vein than the right does when it enters the vena cava.

2. The left renal vein is crossed by and may be compressed by the pelvic colon.

3. The left testicular vein is longer than the right.

4. The terminal venous valve is frequently absent on the left side.

VARICOCOELE[99]

Carry out examination of the groin (see pg 349).

'There is (in this young man) a mass in the left scrotum[100]. It is a soft, irregularly shaped mass, above the testicle which can be felt separately. The cord structures can be felt around and through the swellings, which have the texture of the characteristic 'bag of worms'. The mass is compressible, enlarges and becomes firmer when the patient leans forward, and disappears when the patient lies down. It does not transilluminate. This is a varicocoele, common and usually asymptomatic in young men, but needing investigation if it appears suddenly in middle or old age.'

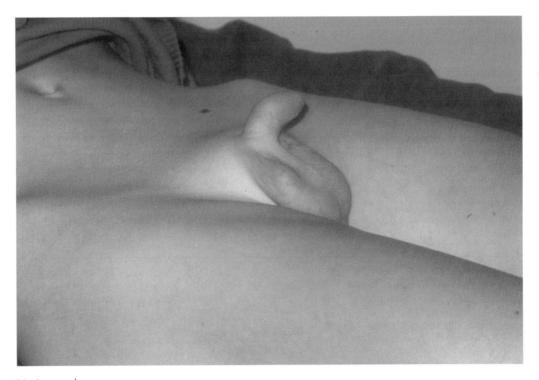

Varicocoele

Testicular tumour
[101] Testicular cancer

Epidemiology: Commonest solid tumour in young males, peaking at 25–35 years with a later peak over 60. Commoner in Caucasians.

Aetiology/Predisposing factors
Family history
Cryptorchidism (undescended or maldescent)
Cryptorchidism in the opposite testicle (10%)
Trauma
Mumps
Higher socio-economic group

Types of testicular cancer
Seminoma
Nonseminomatous germ cell tumours (NSGCTs)
 Embryonal cell carcinoma
 Teratoma
 Choriocarcinoma (<1% of testicular tumours)
 Mixed cell tumour

All except choriocarcinoma show slow regional lymphatic spread to the paraaortic nodes, usually to the same side, although right testicular cancers may occasionally spread to the left paraaortic nodes.
Choriocarcinoma shows early haematological spread.

Staging
TNM (in the US) or Royal Marsden Hospital system (in the UK)

Royal Marsden Staging System	5yr Survival rate (%)	
	Seminoma	NSGCTs
I-tumour confined to the testis	100	100
II- abdominal lymph node involvement (<2cm, 2–5cm, >5cm diameter)	93	95
III-lymph nodes above the diaphragm involved	90	
IV- extralymphatic or visceral metastases		} 65

Symptoms
Painless mass in scrotum with dragging sensation, gynaecomastia, haemoptysis (if pulmonary involvement)

Tumour markers
Serum alpha fetoprotein (AFP) -increased with NSGCTs but never with seminomas
Human chorionic gonadotrophin (HCG) -increased with NSGCTs but only in 7% of seminomas
Other tumour markers include lactate dehydrogenase, placental alkaline phosphatase and gamma glutamyl transpeptidase.

Management
NEVER ASPIRATE OR TRUCUT the mass as this risks scrotal skin seeding.
Chest X-ray: shows 90% of pulmonary metastases.
CT abdomen: reveals retroperitoneal lymphadenopathy.
Exploratory surgery: Clinical diagnosis of testicular neoplasm indicates orchidectomy through an inguinal incision.
Principles of surgery include:
 Early cross-clamping of the cord to avoid proximal haematological and lymphatic spread on handling the testicle.
 Avoidance of scrotal incision to prevent seeding of tumour cells into scrotal skin.

TESTICULAR TUMOUR[101]

Carry out examination of groins (see pg 349).

'There is a firm, non-tender mass in the left scrotum. The testicle cannot be felt separately, but the epididymis can. The mass is not transilluminable (although there may be an associated hydrocoele). The diagnosis is of a testicular mass[102]. I would like to examine the opposite scrotum and the abdomen and supraclavicular area for lymphadenopathy[103].'

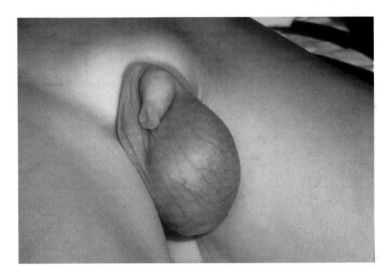

Left testicular tumour

Seminoma
Radiosensitive. Chemosensitive
Radical orchidectomy and retroperitoneal irradiation is the mainstay of treatment
Stage IIc, III and IV adjuvant combination chemotherapy usually involving cysplatin, bleomycin and vinblastine or etoposide.
NSGCTs
Stage I: radical orchidectomy and close follow-up.
Stage II and above: radical orchidectomy and adjuvant chemotherapy as described for seminomas above.
Residual abdominal retroperitoneal mass on CT after treatment: radical lymph node dissection.
Retroperitoneal lymph node dissection is controversial
Advantages: Allows accurate staging of patients
Disadvantages: High morbidity and complications e.g. retrograde ejaculation and infertility
                 Up to 1/3 of resected masses are fibrotic with no signs of residual or recurrent tumour.
[102] To prevent distress or misunderstanding, beware saying 'tumour', 'carcinoma' or 'cancer' in front of the patient. If pressed, say you would be concerned to exclude a malignancy or a neoplastic process, unless you are out of earshot of the patient.
[103] Abdominal nodes, being retroperitoneal, are rarely palpable. Gynaecomastia may occur. Haemoptysis is a sign of pulmonary metastases.

Absent testicle

[104] This could be due to previous exploration or attempted (and failed) orchidopexy in an undescended testicle. Alternatively it could be the scar of the orchidectomy after trauma, tumour or torsion.

[105] Management of the apparently missing testicle in a child

1. Is it retractile rather than truly missing?
Parents report seeing it during bath-time
Scrotum normally developed
Testicle can be felt in the inguinal canal and coaxed into the scrotum on examination
No further intervention is needed – testicle likely to descend normally by puberty. Follow up to check.
2. Is it undescended in the normal line of descent? (86%)
These carry increased risk of torsion, malignancy, decreased sperm production and concern to the child. Therefore these should be replaced in the scrotum (orchidopexy) in early childhood ('2 in the bag by the age of 2'). 80% of undescended testicles are palpable and for these, the treatment is orchidopexy. 20% of undescended testicles are impalpable and of these a third are absent, a third are in the canal and a third are intraabdominal. Laparoscopy is the investigation of choice.
Since surgery is always indicated, investigations such as ultrasound (unreliable), MRI and CT (Need anaesthetic) and laparoscopy (two thirds are unnecessary and leads to open surgery) are not indicated. Alternatively, open exploration is via a high inguinal incision allowing first the inguinal canal, then the abdominal cavity to be explored.
If a testis is located and is dysplastic it must be removed. If normal it must be replaced in the scrotum. Testicular biopsy is not indicated. Cord length is a limitation in orchidopexy, and a two-stage approach may be needed. Alternatively, the Fowler Stephen's procedure is ligation of the testicular vessels leaving the testicle dependent upon collateral supply to the vas deferens. The orchidopexy is carried out later, but success rates are about 50%. Free transfer with microvascular anastomosis is also possible.
3. Is it maldescended or ectopic? (not in the normal line of descent – see fig below (2%)
Management is as for undescended testicle.

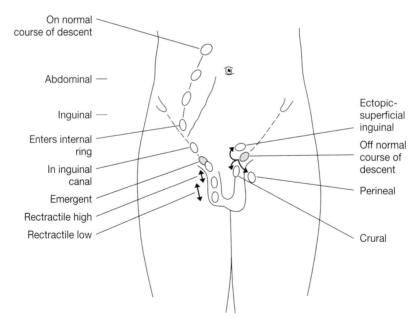

Ectopic positions possible for an incompletely descended or maldescended testicle

ABSENT TESTICLE

Carry out examination of the groin (see pg 349).

Case 1

'There is (in this middle-aged/elderly man), a bilaterally empty scrotum with no evidence of either testicle. There is no evidence of an ectopic or undescended testicle, the scrotum is normally developed, and there is a groin/scrotal scar. This patient has had bilateral orchidectomy, the commonest indication being metastatic prostatic carcinoma.'

Case 2

There is (in this child/young man), an empty, underdeveloped scrotum on the left with a normal testicle on the right. There is/is no evidence of the left testicle in the line of descent of the testicle or in any of the normal sites for an ectopic testicle. There is a groin scar on the left[104]. The differential diagnosis in this patient is an undescended testicle or a unilateral orchidectomy, most commonly the result of trauma, torsion or testicular cancer. The underdeveloped scrotum suggests that this is an undescended testicle[105].

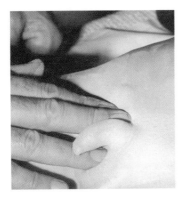 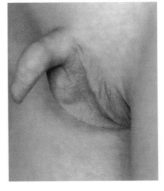 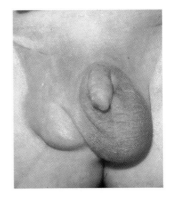

Undescended testicle
This 7-year-old boy had a normally placed left testicle, an empty right scrotum and a bulge in the right groin (seen above the Examiner's index finger) which could not be coaxed into the scrotum

Retractile testicle
The right testicle is normally placed, and the left testicle can be seen at the top of the empty right hemi-scrotum emerging from the superficial ring. It could be coaxed into the scrotum

Ectopic/maldescended testicle
The right testicle is abnormally located in the perineum

[107] **Ileostomy**

The ileostomy was a common case and was seen by over 1 in 20 of the candidates surveyed.

Indications

- **Temporary**: to protect an ileorectal anastomosis; persistent low intestinal fistula; right-sided colonic trauma; preliminary to construction of ileo-anal reservoir
- **Permanent**: panproctocolectomy for: ulcerative colitis; severe Crohn's disease; familial polyposis coli; multiple colonic cancer

Forming an ileostomy

Usually in the right iliac fossa. A circular skin defect 2–3 cm in diameter is excised. A cruciate (trephine) incision is made in the underlying rectus. The peritoneum is incised. The clamped ileum is passed through the incision in the peritoneum. A peritoneal tunnel lessens the risk of herniation and prolapse. The main abdominal wound is closed and dressed. The intestinal clamp is then removed. A 4–5 cm spout is formed by everting the stump and suturing the mucosa to the skin with interrupted absorbable sutures. A bite of the serosa is taken a few cm proximal to the stump with each stitch to evert the stoma. (NB. 500ml/day of high enzyme content fluid is lost from a low output ileostomy. One litre per day in a high output ileostomy.)

[108] There may have been previous operations leaving stomata which have now been closed.

Example 1: a colitic might have a subtotal colectomy leaving a mucous fistula and an end ileostomy. Problems with the rectal stump may lead to a completion proctectomy, leaving an end ileostomy and a scar in the left iliac fossa where the mucous fistula was.

Example 2: a patient with a low rectal cancer might have an abdominoperineal resection, leaving a colostomy. Subsequently if he developed another tumour in the right colon he might proceed to a completion colectomy leaving an end ileostomy with a scar in the left iliac fossa at the site of the previous colostomy.

[109] Surgeons often leave a loop ileostomy to protect delayed reconstructive procedure.

Example 1: a patient with ulcerative colitis has an emergency left hemicolectomy and an end colostomy. Later when things have settled down his colon is rejoined with a low left sided anastomosis. At this operation the surgeon elects to defunction the bowel with a loop ileostomy, planning to close it after the anastomosis has healed. In the meantime the patient would have a right sided loop ileostomy with a scar where the old colostomy used to be.

Example 2: A perforated left sided colonic cancer is treated with an emergency Hartmann's procedure leaving a colostomy. At a later date the Hartmann's procedure is reversed (the colon is rejoined to the rectal stump). At this operation the surgeon elects to defunction the bowel with a loop ileostomy, planning to close it after the anastomosis has healed. In the meantime the patient would have a left-sided loop ileostomy with a scar in the right iliac fossa where the old colostomy used to be.

ILEOSTOMY[107]

Spot diagnosis or examination of abdomen (see pg 339) or stoma (see pg 353).

Case 1

'There is a stoma in the right iliac fossa. There is one lumen which is small in calibre. There is a 2–3 cm spout and the contents of the bag are green and fluid. There is a midline scar and there are/and there are no scars of other, previous stomata in the left iliac fossa[108]. This is an end ileostomy, most commonly performed after panproctocolectomy for ulcerative colitis, familial polyposis coli or multiple colonic cancer. I would like to know if this patient has an anal orifice and rectal stump (in which case reconstruction may be planned) or a perineal scar (in which case this is a permanent end ileostomy).'

Case 2

'There is a stoma in the right iliac fossa. There are two lumens, both of small calibre, the lower of which has a spout. The contents of the bag are green and fluid. There is a midline scar and there are/are no scars of other, previous stomata in the left iliac fossa[109]. This is a loop ileostomy, most commonly formed to achieve temporary diversion to protect a distal anastomosis, a low intestinal fistula, achieve bowel rest in severe inflammatory disease or preliminary to construction of an ileo-anal reservoir.'

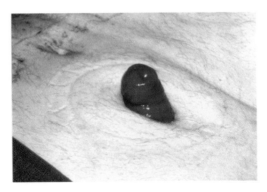

End ileostomy in right iliac fossa with a spout

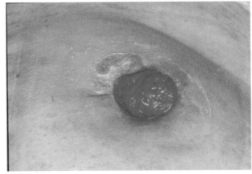

Ileostomy with some para-stomal excoriation

¹¹⁰ **Colostomy**

The colostomy was a common case and was seen by over 1 in 20 of the candidates surveyed.

Indications

- **Temporary**: to protect distal anastomosis; to achieve bowel rest (e.g. for perineal Crohn's); if primary anastomosis is not possible after resection (e.g. in the presence of perforation, sepsis, ischaemia or obstruction)
- **Permanent**: after abdomino-perineal resection for low rectal tumours

Types of colostomy

- **Loop colostomy**: used for diversion; not resection; usually in right transverse colon, proximal to the middle colic artery; a colostomy bridge is passed around loop of colon through small avascular window in mesocolon; loop is brought out through the abdominal wall incision; the bridge is secured, laparotomy wound (if present) closed then stoma opened and formed.
- **End colostomy and rectal stump (Hartmann's procedure)**: if a primary anastomosis is contraindicated; after resection, colostomy is brought out using the proximal end of colon; the distal end (usually rectal stump) is oversewn and left in the abdomen. This is difficult to rejoin later, as the rectal stump is hard to find.
- **End colostomy and mucous fistula**: used in similar circumstances to a Hartmann's but instead of dropping the rectal stump back into the abdomen, it is brought out as a separate stoma which, being an efferent limb, only produces mucus. This makes the distal limb more accessible when the bowel is rejoined later.
- **Double-barrelled colostomy**: used after resection when both limbs of the stoma can be brought to the skin surface adjacent to each other (e.g. mid-sigmoid perforation or volvulus). After resection, the proximal and distal limbs of the colon are sutured together along antimesenteric border. This is as easy to close as a loop colostomy at a later date.
- **Closure of colostomies**: best left for six weeks until inflammation and oedema have settled, so minimising the risk of a leak. After 10–12 weeks, mobilisation of the bowel may become more difficult because of fibrous adhesion formation.
- **Output of colostomies**: mid-transverse colon- 200–300 ml/day, significant enzyme content; low colostomy- 100 ml/day, virtually no enzyme.

Alternative methods of colostomy management

- **Irrigation**: flushing fluid into colon via stoma (no appliance needed); patient needs suitable bathroom facilities; not satisfactory for Crohn's.
- **Colostomy plug**: foam plug which clips to a flange; plug fills lumen and blocks bowel for 8–12 hours.

¹¹¹ Typically after abdominoperineal resection of a low rectal tumour.

¹¹² Typically after a Hartmann's procedure where primary anastomosis was contraindicated due to sepsis or peritonitis.

¹¹³ In which case reconstruction may be planned.

¹¹⁴ In which case this is a permanent end colostomy.

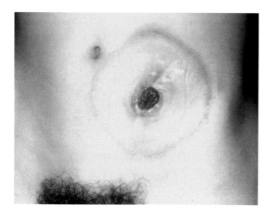

End colostomy in left iliac fossa

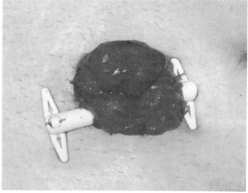

Defunctioning loop colostomy in the right iliac fossa with bridge (usually removed 7–10 days post-operatively)

COLOSTOMY[110]

Spot diagnosis or examination of abdomen (see pg 339) or stoma (see pg 353).

Case 1

'There is a stoma in the left iliac fossa. There is one lumen which is large in calibre. There is no spout and the contents of the bag are brown and semi-solid. There is a midline scar and there are/are no scars of other, previous stomata in the right iliac fossa. This is a colostomy, which may be permanent[111] or temporary[112]. I would like to know if this patient has an anal orifice and rectal stump[113] or a perineal scar[114].'

Case 2

'There are two stomata in the left iliac fossa. One has the typical appearance of a colostomy (large lumen, no spout, brown semisolid bag contents) and the other has the typical appearance of a mucus fistula (large lumen, no spout, no bag, dry and recessed). There is a midline scar. This patient has had a large bowel resection during which primary anastomosis was contraindicated, and a mucus fistula was formed from the rectal stump to facilitate future reconstruction.'

Case 3

'There is a stoma in the left or right iliac fossa or in the epigastrium of the abdomen. There are two adjacent large calibre lumens and no spout, and there are brown semisolid products in the bag. This is a loop colostomy, which is usually used for diversion rather than resection. It is often sited in the right transverse colon, proximal to the middle colic artery, but can also be formed from the sigmoid colon. Indications include decompression of an emergency obstruction, prophylactic decompression before radiotherapy of a stenosing rectal tumour, or alleviation of obstructive symptoms in a patient not fit for major surgery.'

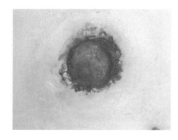

Necrosis

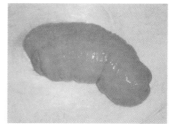

Prolapsed stoma

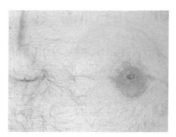

Stenosed stoma

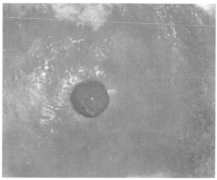

Peristomal rash

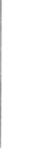

Parastomal hernia

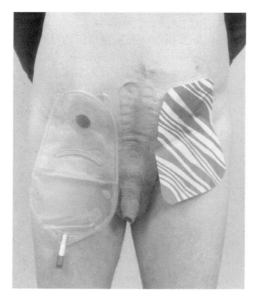

Ileal conduit (on the right) and colostomy
(on the left) after pelvic clearance

UROSTOMY[115]

Spot diagnosis or examination of abdomen (see pg 339) or stoma (see pg 353).

Case 1
'There is a small stoma in the right iliac fossa. It has no spout, a single lumen, no evidence of a bag, no discharge, and there is a catheterisation kit lying next to the patient. This is a continent urinary stoma, usually formed by the Mitrofanoff method.'

Case 2
'There is a stoma in the right iliac fossa. It has a spout, a small calibre, a single lumen, and there is urine in the bag. This is an ileal conduit.'

Case 3
'There is a catheter running from a stoma in the suprapubic region to a bag of urine. This is a suprapubic urinary catheter.'

---

[115] **Urostomy**
Principle of urinary diversion:
Ureters are attached to the ileum and a conduit is created to the outside.
Techniques available include:
Urethral closure with a Mitrofanoff. The Mitrofanoff is the commonest procedure for creating a continent pouch, where the appendix is used to create a continent valve. The ileum and sigmoid colon have also been used. Intermittent self-catheterisation is required to empty the pouch, and the stoma is placed in a position that allows comfortable self-catheterisation.
Neobladder formed from ileum with Mitrofanoff diversion or indwelling suprapubic catheter.
Formation of a neourethra using a segment of bladder to provide a catheterisable conduit just above the pubic symphysis
Ileal conduit, which is an incontinent pouch that requires a bag to collect the urine. Early pouches were incontinent, attaching the ileum, ureters or bladder to the abdominal surface with closure or excision of the bladder.

Percutaneous endoscopic gastrostomy (PEG)

[116] **Gastrostomies**

Can be used for either gastric decompression or feeding.

Percutaneous Endoscopic Gastrotomy

This is the method of choice.

Indications

Feeding in patients with neurological impairment, oropharyngeal tumours or facial trauma.

Gastric decompression in patients with carcinomatosis, radiation enteritis or diabetic gastropathy obstruction.

To supplement nutrition in inflammatory bowel disease.

To establish a route for recycling bile in those with malignant biliary obstruction.

Procedure (see opposite)

After passing the endoscope, the anterior abdominal wall is transilluminated.

The abdominal wall is indented with the finger and the indentation observed from inside to select the insertion site.

After infiltration with local anaesthetic, a needle is passed through the abdominal wall into the lumen of the stomach.

A wire is passed through the needle and grabbed by a snare passed through the endoscope.

The endoscope is withdrawn with the snare and the wire until the wire comes out of the mouth.

The wire is then attached to the gastrostomy tube and pulled in a retrograde manner down the oesophagus, into the stomach and out of the abdominal wall where it is secured.

The position is checked by endoscopy.

Open gastrostomy

If the passage of an endoscope is prevented by tumour or stricture, an open procedure such as the Stamm gastrostomy is performed. This involves an upper midline laparotomy incision and insertion through a gastrostomy of a Malecot or mushroom catheter. The catheter is brought out of a stab incision in the left hypochondrium. The stomach is then sutured to the inside of the anterior abdominal wall.

Jejunostomy

This is often used after major upper gastrointestinal surgery as it enables nutrition to be infused at the jejunal level, and avoids gastric stasis. Many techniques are available, the commonest being the Witzel jejunostomy. In this (open) method, the jejunostomy is sited 30cm distal to the ligament of Treitz on the antimesenteric border. The catheter is fastened at the point of entry through the mucosa and then tunnelled in a seromuscular groove. The tunnel is closed and the jejunostomy sutured to the anterior abdominal wall.

PERCUTANEOUS ENDOSCOPIC GASTROSTOMY (PEG)[116]

Spot diagnosis.

'There is a feeding tube attached to a bag of enteral nutrition entering the epigastrium. This is a feeding gastrostomy, probably performed percutaneously with endoscopic assistance (PEG).'

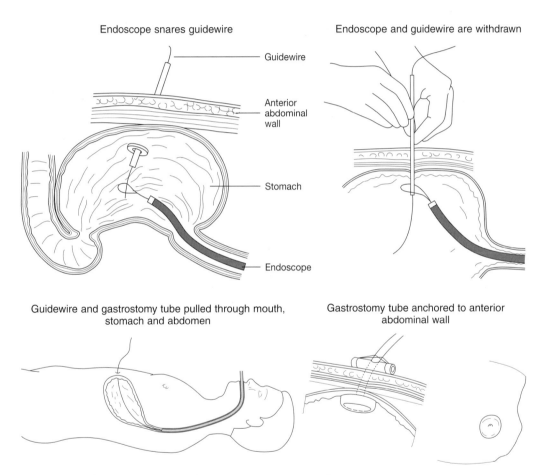

Placement of percutaneous endoscopic gastrostomy tube

393

An abdominal mass

[117] Abdominal mass (not including liver, spleen or kidney) was a very common case: seen by over 1 in 10 of the candidates in our survey.

Solid tumours which may cause generalised abdominal distension

Hepatomegaly

Splenomegaly

Pancreatic carcinoma

Retroperitoneal lymphadenopathy

Retroperitoneal sarcoma

Nephroblastoma (in children)

Fibroids

Large colon cancers

Polycystic kidneys

Carcinoma of kidneyCarcinoma of liver Perinephric abscess

Ganglioneuroma (in children)

AN ABDOMINAL MASS

Carry out examination of abdomen (see pg 339).

Common abdominal masses are summarised in the diagram below.
When examining an abdominal mass, note the following:
> Position
> Shape
> Surface
> Edge
> Composition (consistency, fluctuation, fluid thrill)
> Resonance
> Pulsatility
> Tenderness
> Association with enlargement of palpable organs.

The traditional 'six F's' is a useful list of common causes of generalised distension:
Foetus, Flatus, Faeces, Fat, Fluid (free or encysted), and Fibroids and other solid
tumours[117].

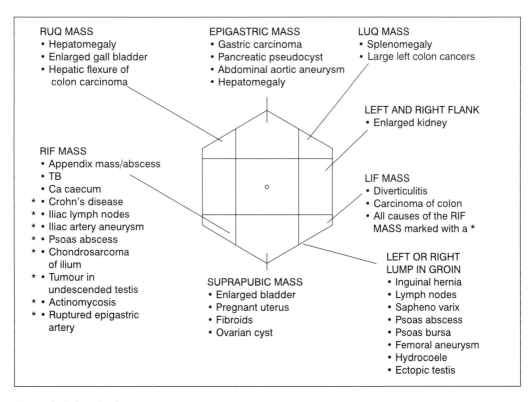

RUQ MASS
• Hepatomegaly
• Enlarged gall bladder
• Hepatic flexure of
  colon carcinoma

EPIGASTRIC MASS
• Gastric carcinoma
• Pancreatic pseudocyst
• Abdominal aortic aneurysm
• Hepatomegaly

LUQ MASS
• Splenomegaly
• Large left colon cancers

LEFT AND RIGHT FLANK
• Enlarged kidney

RIF MASS
• Appendix mass/abscess
• TB
• Ca caecum
* • Crohn's disease
* • Iliac lymph nodes
* • Iliac artery aneurysm
* • Psoas abscess
* • Chondrosarcoma
    of ilium
* • Tumour in
    undescended testis
* • Actinomycosis
* • Ruptured epigastric
    artery

LIF MASS
• Diverticulitis
• Carcinoma of colon
• All causes of the RIF
  MASS marked with a *

SUPRAPUBIC MASS
• Enlarged bladder
• Pregnant uterus
• Fibroids
• Ovarian cyst

LEFT OR RIGHT
LUMP IN GROIN
• Inguinal hernia
• Lymph nodes
• Sapheno varix
• Psoas abscess
• Psoas bursa
• Femoral aneurysm
• Hydrocoele
• Ectopic testis

Sites of abdominal mass

Jaundice

Liver disease was a Top Five Case: seen by over a fifth of the candidates in our survey. Accounted for 8.6% of the cases in this bay. Jaundice alone was a very common case and was seen by over one in 10 of the candidates in our survey.

[118] **Classification of jaundice**

	Pre-hepatic	Hepatic jaundice	Post-hepatic (obstructive) jaundice*

Causes	Spherocytosis
	Haemolytic anaemia
	Pernicious anaemia
	Incompatible blood
	  transfusion
		Hepatitis
		Cirrhosis
		Drugs
		Toxins (e.g.
		  phosphorus,
		  chloroform)
		Liver tumours
		  (primary or
		  secondary)
			Obstruction in the lumen-gallstones
			Obstruction in the wall- atresia, traumatic
			  stricture, tumour of bile duct, chronic
			  cholangitis, sclerosing cholangitis
			External compression- pancreatitis, tumour of
			  pancreas

Jaundice	Mild jaundice
	Bilirubin rarely
	  >100 mmol/l
	  unconjugated
		Variable jaundice
		May be conjugated
		  or unconjugated
			Variable jaundice
			Bilirubin may exceed 1000 mmol/l conjugated

Urine	Normal colour Bilirubin not present Urobilinogen raised	Dark Bilirubin may be present	Dark Bilirubin present
Stool	Normal colour Increased urobilinogen	Normal colour	Pale stools Stercobilinogen down
Alkaline Phosphatase	Normal	Mildly raised Very high in 1° biliary cirrhosis	Very high

Amino Transferases	Normal	Typically very high
		  especially in acute
		  viral hepatitis or
		  cirrhosis
			Normal or moderately raised

Prothrombin time	Normal	Prolonged and not
		  correctable with
		  vitamin K
			Prolonged but correctable with vitamin K

History of a jaundiced patient

- Recent travel; drug addiction; joint pains; anorexia; malaise. **Suggests hepatitis**.
- Alcohol addiction. **Suggests cirrhosis**.
- Fat intolerance; recurrent right upper quadrant pain. **Suggests gallstones**.
- Weight loss; constant epigastric boring pain. **Suggests malignancy**.
- Family history of blood disorders. **Suggests haemolytic disorders**.
- Bruising tendency. **Suggests hepatocellular damage**.
- Pale stool, dark urine; pruritus. **Suggests obstructive jaundice**.

JAUNDICE[118]

Carry out abdominal examination (see pg 339).

'This patient looks frail and unwell and is obviously jaundiced. His skin and especially his conjunctiva have a deep yellow-orange hue. He has finger clubbing, palmar erythema and leukonychia. There are more than six spider naevi on the chest, and has gynaecomastia. There is ascites, hepatosplenomegaly and distended superficial abdominal veins. This patient has stigmata of chronic liver disease.'

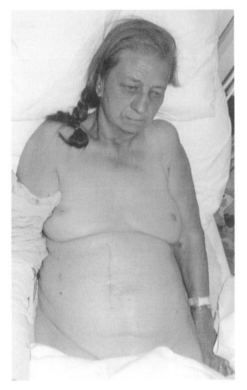

Hepatic jaundice due to metastatic liver disease

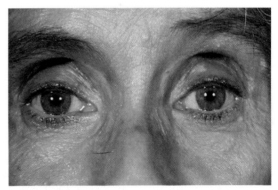

Jaundiced sclera and xanthelasma which is associated with chronic cholestasis

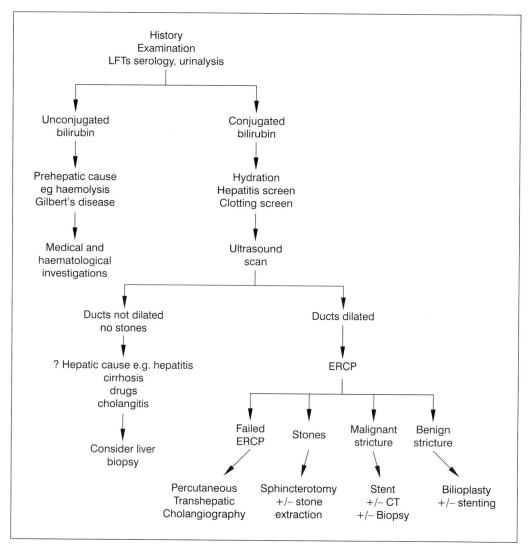

Investigation of the jaundiced patient

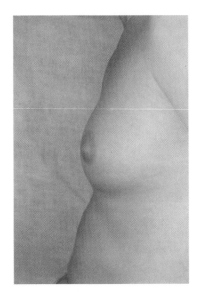

Gynaecomastia

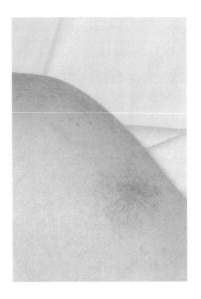

Spider naevus

Scratch marks

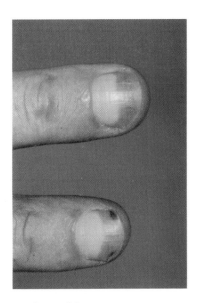

Leukonychia

[119] **Ascites**

Causes

- Increased portal venous pressure:

Prehepatic	Portal venous thrombosis; compression of portal vein by lymph nodes
Hepatic	Cirrhosis of the liver; multiple hepatic metastasis
Post-hepatic	Budd-Chiari syndrome (thrombosis of hepatic vein)
Cardiac	Constrictive pericarditis; right heart failure
Pulmonary	Pulmonary hypertension; right heart failure

- **Hypoproteinaemia**

    Kidney disease associated with albuminuria

    Cirrhosis of the liver

    Cachexia of wasting diseases, malignancy and starvation

    Protein-losing enteropathies

- **Chronic peritonitis**

Physical	Post-irradiation; talc granuloma; tuberculous peritonitis
Infection	Tuberculous peritonitis
Neoplasms	Peritoneal metastases; mucus-forming tumours (pseudomyxoma peritonei)

- **Chylous ascites**

    Congenital abnormalities

    Trauma

    Primary or secondary lymph gland disease

Causes of portal hypertension

World-wide, post viral hepatitis is the most common cause. In developed countries, alcoholic cirrhosis is the principal cause.

<u>Pre-sinusoidal</u>

- **Extrahepatic**: portal vein thrombosis; splenic vein thrombosis; arteriovenous fistula; tropical splenomegaly; immunological (lupoid); occlusion by tumour or pancreatitis
- **Intrahepatic**: schistosomiasis; chronic active hepatitis; early primary biliary cirrhosis; congenital hepatic fibrosis; sarcoidosis; toxins; idiopathic

<u>Sinusoidal</u>

- Cirrhotic: post-viral hepatitis; alcoholic; metabolic (e.g. Wilson's disease); drugs (e.g. methotraxate); cryptogenic
- **Non-cirrhotic**: acute alcoholic hepatitis; cytotoxic drugs; vitamin A intoxication

<u>Post-sinusoidal</u>

Budd-Chiari syndrome (tumour invasion of hepatic vein); veno-occlusive disease; caval abnormality; constrictive pericarditis.

ASCITES[119]

Carry out abdominal examination (see pg 339).

'There is a generalised swelling of the abdomen and the umbilicus is everted. The flanks are stony dull to percussion but the centre is resonant[120]. The dullness is shifting and a fluid thrill can be demonstrated[121]. This is ascites.'

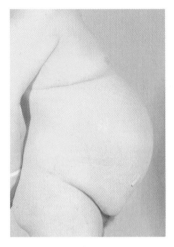

An alcoholic with gross ascites (note everted umbilicus and site of previous ascitic tap)

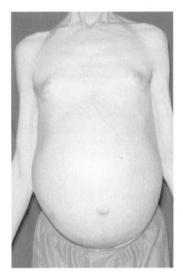

Dilated abdominal wall veins seen in portal hypertension

Technique for aspiration of ascites

Explain what you are going to do to the patient, and obtain their consent.

The patient lies supine, with a pillow under the left hip to make them tilt slightly towards the right.

The right side of the abdomen is percussed, and the point at which the dull tone becomes resonant is noted and marked.

Using aseptic technique, a sterile tray is set out, the area prepped and the skin infiltrated with local anaesthetic. The site is two fingerbreadths superior to and medial to the anterior superior iliac spine in the right iliac fossa. Check that this is below the point marked earlier where the percussion note became resonant.

A diagnostic tap can be performed using a 50 ml syringe with a green needle and distributing the fluid aspirated into three sterile specimen pots (like those used for MSSUs) for cytology, biochemistry and microbiology. Try to get at least 20 ml into the cytology specimen pot to increase the cell yield.

A therapeutic tap can be performed by inserting a grey Venflon attached to a three way tap, and using a 50 ml syringe to repeatedly aspirate and discharge the contents via the three way tap into a sterile jug.

As the fluid volume reduces, withdraw the needle and cover the puncture site with a sterile dressing.

Beware withdrawing large amounts of fluid from frail patients: hypovolaemia can result from the ascites reaccumulating at the expense of the circulating volume. Intravenous salt poor albumin infusion (20% Human Albumin Solution) has been used to counteract this, but this has provoked controversy in recent years and is frowned upon by some units.

[120] Due to floating, gas-filled bowel.

[121] In tense, large ascites.

Hepatomegaly

Common case: seen by more than 1 in 20 of the candidates in our survey.

[122] **Causes of enlargement of the liver**

<u>Smooth, generalised enlargement, without jaundice</u>

Congestive heart failure

Cirrhosis

Reticuloses (eg lymphoma)

Hepatic vein obstruction (Budd-Chiari syndrome)

Amyloid disease

<u>Smooth generalised enlargement, with jaundice</u>

Infective hepatitis

Biliary tract obstruction (gallstones, carcinoma of pancreas)

Cholangitis

Portal pyaemia

<u>Knobbly generalised enlargement, without jaundice</u>

Secondary carcinoma

Macronodular cirrhosis

Polycystic disease

Primary hepatic carcinoma – (hepatoma)

<u>Knobbly generalised enlargement, with jaundice</u>

Extensive secondary carcinoma

Cirrhosis

Localised swellings

Riedel's lobe

Secondary carcinoma

Hydatid cyst

Liver abscess

Primary multicentric hepatic carcinoma

Causes of cirrhosis of the liver

Alcohol, hepatitis B and hepatitis C account for 50% of cases of cirrhosis in this country. These and other causes are listed below.

- **Portal**: alcoholic; nutritional (protein deficiency); post-hepatic; idiopathic
- **Congenital**: haemochromatosis; Wilson's disease; α1-antitrypsin deficiency; galactosaemia; type IV glycogen storage disease
- **Drug-induced**
- **Idiopathic**
- **Biliary**: primary biliary cirrhosis; secondary biliary cirrhosis
- **Cardiac**: congestive cardiac failure
- **Other**: chronic active hepatitis; schistosomiasis; sarcoidosis; viral hepatitis

HEPATOMEGALY[122]

Carry out examination of the abdomen (see pg 339).

'There is a mass palpable in the left hypochondrium and epigastrium. It descends from below the right costal margin and costal angle. It moves with respiration and I cannot get above it. It is dull to percussion up to the level of the 8th rib in the mid-axillary line. The surface is smooth/knobbly. This is an enlarged liver.'

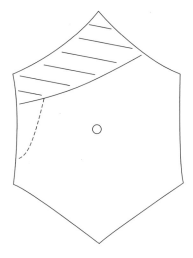

Hepatomegaly. The dotted line indicates the site of Riedel's lobe, a normal anatomical variation

Splenomegaly

A very common case: seen by over 1 in 10 of the candidates in our survey.

[123] Causes of splenomegaly

<u>Cellular proliferation</u>

Myeloid and lymphatic leukaemia

Pernicious anaemia

Polycythaemia rubra vera

Spherocytosis

Thrombocytopaenic purpura

Myelosclerosis

Mediterranean anaemia

<u>Infection</u>

Viral (glandular fever)

Bacterial (typhoid, typhus, TB, septicaemia)

Protozoal (malaria, kala-azar)

Spirochaetal (syphilis, Leptospirosis)

<u>Congestion</u>

Portal hypertension (cirrhosis, portal vein thrombosis)

Hepatic vein obstruction

Congestive heart failure (cor pulmonale, constrictive pericarditis)

<u>Infarction</u>

Embolic (bacterial endocarditis, left atrium, left ventricle)

Thrombotic (splenic artery or vein thrombosis in polycythaemia and retroperitoneal malignancy

<u>Cellular infiltration</u>

Amyloidosis

Gaucher's disease

<u>Collagen diseases</u>

Felty's syndrome

Still's disease

<u>Space-occupying lesions</u>

Lymphoma

True solitary cysts

Polycystic disease

Hydatid cysts

Angioma

Lymphosarcoma

If you have trouble remembering long lists, try to just remember the seven headings and the first example of each.

SPLENOMEGALY[123]

Carry out examination of the abdomen (see pg 339).

'There is a mass in the left hypochondrium. It appears from below the top of the left tenth rib and extends along the line of the rib towards the umbilicus. It is firm and smooth and has a notch on its upper edge (superomedial aspect). It moves with respiration, is dull to percussion and I cannot get above it. It is not ballotable. This is splenomegaly.'

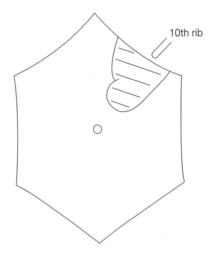

10th rib

Splenomegaly. The notch is not always palpable

Enlarged kidney

Very common case: seen by over 1 in 10 of the candidates in our survey.

[124] **Causes of an enlarged kidney**

Hydronephrosis (may be bilateral)

Pyonephrosis

Perinephric abscess

Carcinoma or nephroblastoma (occasionally bilateral)

Solitary cysts

Polycystic disease (usually bilateral)

Hypertrophy

A mobile or low lying kidney may be easily palpable and so seem to be enlarged.

Differences between a spleen and a kidney on examination

A kidney is ballotable and reduces into the loin

The kidney moves vertically, not diagonally with respiration

The kidney is dull to percussion

The spleen has a notch

Clinical signs of chronic renal failure

Uraemia (yellow tint to skin)

Brown line on fingernails

Anaemia (decreased erythropoietin)

Hypertension

Fluid overload (high JVP, oedema)

Signs of renal support (AV fistula/shunt, peritoneal dialysis catheter)

Nephrectomy scar

Causes of chronic renal failure

Glomerulonephritis

Pyelonephritis

Diabetes mellitus

Hypertension

Clinical signs of polycystic kidneys

Bilaterally enlarged kidneys

Signs of chronic renal failure

AV fistula shunt on arm

Hypertension

Urine containing blood, protein, casts

Cysts will occur in other organs eg berry aneurysms, liver cysts

Other affected family members (childhood variant is autosomal recessive, adult variant is autosomal dominant)

Complications of polycystic kidneys:

Hypertension

UTIs

Haemorrhage into a cyst

Subarachnoid haemorrhage (association)

[125] This means it can be bounced between your hands, one on the anterior abdominal wall and the other behind the renal angle, rather like a ball being patted between the hands. This sign is diagnostic of a renal mass and depends upon the mass reducing into the loin.

[126] Look for other signs of kidney transplantation following a long stint of renal failure e.g. AV fistula.

ENLARGED KIDNEY[124]

Carry out examination of the abdomen (see pg 339).

'There is a mass in the right/left flank. It is smooth and hemi-ovoid, moves with respiration and is not dull to percussion. It can be felt bimanually and is ballotable[125]. I can reduce it into the loin. This is an enlarged kidney.'

Transplanted kidney

Carry out examination of the abdomen (see pg 339).

'There is a mass in the left iliac fossa with an overlying scar. It is smooth, ovoid, non-tender, and dull to percussion. There is a/is no nephrectomy scar on the same side. This is a transplanted kidney[126].'

Abdominal cysts

Cystic swellings which may cause abdominal distension

Ovarian cysts	Hydronephrosis
Polycystic kidney	Urinary bladder
Pancreatic cysts	Mesenteric cysts
Hydatid cysts	

[127] Pseudocysts are most commonly a complication sequelae of severe pancreatitis, a debilitating and prolonged disease which tends to leave patients exhausted and malnourished.

[128] Pancreatic pseudocyst

<u>Definition</u>: a collection of serous fluid in relation to the pancreas following acute pancreatitis.

<u>Site</u>: the most common site is the lesser sac as a result of the blockage of the gastroepiploic foramen by inflammatory adhesions. Pseudocysts may occur anywhere adjacent to, or sometimes within, the pancreas.

<u>Incidence</u>: Routine ultrasound or CT will detect pseudocysts in up to 30% of patients with acute pancreatitis, and all but 5% resolve spontaneously.

<u>Management</u>: due to the natural history described above, conservative management is the treatment of choice.

<u>Indications for drainage include</u>:

Persisting pancreatic inflammation with hyperamylasaemia.

Palpable abdominal swelling which may compress the stomach or duodenum and cause vomiting.

Infection or haemorrhage of the cyst.

<u>Methods of drainage</u>: Percutaneous under CT or USS control – often reaccumulate.

Endoscopic drainage through the posterior wall of the stomach.

Open pseudocysto-gastrostomy where an incision from the posterior wall of the stomach to the cyst is formed then the sac is sutured to the gastric wall.

Open pseudocysto-jejenostomy for inferior cysts involves formation of a Roux loop.

[129] Mesenteric cysts

These are cysts of clear fluid found in the mesentery arising from vestigial remnants of reduplicated bowel. They may be found by chance, being symptomless, or cause abdominal distension or recurrent colicky pain. Like all cysts they can rupture, twist, and have intraluminal bleeding. Twisting is rare because they are fixed within the small bowel mesentery.

ABDOMINAL CYSTS

Carry out examination of the abdomen (see pg 339).

Case 1

'There is (in this thin[127], middle-aged patient) a firm tender/non-tender, non pulsatile mass in the epigastrium with an indistinct lower edge. The upper limit is not palpable. It is resonant to percussion and moves slightly with respiration. It is not possible to elicit fluctuation or a fluid thrill. The patient is/is not jaundiced and is/is not on total parenteral nutrition. This is a pancreatic pseudocyst[128].'

Case 2

'There is a smooth, mobile, spherical swelling in the centre of the abdomen. It moves freely diagonally from the right hypochondrium to the left iliac fossa (at right angles to the root of the mesentery), but only slightly from the left hypochondrium to the right iliac fossa (parallel to the root of the mesentery). It is dull to percussion and is fluctuant with a fluid thrill (if fixed). This is a mesenteric cyst[129].'

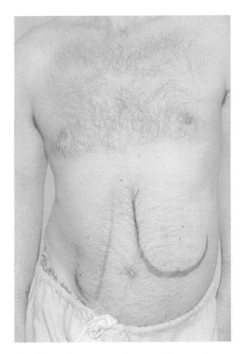

Outline of pancreatic pseudocyst in a man who had a laparotomy (note scar) for acute abdominal pain which turned out to be pancreatitis

Enlarged gall bladder
[130] **Causes of a large gall bladder**
<u>With jaundice</u>
Carcinoma of head of pancreas
Carcinoma of ampulla of Vater
Gallstone formed in situ in common bile duct
Mucocoele due to stone in Hartmann's pouch and stone in common bile duct.
Common bile duct cholangiocarcinoma
<u>Without jaundice</u>
Mucocoele
Empyema
Carcinoma of gallbladder
Acute cholecystitis

An enlarged gall bladder is usually due to obstruction of the cystic duct or common bile duct.
Obstruction of the cystic duct is usually by a gallstone and rarely by an intrinsic or extrinsic carcinoma. The patient is not jaundiced and the gall bladder will contain bile, mucous (a mucocoele) or pus (an empyema)
Obstruction of the common bile duct is usually by a stone or a carcinoma of the head of the pancreas. The patient will be jaundiced. Courvoisier's law states:
'In the presence of jaundice, the palpable gall bladder is unlikely to be due to stones'
This is because previous inflammation will have made the gall bladder thick and non-distensible. The exceptions are:
Stones which form in the bile duct.
Stones in the cystic duct as well as a stone or carcinoma in the bile duct.

ENLARGED GALL BLADDER[130]

Carry out examination of the abdomen (see pg 339).

'There is a mass in the left upper quadrant below the tip of the right ninth rib. It is smooth, hemi-ovoid, dull to percussion and moves with respiration. I cannot feel a space between the lump and the edge of the liver. This is an enlarged gall bladder.'

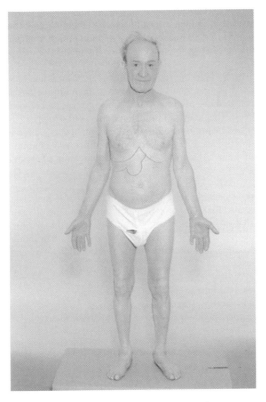

Enlarged gall bladder in a man with painless jaundice

[131] Pleural effusion

Altogether thoracic cases accounted for 3.9% of the cases in this bay and were seen by 9.6% of the candidates in our survey.

Causes

Exudate (>30g/l protein)

Neoplastic (primary or secondary)

Inflammatory: pneumonia/TB; PE; trauma; rheumatoid arthritis; SLE; subphrenic abscess; pancreatitis.

Transudate (<30mg/l protein)

Heart failure; liver cirrhosis; nephrotic syndrome

Meig's syndrome (ovarian fibroma)

Management of pleural effusion

1. Determine underlying cause, and treat as appropriate

2. Aspiration of pleural effusion

Get an AP and lateral X-ray, and percuss out the level of the effusion.

Explain the procedure to the patient and obtain consent.

Sit the patient erect, leaning forward, with their arms folded on a table in front of them.

The site of aspiration is usually in the eighth intercostal space in the posterior axillary line (see fig opposite). Mark the site, and determine that it is below the level at which the percussion note changed from resonant to dull.

Using aseptic technique, set up a tray, prep the site and infiltrate with local anaesthetic.

A diagnostic tap can be performed using a 50 ml syringe with a green needle and distributing the fluid aspirated into three sterile specimen pots (like those used for MSSUs) for cytology, biochemistry and microbiology. Try to get at least 20 mls into the cytology specimen pot to increase the yield of cells.

A therapeutic tap can be performed by inserting a grey venflon attached to a three-way tap, and using a 50 ml syringe to repeatedly aspirate and discharge the contents via the three-way tap into a sterile jug.

As the fluid volume reduces, withdraw the needle and cover the puncture site with a sterile dressing.

3. Chest drain insertion (see pg 415)

4. Pleurodesis

In the case of recurrent or resistant pleural effusion, such as in untreatable malignancy, pleurodesis can be carried out in several different ways. Thoracoscopic pleurectomy, where the pleura is stripped from the lung leaves an oozing, raw surface that sticks to the chest wall and heals fused to it, thus obliterating the pleural space. Chemical pleurodesis involves instilling either down the chest drain or thoracoscopically irritating chemicals (such as talc or tetracycline) that induce a fibrous reaction into the pleural space.

Chest X-ray signs of pleural effusion

First 300 mls not visualised on PA view

Lateral decubitus views may detect as little as 25 ml.

Hemidiaphragm and costophrenic sinuses obscured.

Meniscus shaped semicircular upper surface with lowest point in midaxillary line.

Associated collapse of ipsilateral lung.

Massive pleural effusion

Enlargement of ipsilateral hemithorax

Displacement of mediastinum to contralateral side

Severe depression/flattening/inversion of ipsilateral hemidiaphragm; visible air bronchogram.

PLEURAL EFFUSION[131]

Carry out respiratory examination (see pg 346).

'The pulse is regular and the jugular venous pressure is not elevated. The trachea is central (or deviated away from the abnormal side) and the expansion is normal. The percussion note is stony dull at the right base with diminished tactile fremitus and vocal resonance and diminished breath sounds. There is (may be) an area of bronchial breathing above the area of dullness. The diagnosis is a right pleural effusion.'

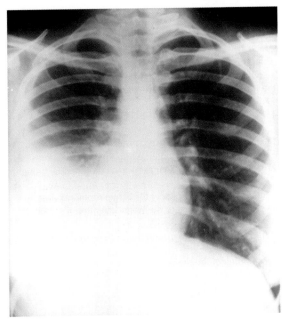

Right pleural effusion

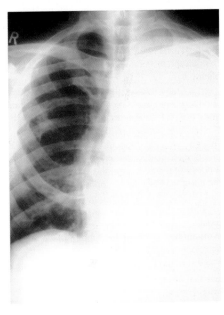

'White out' of left hemithorax due to a large pleural effusion

Chest drain insertion

If the pleural effusion is causing symptoms of breathlessness, and reaccumulates after aspiration, a chest drain may be inserted. Bear in mind these anatomical facts:

- The left hemidiaphragm with the spleen beneath it rises to the fifth rib at rest
- The right hemidiaphragm with the liver beneath it rises to the fourth space
- Either hemidiaphragm may be raised due to collapse or phrenic nerve damage due to pathology of that lung
- The intercostal bundle of nerves, arteries and vein, runs inferior to each rib, so placing the drain just superiorly to the rib avoids damage to these structures.

Select the size of drain (30F for pus or blood, 20–24 F for fluid or air) and make sure the underwater seal bottle is ready.

Check the chest X-ray and check the side is correct (beware mediastinal shift).

Explain the procedure to the patient and obtain consent.

Sit the patient up at 45 degrees with the ipsilateral arm behind their head (they are often not comfortable lying flat).

The safest site is the fifth intercostal space in the anterior axillary line.

Using an aseptic technique, set up a tray and prep and drape the site.

Infiltrate just above the sixth rib with local anaesthetic. The syringe fills with fluid when aspirated as it enters the pleural space.

Make a generous stab incision in the line of the intercostal space with a scalpel after an appropriate pause for the local anaesthetic take effect (this is a minithoracotomy).

Deepen the incision with a combination of blunt and sharp dissection using scissors or a haemostat until the pleura is reached.

Insert a finger into the thoracic cavity to confirm that the lung is not adherent to the parietal pleura at this site and there is a clear, safe path for your chest tube.

Insert a purse string or mattress suture across the incision (non absorbable) and tie it loosely, to be used for closure after removal of the chest drain.

Take the selected drain and REMOVE THE TROCAR. A trocar should never be used. Instead, insert a haemostat into one of the perforations in the chest drain to stiffen it and make it easier to guide into the hole, making sure it does not protrude from the end (see fig a, opposite). This should be withdrawn as soon as the drain is through the chest wall (see fig b, opposite).

Slide the chest drain in through the tract made by your finger, directing it apically for a pneumothorax, basally for a pleural effusion. Connect the drain to the underwater seal and make sure the water level 'swings' with each breath.

With another stitch, tie the tube in place and place a sterile gauze dressing around the exit site of the drain (see fig c, opposite).

Make sure to check the chest X-ray to confirm correct positioning of the drain.

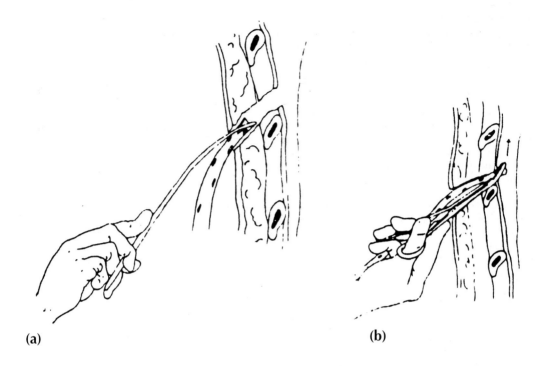

(a)

(b)

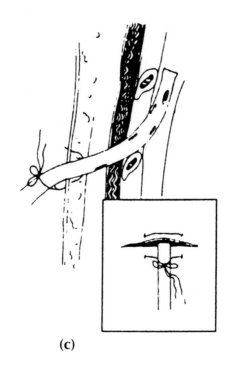

(c)

Insertion of chest drain

Pneumothorax

[132] **Definition**: Accumulation of air in the pleural space.

Pathophysiology: Disruption of visceral pleura/trauma to parietal pleura.

Symptoms: Dyspnoea in 80–90%. Pleuritic back/shoulder pain.

Causes of pneumothorax: Remember the mnemonic 'THE CHEST SET'

T rauma: Penetrating trauma

              Blunt trauma   a) rib fracture

                                  b) increased intrathoracic pressure against closed glottis, lung contusion/laceration

                                  c) bronchial rupture

H oneycomb lung (pulmonary fibrosis, cystic fibrosis, sarcoidosis, sclerodermarheumatoid lung)

E mphysema, Esophageal rupture

C hronic obstructive pulmonary disease

H yaline membrane disease

E ndometriosis – catamenial pneumothorax = recurrent spontaneous pneumothorax during menstruation associated with endometriosis of the diaphragm (Usually right-sided)

S pontaneous, Scleroderma

T uberous sclerosis

S arcoma (osteo), Sarcoidosis

E osinophilic granuloma

T uberculosis and fungus

X-ray signs of simple pneumothorax

White margin of visceral pleura separated from parietal pleura.

Absence of vascular markings beyond visceral pleural margin.

X-ray signs of tension pneumothorax

Displacement of mediastinum away from affected side.

Deep sulcus sign – on frontal view larger lateral costodiaphragmatic recess than on opposite side.

Diaphragmatic inversion.

Total/subtotal lung collapse.

Collapse of SVC/IVC/right heart border.

Management of simple pneumothorax

Treatment is not required in a healthy individual with a small pneumothorax.

Chest drain (see pg 414, pleural effusion) indicated if:

    Larger pneumothorax associated with dyspnoea

    Increasing in size

    Not resolving after one week

    Pneumothorax complicating underlying severe chronic bronchitis with emphysema

    Pneumothorax exacerbating acute severe asthma

Pneumonectomy (see pg 413, pleural effusion) indicated in recurrent spontaneous pneumothorax.

Tension pneumothorax

Definition: A pneumothorax with a one-way valve air leak. Each breath tends to enlarge the pneumothorax, displacing the mediastinum. Tension pneumothorax is a medical emergency and should be diagnosed on clinical grounds and treated immediately, not delayed while an X-ray is arranged.

Clinical signs: SOB, Shock, Tracheal deviation, reduced breath sounds, neck vein distension, hyperresonance.

Treatment: Decompress urgently with cannula in 2nd intercostal space in midclavicular line. This only buys time while a chest drain is inserted.

Chest drain in 5th intercostal space, anterior axillary line (see pg 414, pleural effusion). Oxygen, monitoring.

PNEUMOTHORAX[132]

Carry out respiratory examination (see pg 346).

'The right side of the chest (of this tall thin young adult male or old emphysematous man) expands poorly compared with the other side. The percussion note on the right side is hyper-resonant, the tactile fremitus, vocal resonance and breath sounds are all diminished. The trachea is central (deviation suggests a very large pneumothorax or a tension pneumothorax, not likely to be sitting untreated in the exam!). This is a right-sided pneumothorax.'

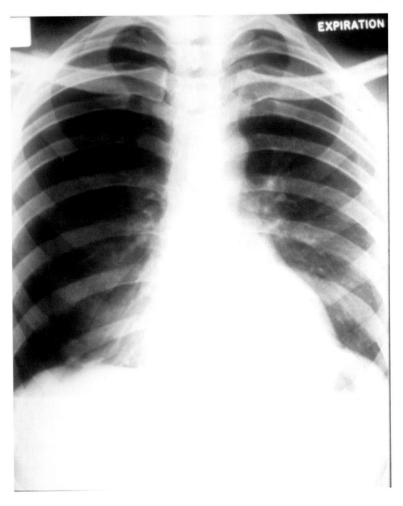

Simple pneumothorax on the right. Trace the lung margin and note where the lung markings stop. There is no mediastinal shift. See also pg 420

Thoracotomy scars
[133] **Thoracotomy incisions**

Posterolateral thoracotomy

Exposes lungs, oesophagus and thoracic aorta on the left.

Incision runs from a posterior point midway between the spinous processes of the vertebrae and the medial border of the scapula, and extending forwards in the line of the ribs two to three fingerbreadths below the tip of the scapula as far as the midaxillary line. The intercostal space that is opened is chosen according to the procedure: above the fifth rib for an upper lobectomy, above the sixth rib for a lower lobectomy, pneumonectomy, Ivor Lewis (two phase) oesophagectomy or middle lobectomy on the right, above the seventh rib for access to the lower oesophagus. A thoracic incision can be extended across the cartilage of the costal margin and down into the diaphragm as a thoracoabdominal incision.

Midline sternotomy

Exposes the anterior mediastinum and the pericardium.

Incision is from 1cm below the suprasternal notch to approximately 6cm below the xiphisternum. The sternum is divided with an air driven vertical saw with a guarded tip (or an oscillating saw in a re-operation, to avoid the right ventricle firmly adherent to the sternum).

Right parasternal incision

Used for aortic and mitral valve procedures. Involves dislocation of the costosternal junction of two or more ribs.

Upper hemisternotomy (sternal incision T-cut)

This can be used for aortic and mitral valve procedures. The main advantage is in leaving half the sternum intact for stability; it also avoids an intercostal incision and the possibility of a chest wall hernia.

Anterior thoracotomy

Valuable for limited intrathoracic procedures e.g. lung biopsy thoracoscopy, mediastinal node biopsy or pericardial fenestration.

Anterior mediastinostomy

Used for mediastinoscopy can yield valuable information in the diagnosis of mediastinal tumours and the staging of thoracic disease.

Indications for an emergency thoracotomy in trauma.

1.5 litres of blood drain immediately chest drain is inserted.

Blood loss continues at >200 ml/hr.

Medial penetrating wound (front or back).

EMD or cardiac arrest with hypovolaemia (for internal cardiac massage).

When not to do an emergency thoracotomy

No qualified experienced surgeon present.

No electrical cardiac activity.

[134] **X-ray signs of pneumonectomy**

Early signs (within 24 hours)

Partial filling of thorax.

Ipsilateral mediastinal shift and diaphragmatic elevation.

Late signs

Complete obliteration of space

NB. Depression of diaphragm/shift of mediastinum to contralateral side indicates a bronchopleural fistula/empyema/haemorrhage.

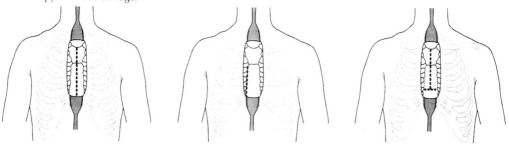

Median sternotomy   Right parasternal   Upper hemisternotomy (T-cut)

THORACOTOMY SCARS[133]

Spot diagnosis or carry out respiratory examination (see pg 346).

'There is a midline sternotomy scar indicating previous cardiothoracic surgery. The commonest operations performed through this scar are coronary artery bypass surgery and aortic or mitral valve replacement. I would like to do a cardiovascular examination, look at the legs for vein harvest scars and see the chest X-rays.'

'There is a posterolateral thoracotomy scar indicating previous thoracic surgery. The commonest operations performed through this scar are partial or total pneumonectomy and oesophageal surgery. I would like to perform a respiratory examination and see the chest X-rays[134].'

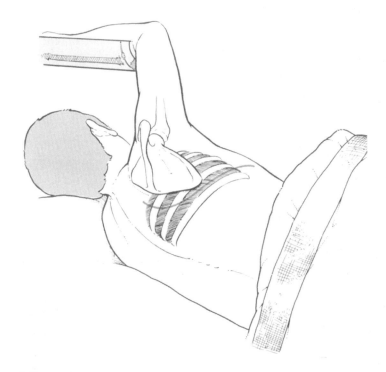

Posterolateral thoracotomy

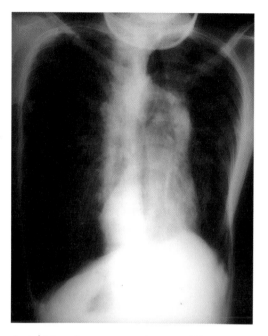

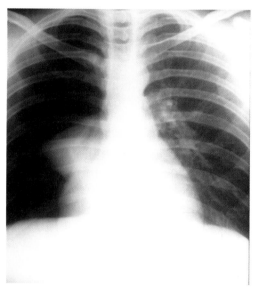

A right tension pneumothorax with mediastinal shift in a patient with cystic fibrosis

Complete right pneumothorax. Note loss of lung markings on the right and collapsed lung near the right heart border. Although this is a complete pneumothorax, it is not a tension pneumothorax as the mediastinum is not shifted

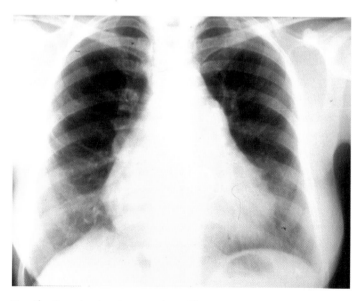

Prosthetic mitral valve on chest X-ray

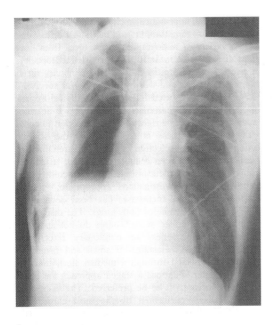

a

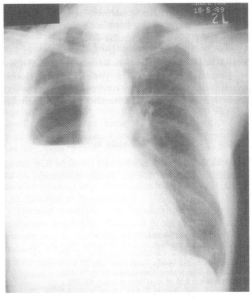

c

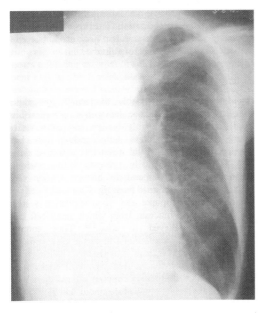

b

Sequence of chest X-rays showing progress following pneumonectomy. a) Immediate postoperative film shows the hemithorax containing only air and reduced in volume by mediastinal shift and elevation of the diaphragm. b) Three days later the pneumonectomy space now contains a fluid level as air is absorbed and an exudate accumulates. If the volume of air starts to increase beware of a blown bronchial stump. c) By 4–6 weeks there is complete opacification of the space.

DEXTROCARDIA[135]

Perform examination of the heart (see pg 276).

'The pulse is regular, at 70 beats per minute and of good volume. The jugular venous pressure is not raised. The apex beat is not palpable on the left side, but can be felt in the fifth right intercostal space in the midclavicular line. The patient has dextrocardia. I would like to listen to the chest[136] and feel for a liver[137].'

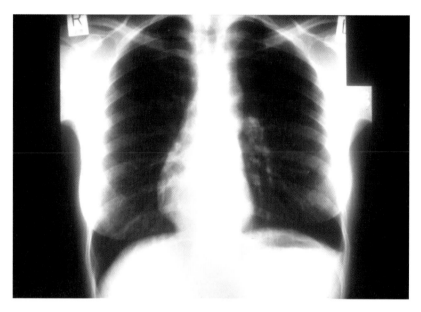

Dextrocardia
Note that although the heart shadow is on the right, the gastric bubble under the diaphragm is still on the left as normal. This is not the case in situs inversus

---

Dextrocardia

[135] Consider this diagnosis if you cannot feel an apex beat and then have difficulty hearing the heart sounds. As you move the stethoscope to the right, the heart sounds get louder. After auscultation, repeat the identification of the apex beat on the right side exactly as you would on the left (see examination of the heart, pg 276).

[136] **Kartagener's syndrome**: dextrocardia, bronchiectasis, situs inversus, infertility, dysplasia of frontal sinuses, sinusitis and otitis media. Patients have ciliary immotility. One of the candidates in our survey was asked why one would refer a patient with dextrocardia to an ENT surgeon – the answer is if they have Kartagener's syndrome they will have the aforementioned problems with their sinuses and middle ear.

[137] If **situs inversus** (lateral transposition of the viscera of the thorax and the abdomen) is present the patient is usually otherwise normal. Dextrocardia without situs inversus is usually associated with cardiac malformation. Dextrocardia may occur in Turner's syndrome, a sex chromosome abnormality (usually XO) which results in short, infertile, often mentally retarded phenotypic girls who occasionally display characteristic features such as webbed neck or wide spaced nipples.

PEUTZ-JEGHERS SYNDROME[138]

Spot diagnosis.

'There are small brownish-black pigmented macules on the lips, around the mouth, and sometimes on the eyes, nose and buccal mucosa (but not on the tongue). There are also (maybe) similar lesions on the hands and fingers. If this pigmentation is associated with intestinal polyposis the diagnosis is Peutz-Jeghers syndrome.'

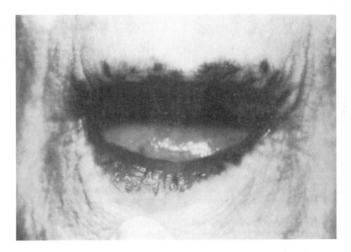

Circumoral pigmentation in Peutz-Jeghers syndrome

---

[138] **Peutz-Jeghers syndrome**
This is an autosomal dominant inherited syndrome consisting of the characteristic pigmentation around the lips associated with characteristic intestinal polyps. The polyps are most common in the small intestine but can occasionally occur in the colon. These are hamartomas: polyps with a very low malignant potential. Complications include intestinal obstruction or intussusception (causing recurrent colicky abdominal pain), bleeding (resulting in iron deficiency anaemia or frank gastrointestinal haemorrhage). Malignant transformation is rare.
See Osler Weber Rendu syndrome for comparison (pg 317).

[139] **Pilonidal sinus**

A pilonidal sinus is a subcutaneous sinus which contains hair, most commonly found in the natal cleft associated with chronic inflammation and acute abscess formation. The condition is common and affects young adults. There are rare variants of the pilonidal sinus in other sites (e.g. the webs of barbers' fingers, the axilla, the lumbar region in children). The latter are congenital and extend to the neural canal and dura.

Pathology

Perianal pilonidal sinuses are thought to be an acquired condition, starting at the onset of puberty when the hair follicles become distended and inflamed. The sinus usually consists of a midline opening or openings in the natal cleft about 5cm from the anus. The primary track (lined with squamous cell epithelium) leads to a subcutaneous cavity containing granulation tissue and usually a nest of hairs. Secondary openings can be seen often 2.5cm lateral from the midline pits.

Clinical features

Patients are usually between the age of puberty and 40 years (75% male). Patients are often dark and hairy and may be obese. 50% present as emergencies with an acute pilonidal abscess. The rest have intermittent discomfort and discharge. Examination reveals the characteristic midline pit or pits which may have hair protruding. Lateral pits may be present.

Treatment

Incision and drainage

An acute pilonidal abscess needs incision or excision and drainage under general anaesthetic with follow-up. Later treatment of the pilonidal sinus may be required when the abscess cavity has healed if there are residual problems (one-third of patients require further treatment).

Excision of pits and laying open of sinus

This is usually done under GA. The midline pits and lateral openings are excised with a small area of surrounding skin. The cavity is curetted and packed loosely with a gauze ribbon. Frequent changes of dressing and close supervision are needed post-operatively. Regular rubbing with a finger avoids premature closure. Meticulous hygiene and shaving are important. Shaving may be stopped once the wound has healed.

Excision with primary suture

Some surgeons recommend excision of sinus with primary suturing of the defect. The advantages and disadvantages are shown in the table below. The proportions of wounds healed at two months are similar for both forms of treatment.

Advantages and disadvantages of laying open (versus primary closure) of pilonidal sinus

- Advantages: effective in most hands; shorter period in hospital; healing by secondary intention leaves broad, hairless scar which reduces recurrence
- Disadvantages: slower healing; open wound delays return to work; active wound care with frequent wound dressing

Recurrence

Occurs in up to 50%. Causes include:
- Neglect of wound care (e.g. shaving, finger treatment)
- Persisting poorly drained tracks
- Recurrent infection of hair follicle
- Midline scars

PILONIDAL SINUS[139]

Spot diagnosis.

'There is, in this hirsute young man, a small, tender swelling in the midline just above the natal cleft. In the line of this swelling are three tiny pits, one with hair protruding from it and at least two producing discharge on gentle palpation. There is also a pit 1cm lateral to the midline on the right. This is an inflamed pilonidal sinus.'

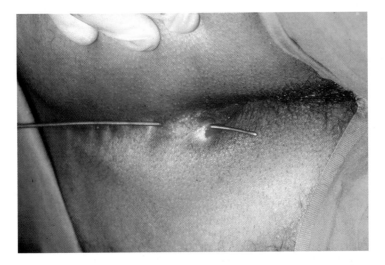

Midline and lateral openings of pilonidal sinus at the top of the natal cleft demonstrated by a probe

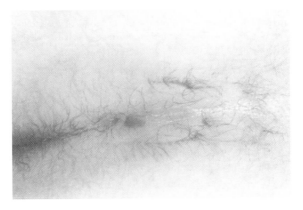

Pilonidal sinus with discharge

Crohn's disease and ulcerative colitis

Crohn's fistulae were a common case: seen by over 1 in 20 of the candidates in our survey.

[140] **Inflammatory bowel disease**

Inflammatory bowel disease is a chronic gastrointestinal inflammation without identifiable cause.

Crohn's disease

Although most commonly found in the terminal ileum, Crohn's disease may occur anywhere in the alimentary canal, from mouth to anus. It may be confined to the large bowel, or there may be involvement of both the small and large intestine. Perianal involvement is seen in 75% of patients.

Ulcerative colitis (U.C.)

This is a mucosal disease that almost invariably involves the rectum and then spreads more proximally in a continuous manner. Only 15% of cases extend more proximally than the splenic flexure. (This group has a greater risk of complications including cancer.) In a few cases, the ileum is also affected (backwash ileitis).

Epidemiology

Both Crohn's disease and U.C. are more common in developing countries and younger adults.

Aetiology

Unknown. Family history in 20–30%. ?post-infective ?autoimmune ?environmental ?dietary factors

Pathology

Crohn's disease: can affect the GI tract from mouth to anus, 70% involving small bowel. Perianal involvement ion 50–70%. Skip lesions of abnormal areas with intervening normal mucosa. Whole thickness of bowel affected. Cobblestone appearance of mucosa, fatty encroachment on serosa. Fistulation common to adjacent organs. Non-caseating epithelioid granulomas in 60–70% of patients.

Ulcerative colitis: occurs in the rectum and extends continuously proximally. Can affect entire colon with 'backwash ileitis' but no other area of GI tract affected. Inflammation limited to mucosa, not transmural. Serosa not affected. Inflammatory pseudopolyps and small shallow ulcers. Granulomas not typical.

Clinical features

Typical features of Crohn's disease

- Stricture formation leading to chronic intestinal obstruction
- Local perforation
- Abscess
- Fistula to exterior or other organs
- Colitis leading to diarrhoea, mucus and bleeding
- Anal fissure, ulcers, infections and skin tags
- Extra-intestinal manifestations (see pg 428)
- Anorexia, weight loss, malnutrition, anaemia, nausea

Typical features of UC

- Bloody diarrhoea with mucus, urgency and incontinence
- Constipation in cases of limited proctitis
- Cramping abdominal pain
- Anorexia, weight loss, malnutrition, anaemia, nausea
- Extra-intestinal manifestations (see pg 428)
- It is important to recognise patients with severe acute colitis: severe local symptoms; frequency more than 10 stools/24 hours with blood; wasting, pallor, tachycardia, pyrexia; tender, distended abdomen; these patients may progress to acute toxic dilatation of the colon and perforation.

CROHN'S DISEASE[140]

Carry out abdominal examination (see pg 339).

'There is (in this thin young woman) multiple laparotomy scars suggest a chronic, relapsing abdominal condition which has led to crises requiring surgical intervention on several occasions. The scars are suggestive of poor healing complicated by infection, as they are irregular, wide and puckered. There is an enterocutaneous fistula discharging from a scar in the right iliac fossa. There are swollen lips and multiple mouth ulcers, and the patient gives a history of chronic diarrhoea. The perineum has a characteristic dusky blue discoloration, and there are multiple oedematous anal tags, fissures and ulceration around the anus. There is evidence of surgery on previous fistulae/there is a Seton suture in situ. The diagnosis is Crohn's disease.'

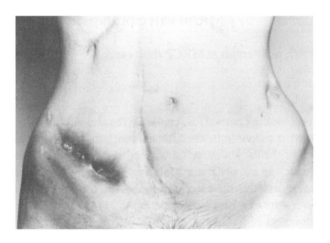

Multiple abdominal scars and fistulae in Crohn's disease

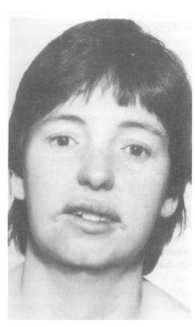

Patient with swollen lips in Crohn's disease

Extra-intestinal manifestations of inflammatory bowel disease
Related to disease activity
- **Skin**: pyoderma gangrenosum; erythema nodosum
- **Mucous membranes**: aphthous ulcers of the mouth and vagina
- **Eyes**: Iritis
- **Joints**: Activity-related arthritis of large joints

Unrelated to disease activity
- **Joints/liver**: sacroiliitis; ankylosing spondylitis
- **Biliary tree**: chronic active hepatitis; cirrhosis; primary sclerosing cholangitis, bile duct carcinoma
- **Integument**: amyloidosis in Crohn's disease; fingernail clubbing

Investigations

Sigmoidoscopy, Colonoscopy, Barium enema, small bowel enema/barium meal, FBC, ESR, serum albumin, stool microscopy and culture.

Barium enema findings

Crohn's disease

Discontinuous distribution ('skip lesion'); rectal sparing common; 'cobblestone' appearance of mucosa; 'Rosethorn' spiculation ulcers; fistulae; strictures.

Ulcerative colitis

Featureless 'hosepipe' colon; decreased haustrae; affects rectum and spreads proximally; mucosal distortion; small ulcers and pseudo-polyps; shortened colon.

Medical management

Anti-inflammatory medication: five amino salicylic acid preparations, steroids, both either oral or as foam enemas and suppositories.

Symptomatic control: Anti-diarrhoeal agents, replacement of fluid and electrolytes

Indications for surgery
- To restore health in patients with chronic disease, (e.g. in nutritional failure)
- To eliminate the risks of side-effects of steroids in patients requiring long term high doses of steroids
- Premalignant change on colonoscopic surveillance
- Patients at high risk of developing cancer (ulcerative colitis with early onset, extensive colonic involvement and continuous symptoms)
- To treat complications (usually emergency surgery) e.g. perforation, severe haemorrhage, toxic dilatation (>6 cm megacolon), stricture causing obstruction, fistulation or abscess formation, sepsis. Acute severe attack, need to defunction diseased bowel with an ileostomy

Principles of surgery

In Crohn's disease, surgery should be as limited as possible and be reserved for patients with a specific operable problem, as it cannot be 'cured' by surgery and postoperative complications are common.

In UC, radical surgery is often employed, because removal of the diseased segment often cures the patient. Furthermore, patients are at risk of lethal toxic megacolon and have a tenfold increased risk of developing carcinoma in long-standing disease. The most common operations performed for UC are proctocolectomy with ileostomy, sphincter-preserving proctocolectomy with ileal pouch, colectomy with ileorectal anastomosis and subtotal colectomy with ileostomy and mucous fistula.

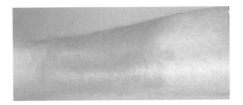

Erythema nodosum secondary to Crohn's disease

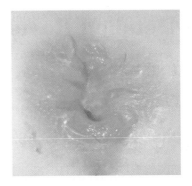

Perianal Crohn's disease showing multiple tags and fissures

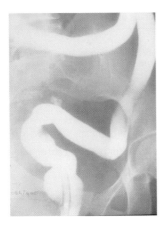

Barium enema showing 'Hosepipe' colon in ulcerative colitis

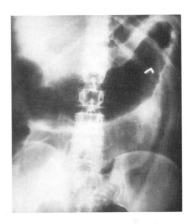

Plain abdominal X-ray showing toxic megacolon

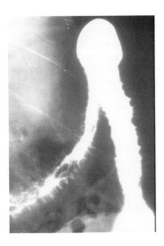

Barium enema of Crohn's disease showing stricturing and 'rose thorn' ulcers

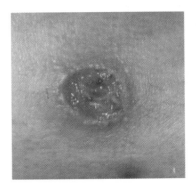

Pyoderma gangrenosum is associated with inflammatory bowel disease

D   Detailed Results of Survey

THE TRUNK BAY

Total of 128 cases reported in the survey.

TOP 5 CASES (accounted for 65.6% of all Trunk cases)

Type of case	Number seen in survey	Breakdown and details of cases
Groin hernias	25	21 Inguinal 1 Femoral 3 Unspecified (assumed groin) Five seen in Superficial Lesions bay. Questions included differential diagnoses, different types of hernia, different types of repair.
Scrotum	17	13 Hydrocoele 1 Testicular tumour 1 Bilateral orchidectomy for prostate cancer 1 Epididymal cyst 1 Tuberculosis of testicle and epididymis Questions included management of hydrocoele, tumour markers.
Stomas	16	5 General (site not specified) 4 Ileostomy 3 Colostomy 1 Urostomy 2 Ileal conduits 1 PEG post strike Questions included types of stoma, sites, indications, complications, 'work out what the operation was' TPN indications, problems with resecting terminal ilium, and discussion about other features in the patients such as Hickman line for chemotherapy, radiotherapy skin changes, supraclavicular lymph nodes.
Hernias (other than groin)	15	7 Incisional 5 Paraumbilical 2 Spegalian (1 in Superficial Lesions bay) 1 Epigastric
Liver disease	11	6 Jaundice (plus 3 hepatomegaly cases had jaundice) 4 Hepatomegaly (3 with jaundice, 1 with enlarged spleen) 1 T-tube after bile duct exploration 1 post total parotidectomy Questions included investigation of obstructive jaundice, features and complications of liver failure

430

OTHER CASES

Type of case	Number seen in survey	Breakdown and details of cases
Splenomegaly	**10**	1 with enlarged liver Questions included causes of splenomegaly, differentiating kidney from spleen, 'what are these marks?' (radiotherapy ink marks).
Palpable kidney	9	3 Polycystic 2 Transplanted (also a feature in 2 arterio-venous fistula cases – see Circulatory chapter pg xx) 2 Enlarged ?cause 1 Pelvic kidney 1 Hydronephrotic kidney
Abdominal mass (not liver, kidney or spleen)	7	1 Pancreatic pseudocyst 2 Palpable gall bladder 1 Left iliac fossa mass and gastric cancer on OGD 1 Psoas abscess 1 Left iliac fossa mass ?cause
Thoracic cases	**5**	1 Chest drain for pneumothorax 1 Thoracotomy scar 2 Dextrocardia (1 in Circulatory bay) 1 Malignant pleural effusion after mastectomy Questions included principles of chest drain, site of needle decompression of pneumothorax, indication for thoracotomy, why send a patient with dextrocardia to see an ENT surgeon?
Fistulae	**3**	2 Enterocutaneous fistula (at least one Crohn's). 1 Crohn's anus
Abdominal scars	**3**	Describe
Bladder	**2**	1 Ectopic bladder (no other details given) 1 Bladder cancer – pelvic mass, differential diagnosis and imaging
Peutz-Jeghers syndrome	**2**	
Pilonidal sinus	**1**	
Peyronie's disease	**1**	With Dupuytren's contracture
Ovarian cancer	**1**	With ascites

CHAPTER SIX

CLINICAL BAY 5
COMMUNICATION

CONTENTS

COMMUNICATION

A   The Bay

The Communication skills bay is a feature of the MRCS (Eng) clinical examination until December 2002, after which it will be a feature of the MRCS *viva voce* examination. Up to December 2002, the bay lasts 15 minutes, involves one actor and accounts for 5 marks. The MRCS guidelines state that this bay is to 'assess communication skills' and summarises the structure of the bay as follows:

'A written vignette or clinical scenario will be given to the candidate in advance of the bay and the candidate will be allowed to study it for a few minutes. The candidate will then approach the 'patient' or 'relative,' played by an actor, and will either ask questions about a relative or enquire about their own disease (e.g. have I got cancer?). The candidate may be required to get consent for a procedure. The two examiners will observe and determine according to predetermined guidelines (which vary according to the scenario) how the candidates performed. The vignettes will be identical in each centre.'

After December 2002 the testing of the communication skills will take place as part of the *viva voce* examination of the English College. It will be expanded to include an assessment of the candidate's ability to gather and communicate information, for example taking a history and then writing a letter to a GP. Not all the Royal colleges assess communication formally, and the author advises candidates to get up-to-date information from their examining college before sitting the examination (see pg 2 for addresses and websites).

B   The Technique

The Communication skills bay is varied and relies more than any of the other bays on your ability to be a natural, professional communicator. The examiners are looking for someone who, as a registrar, will be able to allay fears, inform patients and deal successfully with complaints on their consultant's behalf. The marking scheme assumes basic knowledge regarding certain common clinical scenarios (e.g. what the complications are of certain operations, what the likely future management is of a recently diagnosed condition, what the prognosis is in certain diseases). The possible scenarios are infinite, and the author of this book will assume that you have picked these things up from your medical training and clinical experience. What the marks in this bay are awarded for, and what this chapter emphasises, are the techniques used for communication.

Below is a suggested plan for interviewing the actor. Although the basic suggested structure is adaptable for most cases, details vary when dealing with specific types of cases such as complaints, obtaining consent or breaking bad news, and these are referred to separately.

Structure of the interview
When being taught how to present a talk at a conference, I was once told you have to say what you're going to say, then say it, then say what you've said. In other words, do an introduction, present the talk, then do a summary. This sounds dreadfully repetitive, but anyone who has ever been to a surgical conference will know how much clearer the presentations are of those lecturers who follow this advice. The story is the same in this bay. After introductions are over, the plan is to get the actor's information first, then say what you're going to say, then say it, then, after checking that the actor has no more queries, say what you've said. Finally confirm what the actor can expect to happen next and make sure the lines of communication remain open. Throughout, it is important to empathise with the actor and say you're sorry for any pain or distress caused by your news or past events.

1. Starting the interview

Greeting
Say good morning/good afternoon/how do you do.
Shake hands.
Smile/look friendly and accommodating even in the face of hostility.

Introductions

Say who you are.
'I'm Dr Parchment Smith.'
Confirm who they are and their relationships to the patient if appropriate.
Say what you had to do with the case and what you are there for.

Make the actor comfortable

'Take a seat, sir.'
Speak respectfully; e.g. Sir, Madam, Mr Angry.
If at a desk, sit two chairs across a corner of the desk, so you don't have the desk between you.
Do not stand if the actor is sitting – get a chair so you are both on the same level.

2. Gather information from the actor

After the introduction, your first task is to gather information from the actor including their impression of what has happened so far, what they understand, what their concerns are and what they want done, and (if applicable) why they are angry. In this section of the interview you must LISTEN and let the actor vent without interruption. Let them talk until they run out of steam, gently asking them questions in gaps to get all their worries out of them. Use *open questions* at the beginning of this section 'Tell me what happened' and *closed questions* to clarify points they have made 'So who eventually told you which ward your mother had gone to?' Use *facilitation* by nodding your head and repeating the last statement 'So you went up to the ward to find her – what happened then?'

You can tell when the actor has said all he/she wants to say when
a) they stop and
b) say 'that's everything' when you ask if there are any concerns, or,
c) in the case of the ranters, who could go on forever in a tirade, when they start repeating themselves and are running out of steam.

This stage will vary greatly in length depending on the scenario. It tends to last the longest in actors portraying dissatisfied patients or relatives with a complaint, who may speak if uninterrupted for five or ten minutes. Alternatively, in a 'breaking bad news' scenario the actor may just say 'Well, I know I've had some cells taken away from this lump in my breast and I'm coming today to find out if it is cancerous or not.'

3. Empathise with the actor

During the second section of information gathering and throughout the rest of the interview it is important to put yourself on the side of the actor. Nod sympathetically, listen with interest, look sad and shocked at appropriate intervals. Saying things like
'I see what you mean.' 'That must have been awful for you and the family,' etc. will give the actor the impression that he/she is speaking to a sympathetic ear. This will almost certainly calm him/her down, as he/she is expecting hostility if he/she came in hostile.

Beware, however, not to go too far. Never criticise directly the actions of a colleague, however negligent it may be portrayed by the actor, be it GP, nurse or doctor. This seems like the easy way to get on the actor's good side but its consequences are nearly as disastrous in the examination as in real life. Useful phrases if pressed to do so include 'I'm afraid I'm not allowed to comment on the actions of that doctor, but I can see how frustrated you must have been by them.' In other situations not involving complaints, listen to the actor's understanding of the situation and be equally empathetic.

4. Summarise the actor's input and confirm you are dealing with the correct issues

It is important to listen carefully to the content of the actor's report and try to organise the key factors in your own mind so that you can summarise them and present them back to make sure you have got all the information.

For example, in a complaint case, while you are listening to the actor vent their anger, complaint or frustrations, try to identify the key issues. There are usually only two or three things that most upset a relative, and it is often easy for us as doctors to see how those situations arose (a cancelled theatre slot, an understaffed ward, a consultant's holiday). Before making excuses, it is important to make some sense out of the emotional ranting of the 'upset' actor, put it into an order and present it back to the actor. This will give the examiner the impression that you have been listening carefully, taking note of worries and have taken them seriously. It also enables you to separate out each point so that you can deal with them systematically. At the end of the list, check that there are no more problems that you have missed out, and if there are, add them to the list. Be sympathetic when listing the complaints, and make no attempt to minimise the distress felt at this stage. Remember that you are on their side.

5. Outline your plan for the consultation

You are now going to tell the actor the information they need to know.
Tell them this so they know that it is now your turn to speak and are prepared for what they are going to hear. Phrases like 'I've heard what you have to say,' 'Allow me to take your points one by one' or 'I'm going to give you the results and then we can discuss them,' are useful.

6. Give the actor information in a structured way

Sticking to the plan, give the information in a structured way. It may help to number the points and deal with them methodically. Use clear statements avoiding jargon.

When dealing with complaints, take each point in turn and deal with it as best you can. Try to explain the series of events that led to the unsatisfactory outcome and what was done to try to deal with it at the time. Do not make excuses, and accept responsibility for anything that could have been handled better. Emphasise the positive aspects of care given during that time, which demonstrates how the team were trying their best for the patient. Refer to the whole team, including consultants and nurses, as a unit. Make it clear that lessons have been learned and suggest what changes might be made to improve things.
This section usually takes the longest, and you may have to be creative and repeat your points to get the actor to accept them. Be gentle, not confrontational. When you have got through all the points, go on to the next section.

For details on how to structure your answer when breaking bad news and obtaining consent, see pgs 448, 453.

7. Express your sorrow/apologise

It is vital that you say how sorry you are for the pain suffered by the reason for the complaint, or the bad news you have broken. Saying sorry is not the same as accepting responsibility for negligence, and may be all the actor wants to hear.

8. Check the actor has understood the key facts

Once you have finished the discussion, summarise what you have said and check that the actor is satisfied with the explanations in the complaint situation, understands the implications of the bad news, or understands the procedure and complications in the consent scenario. This may involve repeating yourself, but this is no bad thing when you are trying to put your point across or explain a complicated subject.

9. Ask for any other or new worries and deal with them systematically
'Is that all clear, is there anything that worries you in particular that you would like to discuss?' Don't forget to elicit the actor's view 'How do you feel, has this conversation helped you?'

This is usually towards the end of a complaint consultation, but may be just the beginning of a consent or breaking bad news consultation as the fears and worries come pouring out. Again, listen empathetically, list the concerns, re-present them to the actor in a summarised form, and then deal with them fully one at a time. The consultation is not over until all the concerns have been dealt with. If something seems irresolvable, or you do not have the information they are asking for, consider referral to the appropriate service. 'I can arrange for you to discuss that further with the stoma care nurse/breast care nurse/bereavement counsellor/the consultant performing the operation/the oncologist if you wish.' Make up a definite time off the top of your head: 'She has a slot free tomorrow morning if that would be convenient.'

10. Summarise key facts again and outline immediate action

11. Check the actor is happy with this and does not have any outstanding issues
'Is that all right? Is there anything we haven't covered that you would like to discuss with me?'

12. Offer as a future contact
This may be yourself or an appropriate colleague such as a breast care nurse or colorectal nurse specialist. Make sure the patient is clear on how to contact that person. 'Is there anything else I can arrange for you? Remember, if there are any problems just ring the hospital and ask for Mr. Black's secretary and she can make sure one of us gets back to you. Don't forget my name, Cathy Parchment Smith, Mr Black's SHO, just ask for me if you want to speak to me again.'

13. Departure stating next point of contact
Shake hands and say when you'll see them next, or, if no follow-up is planned, how they can get hold of you if they need to.

SUMMARY

1. Starting the interview
2. Gather information from the actor
3. Empathise with actor
4. Summarise actor input and confirm you are dealing with the correct issues
5. Outline your plan for the consultation (say what you are going to say)
6. Give the actor information in a structured way (say it)
7. Express your sorrow/apologise
8. Check the actor has understood the key facts
9. Ask for any other or new worries and deal with them systematically
10. Summarise key facts again and outline immediate action (say what you've said)
11. Check the actor is happy with this and does not have any outstanding issues
12. Offer a future contact
13. Departure stating next point of contact

The following cases use this basic interview structure as a guide and demonstrate how to adapt it to the common scenarios seen in this bay.

C The Cases

DEALING WITH A COMPLAINT

1. Starting the interview

Greeting
'Good morning,' shake hands, smile.

Introductions
Say who you are.
'I'm Dr Parchment Smith.'

Confirm who they are and their relationship to the patient if appropriate
'Are you Mr Angry, son of Mrs Poorly?'

Say what you had to do with the case and why you are there.
'I am one of the surgical doctors on Mr Black's team who helped look after your mother. I understand you have some concerns about her care and I'm here to find out what they are and see if I can help.'

Make the actor comfortable
'Take a seat, sir.'

2. Gather information from the actor
'Mr Angry, I understand you have some concerns about your mother's treatment. Would you tell me about these, please?'

3. Empathise with the actor
'I see what you mean.' 'That must have been awful for you and the family.'

4. Summarise the actor's input and confirm you are dealing with the correct issues
'So as I understand it, Mr Angry, the main problems are threefold. Firstly, your mother had to wait in casualty for over 12 hours, which I can see, must have been very distressing. Secondly, when you got up to the ward you didn't see the consultant which was the main reason your whole family had been waiting there all night. And lastly, you were not informed when your mother was taken to the operating theatre, and since she unfortunately died on the intensive care unit straight afterwards, you and your sisters felt, understandably, that you weren't given the chance to say goodbye. Are those the main problems? Was there any other aspect of the care that you were unhappy with?'

442

5. Outline your plan for the consultation

'I've heard what you have to say, Mr Angry, and I'm going to take those points one by one, if you'll allow me, and try to explain what I think happened to cause all these problems.'

6. Give the actor information in a structured way

'To deal with the first point, Mr Angry, I agree that 12 hours is a ridiculous amount of time for a seriously ill woman to spend in casualty (**empathy**).

You know that the bed crisis is a serious problem in the National Health Service and our team faces this awful situation every day (**reason for problem beyond our control**).

We understand that there are ten new surgical beds due to be opened next year, which might help ease, the situation. However, this doesn't help you or your poor mother who was on a trolley with no ward bed to go to for a considerably long time (**what might be done in the future to avoid it happening again**).

What I will say is that the SHO did her best to try and find a bed. I think you heard her on the phone in casualty discussing with the bed manager the urgency of your mother's case. She even considered sending your mother to the General Infirmary 15 miles away. She discussed this with your sisters who were not keen, and also with the consultant who thought that this would be too dangerous as she was too ill to be moved (**measures taken at the time by team to try to solve the problem**).

In addition, I'm sure you will agree that the staff did everything in their power to make your mother as comfortable as possible in such dire circumstances. The casualty sister freed up a side room for her, and the house officer was able to start all the necessary treatment including a drip and painkillers while in casualty. When a bed did become available, I understand the house officer even helped push your mother's trolley to the ward because there was a shortage of porters (**emphasise the positive care given**).

May I say that the situation was intolerable and I'm deeply sorry for the distress it caused you and your family. (**Apologise unreservedly**) I hope you feel that the staff tried everything they could to get your mother a suitable bed as soon a possible. (**Try to get resolution and agreement from relative before moving on to second point.**)

As to the second point, of your mother not seeing a consultant at two in the morning when she arrived on the ward ....'

7. Express your sorrow/apologise

'I would like to say how sorry I am that you had such an awful experience. I'm sure I speak for all the staff when I apologise for the distressing situation you and your family found themselves in.'

8. Check the actor has understood the key facts

'So in summary, Mr Angry, I think we agree that you and your family went through a terrible time that was made worse by some unfortunate problems here at the hospital for which I apologise. Firstly, the bed situation, you appreciate, was beyond our control, but I hope you understand that we did everything we could under the circumstances. Secondly, Mr Black was mortified that you didn't realise he had seen your mother already in casualty, and I am so sorry you were under the impression that he would be waiting for you on the ward. I'm sure that the student nurse didn't realise her comments would have led to such an impression. And thirdly, what a shame about your sister's mobile phone batteries! If only we could have got through to her to let her know we were taking your mum to theatre, but as you can appreciate now I have explained about her sudden deterioration, our main priority was to get her to the operating theatre as quickly as possible. I'm glad that you have said how kind the junior doctors and nurses were to your mum; I'm sure you realise that we were all trying to do our best for her under difficult circumstances.'

9. Ask for any other or new worries and deal with them systematically

'Has that been at all helpful? Is there anything that worries you in particular that you would like to discuss?'

10. Summarise key facts again and outline immediate action

'So, Mr Angry, I'll leave it with you to contact Mr Black's secretary if your sisters would like to take up his offer of a chat with him.'

11. Check the actor is happy with this and does not have any outstanding issues

'Is that all right? Is there anything we haven't covered that you would like to discuss with me?'

12. Offer your services as a future contact

'Is there anything else I can arrange for you? Remember, if there are any problems just ring the hospital and ask for Mr Black's secretary and she can make sure one of us gets back to you. Don't forget my name, Cathy Parchment Smith, Mr Black's SHO, just ask for me if you want to speak to me again.'

13. Departure stating next point of contact

Shake hands.
'Goodbye, Mr Angry. Don't hesitate to call anytime. Regards to your sisters.'

BREAKING BAD NEWS

1. Starting the interview

Greeting

'Good morning.' Shake hands, smile.

Introductions

'I'm Dr Parchment Smith. Are you Mrs Anxious?'

Say what you had to do with the case and why you are there

'I am one of the surgical doctors on Mr Black's team and I'm here to discuss the results of your tests.'

Make the actor comfortable

'Take a seat, madam. Have you anyone with you here today? Would you like them to come in as well?'

2. Gather information from the actor

'Mrs Anxious, I'd like to start by asking you what you understand so far about what has happened and why you are here today.'

3. Empathise with actor

'Yes that's right. Yes it is quite complicated.'

4. Summarise the actor's input and confirm you are dealing with the correct issues

'Yes, Mrs Anxious, we have got the results of the cells we took from your breast. As you know, we also did a mammogram, and I have those results here also.'

5. Outline your plan for the consultation

'Mrs Anxious, I am going to give you the results of the biopsies and scans and have a chat with you about what we need to do about them. Would you like me to give you the full details of the diagnosis, or is there someone else you would like me to tell?'

6. Give the actor information in a structured way

'The first thing to say is that I'm afraid the results show that the lump is a cancer' (diagnosis). Allow a pause for her reaction. If there is none, ask how she feels.

'Are you OK? It's a shock, I know. How do you feel?'

Check how much information the patient wants to know.

'Would you like me to tell you the details or would you just like to know what happens next for now?'

Depending on the response, give a detailed outline or a summarised outline of the facts. Avoid jargon, and use aids such as repetition or diagrams (see Educating, pg 449).

'The mammograms and the cells we looked at both show that this is cancer of the breast. It is quite a small lump so the best course of action is to remove the lump and some of the glands in the armpit in an operation. We can arrange that for you urgently next week. You will be in hospital for a couple of days, and if the results show that the cancer is cleared by the operation and there is no cancer in the glands in the armpit, then we would hopefully not need to do any more, just check you over in the clinic regularly. You will not need to lose the whole breast unless the results show that there is cancer left after the operation. You will need radiotherapy after the operation. We would also send you to an oncologist after the operation and he would decide if you would benefit from a course of medical treatment after surgery.'

Check that they have understood

'It's a lot of information, am I making sense to you?'

Ask if that's all they want to know

'Is there anything else you would like to know at this stage?'

7. Express your sorrow/apologise

'I can see you're upset. You weren't expecting this news were you? I'm so sorry.'

8. Check the actor has understood the key facts

This may mean repeating yourself.

'So, Mrs Anxious, you understand that the mammogram and the cells show that the lump is cancer of the breast. I have explained that we plan to admit you to hospital on Thursday for an operation to remove the malignant lump, and some of the glands from under your right arm. Before then, tomorrow, you and your husband will meet with Carol, our breast care nurse and have a chest X-ray and scan of the liver for the reasons we discussed. You will be in hospital for at least two days and a night, but, all being well hopefully be allowed home at the weekend. I have explained that we will not know what, if any further treatment is needed until we have examined the lump, so we will discuss that with you on the following Wednesday.'

9. Ask for any other or new worries and deal with them systematically
'Is that all clear? Is there anything that worries you in particular that you would like to discuss?'

10. Summarise key facts again and outline immediate action
'So Mrs Anxious, you have an appointment with the breast care nurse tomorrow and we'll see you on Thursday morning on Ward A2.'

11. Check the actor is happy with this and does not have any outstanding issues
'Is that all right? Is there anything we haven't covered that you would like to discuss with me?'

12. Offer your services as a future contact
'Is there anything else I can arrange for you? Remember, if there are any problems just ring the hospital and ask for Mr Black's secretary and she can make sure one of us gets back to you. Don't forget my name, Cathy Parchment Smith, Mr Black's SHO, just ask for me if you want to speak to me again.'

13. Departure stating next point of contact
Shake hands.
'Goodbye Mrs Anxious. I'll see you on Thursday.'

NOTES ON BREAKING BAD NEWS

1: Getting Started
How?
In person, not by phone or letter
Where?
In a private room/curtains drawn around bed/both sitting down
Who?
Relatives, friend or nurse present as the patient wishes.
What?
Normal courtesies (Say hello, use patient's name, introduce yourself).
Start with a general question to get the conversation going two ways, assess the patient's mental state and make the patient feel you care ('How are you today, Are you up to having a chat for a few minutes?').

2: Finding out how much the patient knows
How much have they been told?
'What have the doctors told you so far about the illness?'
How much have they understood?
'Have you been thinking that the illness might be serious?'
What is their level of understanding?
This will guide you to the level that you have to pitch your information.
Are they talking in simple terms:
'Well, Doctor says I've a growth of some kind and thank goodness, I thought, it's not a tumour or even worse, a cancer.'
or are they very well educated with a good medical knowledge and wide vocabulary:
'My family doctor thought it might be multiple sclerosis, and now Prof Brown tells me the visual-evoked potentials show optic neuritis.'
What are their feelings?
Distressed, anxious, brave but trembly, offhand and defensive, hostile, in denial?

3: Finding out how much the patient wants to know
'Would you like me to give you the full details of the diagnosis?'
'Are you the type of person who wants to know all the details of what's wrong, or would you prefer if I just tell you what's going to happen next?'
'If your condition is serious, how much would you like to know about it?'
'That's fine. If you change your mind or want any questions answered at future visits, just ask me at any time. I won't push information at you if you don't want it.'

4: Sharing Information
Decide on your agenda:
    Diagnosis
    Treatment plan
    Prognosis
    Support
Start from the patient's starting point (Aligning)
Repeat to the patient what they have said to you and reinforce those things they have said which are correct (gives patient confidence that you are taking their point of view seriously and respect them).

Give the information you need to tell clearly (Educating)
Give the information in small chunks with warning shots
    'Well, the situation does appear to be more serious than that.'
Do not use jargon.
    Say tumour AND THEN cancer, not space occupying lesion or malignancy.
Check reception and clarify.
    'Am I making sense? Do you follow what I'm saying?'
Make sure you both mean the same thing.
    'Do you understand what I mean when I say it's incurable?'
Repeat important points.
    'So, as I said, the main facts are'
    'It's a lot of information, but basically'
Use diagrams and written messages.
Use any printed or recorded information available.
Check your level – too complicated or too patronising?
Listen for the patient's agenda
    'Is there anything you particularly want to talk through/are worried about?'
Try to blend your patient's agenda with the patient's.
Be prepared for the 'last minute' query – the hidden question or the patient trying to ' lead' the interview.

5: Responding to the patient's feelings
Identify and acknowledge the patient's reaction.
Allow silence if needed.
Denial is perfectly natural and should be challenged only if causing serious problems for the patient.
Anger and blame need to be acknowledged; exploring the causes can follow later.
Despair and depression must be acknowledged. Allow the patient to express their feelings and offer support.
Awkward questions such as 'how long have I got?' You may have no honest answer and you may have to reply with an open question, an empathic response, or silence in some situations.
Collusion, where relatives ask the doctor not to tell the patient, is a common request. It must be made clear that the duty of the doctor lies first to the patient, but reasons for collusion need to be explored.

6: Planning and follow through
Organising and planning
Planning for the future is a good way to alleviate the bewildered, dispirited, disorganised thoughts of a patient who has just received bad news.
Demonstrate an understanding of the patient's problem list.
Identify the problems that are 'fixable' and those that are not.
Make a plan, putting the 'fixable' problems in order of priority and explain what you are going to do about each one.
Prepare the patient for the worst and give them some hope for the best.
Identify coping strategies of the patient and reinforce them.
    'I think it's brilliant that you and your wife have started attending a support group and I would encourage this as long as you find it helpful.'
Identify other sources of support for the patient and incorporate them.
    'Your daughter was asking if she could come up and help – perhaps you could let her do some of the shopping and housework once a week?'
Make a contract and follow it through
Summarise the plan you have formulated
Check there are no outstanding issues
Outline what will happen next and what the patient is expected to do.
Make sure you leave an avenue open for further communication.
    'So the cancer care nurse will contact you on Monday and we'll see you on Friday to discuss the CT results.'
    'So the oncologist will expect you at Cookridge Hospital a week on Thursday. I haven't made a formal arrangement to see you again, but you know to contact your GP or ring Mr Black's secretary if you have any problems in the meanwhile.'

OBTAINING CONSENT

1. Starting the interview

Greeting
'Good Morning.' Shake hands and smile/look friendly.

Introductions
'I'm Dr Parchment Smith. Are you Mr. Preop?'

Say what you had to do with the case and why you are there
'I am one of the surgical doctors on Mr Black's team.'

Make the actor comfortable
'Take a seat, sir.'

2. Gather information from the actor
'Mr Preop, what have you been told so far about the operation and why you're having it?'

3. Empathise with actor
Listen encouragingly, nodding and saying 'That's right.'

4. Summarise the actor's input and confirm you are dealing with the correct issues
'Yes, Mr Preop, we have found a blockage in the bowel that we need to operate on. The biopsy results were, as you say, proof of cancer of the bowel causing the blockage. You seem convinced that the cancer has spread, but the scans did not show any spread to the liver, so we have no evidence of that at the moment.'

5. Outline your plan for the consultation
'Mr Preop, I would like to explain the operation we are planning to you now including why, when, what and how we are hoping to go about it. I would also like to tell you a bit about the recovery time and discuss the possible complications. Please feel free to stop me at any time if there is something you don't understand. This is also the time to ask me about anything that may be worrying or confusing you. When everything is clear, I will ask for your signed consent.'

6. Give the actor information in a structured way

You should now go through the consent procedure as outlined on pg 453 getting the patient to sign consent only when it is clear that he understands everything. The main areas that should be covered are listed in detail under '**Providing sufficient information'** and include:

Indication for the treatment (diagnosis, prognosis, what would happen if we didn't operate, what the aim of the surgery is, alternatives available).

Details of the surgery (including preoperative preparation, the planned procedure, pain relief such as epidurals and postoperative care such as HDU).

Complications (common ones even if trivial, serious ones even if rare).

Expected outcome and follow-up (chances of success, permanent changes such as stomas, plans for adjuvant therapy and postoperative scans or endoscopy).

The team involved (mention the consultant in overall care, stress that his juniors will be helping and that student nurses or doctors may be present, emphasise the multidisciplinary team, stoma nurse, anaesthetist, ward staff, dietician etc.).

Unforeseen procedures (the patient should be warned that if anything happens which we don't foresee we may have to carry out an unexpected procedure which would occur only if it could not be safely delayed and was in his best interests).

Objections to treatments to be noted (e.g. is he a Jehovah's witness who wishes to decline in advance any blood transfusion?).

Patient's rights (to withdraw consent, to change their mind at any time even after signing, to seek a second opinion).

Once you are sure the patient has understood and does not need more information or more time to think about it, you can ask him to sign the consent form.

7. Express your sorrow/apologise

'I know this must be an anxious time for you, Mr Preop, and I'm sorry to overwhelm you with all this information, but it is important that you understand what we are planning to do. Don't worry, you are in good hands and we will be doing our very best for you.'

8. Check the actor has understood the key facts

'So, Mr Preop, you understand that you will be having a CT scan tomorrow and that on Wednesday you will start a course of Radiotherapy at Cookridge hospital. When that is finished, we will book you in for surgery, and you will have to have those clear-out sachets again. You will come into hospital on a Thursday evening and have surgery on Friday. You understand that we will be removing the bit of bowel with the cancer in it that includes the lowest part of the bowel. So we will be sealing up your back passage and leaving you with a permanent bag on your tummy where your motions will collect and be emptied. The stoma care nurse will be having a chat with you about those details tomorrow. You also understand that we are hoping to cure you with this operation, but cannot be sure that the cancer will not come back. After the operation you will be on the high dependency unit for a couple of days, but if all goes well we would hope to have you home within a fortnight. You have heard me explain a long list of possible complications, including not making it through the operation, infections, pneumonia, heart attack and thrombosis, but you understand that as a relatively young non-smoker, you have a good chance of getting through this operation with no problems. After surgery, when we have analysed the cancer, we will decide if you need chemotherapy, but if it is at an early stage we will not. We will keep you under regular follow-up.'

9. Ask for any other or new worries and deal with them systematically

'Is that all clear? Is there anything that worries you in particular that you would like to discuss?'

10. Summarise key facts again and outline immediate action

'So, Mr Preop, you have a CT booked for tomorrow after your chat with the stoma care nurse, an appointment to see Dr Radio at Cookridge hospital on Wednesday and we'll see you again after your radiotherapy.'

11. Check the actor is happy with this and does not have any outstanding issues

'Is that all right? Is there anything we haven't covered that you would like to discuss with me?'

12. Offer your services as a future contact

'Is there anything else I can arrange for you? Remember, if there are any problems just ring the hospital and ask for Mr Black's secretary and she can make sure one of us gets back to you. Don't forget my name, Cathy Parchment Smith, Mr Black's SHO, just ask for me if you want to speak to me again.'

13. Departure stating next point of contact

'Goodbye, Mr Preop. I'll see you in a few weeks time.'

NOTES ON OBTAINING CONSENT

The GMC gives useful guidelines in **Seeking patient's consent: the ethical consideration** published by the General Medical Council November 1998. These guidelines are summarised below, the original booklet is available from the General Medical Council.

Providing sufficient information which may include:
Details of diagnosis and prognosis.
Prognosis if condition is left untreated.
Options for further investigations if diagnosis is uncertain.
Options for treatment or management of the condition.
The option not to treat.
The purpose of the proposed investigation or treatment.
Details of the procedure including subsidiary treatment such as pain relief.
How the patient should prepare for the procedure.
Common and serious side-effects.
Likely benefits and probabilities of success.
Discussion of any serious or frequently occurring risks.
Lifestyle changes which may be caused by the treatment.
Advice on whether any part of the proposed treatment is experimental.
How and when the patient's condition will be monitored and reassessed.
The name of the doctor who has overall responsibility for the treatment.
Whether doctors in training or students will be involved.
A reminder that patients can change their minds about a decision at any time.
A reminder that patients have a right to seek a second opinion.
Explain how decisions are made about whether to move from one stage of treatment to another (e.g. chemotherapy).
Explain that there may be different teams of doctors involved (e.g. anaesthetists).
Seek consent to treat any problems which might arise and need dealing with while the patient is unconscious or otherwise unable to make a decision.
Ascertain whether there are any procedures to which a patient would object to (e.g. blood transfusions).
Ask patients whether they have understood the information and whether they would like more before making a decision.

Responding to questions
You must respond honestly to any questions the patient raises, and, as far as possible, answer as fully as the patient wishes.

Withholding information
You should not withhold information necessary for decision making unless you judge that disclosure of some relevant information would cause the patient serious harm (not including becoming upset or refusing treatment).
You may not withhold information from a patient at the request of any other person including a relative.
If a patient insists they do not want to know the details of a condition or a treatment, you should explain the importance of knowing the options and should still provide basic information about the treatment unless you think this would cause the patient some harm.
You must record in the medical records if you have withheld treatment and your reasons for doing so.

Presenting information to patients

Discuss treatment options at a time when the patient is best able to understand and retain the information.

Use up-to-date written material, visual and other aids to explain complex aspects of the treatment where appropriate.

Make arrangements to meet particular communication needs (e.g. with translators or deaf-signers).

Discuss the possibility of the patient bringing a friend or relative or making a tape recording of the consultation.

Use accurate data to explain the probabilities of success or the risks of failure.

Ensure distressing information is given in a considerate way, and offer access to counselling services and patient support groups.

Allow patients time to absorb the material, perhaps with repeated consultations or written back-up material.

Involve nursing or other members of the health care team.

Ensure that the patient has an opportunity to review their decision nearer the time.

Who obtains consent?

The responsibility is that of the doctor providing the treatment or undertaking the investigation.

If obtaining consent is delegated to someone other than the doctor providing the treatment the person to whom the task is delegated should be:

Suitably trained and qualified

Have sufficient knowledge of the treatment and understand the risks

Act in accordance with the above GMC guidelines

The doctor providing the treatment remains responsible for ensuring the patient has been given sufficient time and information to make a decision.

Ensuring voluntary decision-making

You may recommend a course of action but you must not put pressure on patients to accept your advice.

Forms of consent

Patients can indicate their informed consent either orally or in writing. Written consent is advised if:

The treatment or procedure is complex, or involves significant risks or side-effects.

Providing clinical care is not the primary purpose of the investigation or examination, or the treatment is part of a research programme.

There may be significant consequences for the patient's employment, social or personal life.

Where the law requires written consent (e.g. some fertility treatments).

The nature of information provided, specific requests by the patient and details of the scope of the consent given should be recorded.

A signed consent is not sufficient evidence that a patient has given or still gives informed consent to the proposed treatment in all its aspects, and their decision must be reviewed close to the time of treatment.

Children and consent

At age 16 a young person can be treated as an adult and can be presumed to have capacity to decide.

Under age 16 children may have the capacity to decide, depending on their ability to understand what is involved.

Where a competent child refuses treatment, a person with parental responsibility or the court may authorise investigation or treatment that is in the child's best interests (except in Scotland).

Where a child is under 16 and is not competent, a person with parental responsibility may authorise treatment, which are in the child's best interest.

Those with parental responsibility may refuse intervention on behalf of an incompetent child under 16, but you are not bound by that refusal and may seek a ruling from the court. In an emergency, you may treat an incompetent child against the wishes of those with parental responsibility. Where you consider it is in the child's best interests provided it is limited to that treatment which is reasonably required in that emergency (e.g. you can give a life-saving blood transfusion to the incompetent child of Jehovah's Witness parents who refuse to consent, but not to a competent Jehovah's Witness who refuses consent, whatever their age).

Pregnant women and consent

The right to decide applies equally to pregnant women as to other patients, and includes the right to refuse treatment where the treatment is intended to benefit the unborn child.

454

The current marking schedule for the MRCS (Eng) gives marks for each of the following five points, and these are what the examiners will be looking for to tick off on their mark sheet as they watch your performance. This may change after December 2002 always check with your college.

1. Starting the interview

<u>Introduction and greeting</u>

>   Say hello, shake hands, say who you are, check who they are, say what you're there for, make the actor comfortable.

2. Data gathering

<u>Open/closed questions</u>

>   Closed questions for gathering information
>   'Have you had radiotherapy?'
>   Open questions to gauge patient wishes and encourage two-way communication
>   'What do you understand about the situation so far?'

<u>Facilitation</u>

>   Nodding head
>   Repeating last statement e.g. 'so you're worried about your family – what worries in particular?'

<u>Clear questions/statements</u>

>   'I'm sorry to have to tell you that your daughter is dead.'
>   'The cells show that the lump is cancer.'

<u>Asks the actor's view</u>

>   'How do you feel about that?'

3. Organised approach

<u>Appropriate pace</u>

Do not rush, interrupt or babble (the commonest mistakes).

Do not allow long awkward gaps where you are obviously at a loss for something to say.

<u>Use of silence</u>

In some cases, e.g. after breaking bad news, you need to give the actor time to respond, to think or simply to sit in a stunned silence for a while. A period of sensitive silence is appropriate in these circumstances.

<u>Redirects if necessary</u>

'Shall we talk about what the plans are at the moment?'

4. Emotional support

<u>Empathy</u>
'I can see this must be difficult for you.'
'It's a lot of information to take in, isn't it?'
<u>Use of touch</u>
Touch arm if appropriate
<u>Conveys concern/interest</u>
'Is there someone here with you today?'
'Would you like to sit here with a cup of tea for a bit before you go back to her?'

5. Body language

<u>Open/listening posture</u>
Lean forward
Don't cross arms or legs
<u>Eye contact</u>
Look at actor and nod

E   Getting out of trouble with an 'Oscar' winning performance

The bay consists of role play with an actor, and as such, more than the other bays, is a fictional performance which you are required to put on to demonstrate your skills of inventiveness. All the features of a 'Hollywood blockbuster' combine to pull off a competent and mark-winning performance. You will need to write your own script off the top of your head, be a convincing actor, inject some drama and tear-jerking pathos. If you're going for an Oscar, you might want to add just a touch of romance and humour!

In real life, consultations with distraught patients may be very difficult because you don't know the patient or the details of the case. But in the exam, the whole performance is in your hands, and you can make up a scenario that shows you and your team off in its best light. Obviously, the following comments only apply to the faintly absurd situation of role-playing with an actor in the exam. You could never use deceitful tactics with patients in your real practice, make up false excuses for team members, and invent appointments you can't guarantee will happen or pretend you were fond of a patient you hardly knew. But it is precisely because the communications bay is so artificial that you can use all these techniques to your advantage in the exam situation.

Make up a good script
It is important that you do not waffle about things about which you know nothing, like the specialist treatment of rare diseases or the selection and complications of chemotherapy regimes. You will not be given all the information you need to answer the actor's questions so you will have to improvise and 'ad lib' when you are stuck for an answer. Try the **'I can't tell you but I know a man who can'** approach, saying things like 'we will be sending you to the regional specialist centre in Birmingham for treatment of your sarcoma, and they will be able to tell you more about the treatment.' Or 'I have made an appointment with the Oncologist on Friday for you and your husband, and they will decide if chemotherapy is for you, and if so which regime and what side-effects you might expect.'

Stick to what you know – if in doubt, cast your mind back to similar patients you have had to deal with and where you got the necessary information. Feel free to make up **glamorous locations and a star supporting cast** based on your own previous experiences. For example 'As you know, we are only a small district general hospital, so as soon as we discovered the seriousness of your mother's condition we sent her to the specialist hospital in the city centre so she could have the necessary haemodialysis.' Or 'I'm glad you asked that; we have a wide range of breast prostheses and the breast care specialist nurse is waiting outside now to discuss what she can offer you after the operation.'

It is also important you do not get drawn into criticisms of your team's (especially your bosses) deficiencies or absences, and cover for them imaginatively. Stories about their participation in the case (**'They wanted to be here themselves tonight but'**) are useful such as 'My consultant is in theatre at the moment, but he has asked me to make a note of anything which you wish to discuss with him and he will be happy to see you and go into it in more detail' or 'The junior doctor concerned is very sorry about what happened, and he has asked me to make it clear to you that he and the consultant would be more than happy to meet with you and go through anything which I do not make clear.'

Convey tear-jerking pathos
In complaints or explaining deaths, one of the best ways to get the actor on your side is to **convey how much the patient meant to the team.** This gives the (almost always accurate) impression that the surgeons, nurses and family were all on the same side, and were all disappointed when things turned out badly. Making up **endearing personal characteristics** (within limits) is a useful tool, as is **identifying particular members of the team** who were closest to the patient and who the family were likely to have heard of or have met. For example 'The doctors and nurses were devastated when she died. She was always so cheerful and uncomplaining, and Sister Green said she was a pleasure to nurse.' or 'We certainly miss her on the ward. She was a very thoughtful lady and was a particular favourite of Dr Brown, the house officer. I know he was especially upset when we couldn't save her.' or 'I'm sure your family are distraught. I know how close you all were, she often used to tell us how you and your brother did everything for her.' Remember how it feels to lose a patient of whom you were very fond in real life, and try to convey the sense of empathy you had in that real situation into this artificially staged one.

Add drama
The relative must be made aware of how much the team has struggled to do their utmost for the patient throughout their dealings with her. Outlining a scenario to demonstrate this, by going through the script **casting your team as the embattled heroes** is a good technique.

'When Mr Black first saw your mother in clinic, he was so shocked by her condition that he wouldn't even let her go home. He got her straight onto Sister Green's ward and Dr Brown the house officer urgently arranged all her investigations that same afternoon including the contrast X-ray that showed the blockage. You will remember that we worked through the night getting your mother into a fit state for surgery. Putting up oxygen masks, putting in drips and antibiotics and moving her to the high dependency unit where the consultant anaesthetist himself saw her and put her on medicine to improve her chest. By morning she was more stable so we got her first on the list in the operating theatre where the whole team worked on her for four hours, trying to take out the cancer and deal with the damage the blockage had caused. Mr Black was very disappointed when he found that the cancer was so extensive, but he said that wasn't going to stop him doing whatever he could to give your mother every chance. Unfortunately, as you know, her poor heart couldn't take the strain of such a major operation after such a bad illness, and she had a massive heart attack that night. The whole team were devastated after working so hard to save her, and we feel for your family, who must be in shock as it was so unexpected.'

Most admissions to hospital, especially emergency surgeries, lend themselves very well to a dramatic tale, and relaying this to the actor, with the emphasis on how events conspired against the heroic efforts of a willing team, will make him feel that **'everything possible was done.'** Keep the story clear, the language simple but the medical facts accurate, like an episode of a TV medical drama programme, and avoid jargon.

Risk a bit of humour

The actors are often aggressive and hostile as they are instructed to be. **There are not many cases where humour is appropriate**, and it is a risky tactic, which must be done sensitively, but if you can get the actor to smile with you, the interview has almost certainly been a success. The best cases for these are those involving children, where you can convey fondness for your patient, empathy with the parent and inject humour to relax the atmosphere by recounting a little (made up, of course!) **story about the bravery of the child**. In my exam, I had to 'counsel' an actor playing a woman whose child had fractured a femur in an accident on his bike. After all the preliminaries and dealing with her questions, but before terminating the interview, I said 'He's really impressing us all with how brave he is. He keeps asking about whether we'll be able to fix his bike – I think he's more worried about that than his leg, bless him.' Hardly Oscar winning comedy, but it raised a smile from my previously distraught actor mum and showed a personal touch which reassured her that people who cared about her 'son' were looking after him.

Easy on the romance
The appropriate use of touch to convey empathy gives you a credit in the marking scheme of the communications bay. However, most people would agree that, to keep it professional, **a reassuring touch on the arm or hand** if the actor seems particularly distraught would be the full extent of the physical contact deemed appropriate. Try to get this in if you can, but don't let it linger uncomfortably long, and be careful not to be too enthusiastic. (I once gave a reassuring squeeze to the groin of an elderly male actor in my communications bay of the 'Care of the Critically Ill Patient' course because he moved his hand to wipe an imaginary tear just as I was lunging for it!)

Unlike the Oscars, romantic gestures have no place in the MRCS examination. Boys especially, be careful that you do not touch the actor in anyway that could be deemed inappropriate (e.g. an Oscar-winner's hug on departure!). Girls may, depending on what you are like in real life with patients, feel it appropriate to be a bit more physical but **be guided by the actor.** A bereaved trembly old lady who collapses in hysterics obviously needs a bit more contact than a stiff, cross, middle-aged businessman with a complaint about the care of his mother.

Avoid overacting
Don't get carried away. Film buffs take painful pleasure in watching the best actress on the televised awards ceremony gripping her Oscar with tears running down her cheeks as she gives a cringeworthy gushing speech in an ill-fitting pink dress. Not the look we're going for here! Stay professional. Don't cry! Don't grip the actor's hands in yours throughout the interview! Don't rabbit on making up elaborate fantasies. Just stick to short bits of make-believe which help you get through the tricky bits.

Try method acting
Some of us, especially girls, absolutely love this bay because we get to pretend, playact, cajole, make up stories and charm grumpy old men, which we are good at because, as women in surgery, we tend to spend our whole working week doing just that. On the other hand, some people (sorry boys, but it seems to be usually you lot!) will almost always find this bay a torture because playacting does not come naturally to them. They will be stiff and artificial, because they feel frankly ridiculous at having to go through this charade which is in so many ways artificial. The worst hurdle is in pretending the actor is a real patient or relative (and, although mine was very good, some actors are apparently, so bad as to be frankly laughable). The best way to get over this is to take a leaf out of Robert De Niro's book and indulge in some method acting yourself. In this technique, you have to suspend disbelief and go into the consultation believing this really is a patient or relative, and you really do have to talk to them as you would at work. When you make up things, such as your breast care nurse outside the door, or the

appointment with the consultant oncologist who will explain all the chemotherapy, tell yourself that this is what really would be happening in a genuine clinic. You may not be able to throw yourself into it and take their hand and make up charming tales about their sweet departed imaginary mother, but at least you will be able to turn in a reasonable performance. And let's face it, not all of us can be Oscar winners.

F Details of the communication cases from our survey

Total 52 cases. Please note that some of the Royal colleges do not include a Communications bay in their examination.

Type of case	Number seen in survey	Breakdown and details of cases
Explain to a relative	32	10 that patient has to have emergency operation 14 that patient has had complication of operation 8 who is anxious about a diagnosis /operation /failed care
Consent patient	13	6 for elective operation 2 addressing specific concern 3 for procedure 2 for emergency operation
Breaking bad news	4	
Investigate presenting complaint	2	
Dealing with complaint	1	(but applies in part to many of above – see list of cases pg 463)

Examples of Communication Cases from our survey

1. A patient with diabetes is admitted with diabetic ketoacidosis, confused with a previous below knee amputation. There is infection in the remaining foot. An X-ray shows gas in the tissues. Explain to the son of the patient the possibility of operation and possible amputation.

2. You are the surgical SHO on call, being asked to speak to a child's mother. The child had an appendicectomy eight days previously (for a perforated appendix) which had been complicated by postoperative swinging pyrexia. The child recovered from this and was discharged seven days post-operatively. He re-presented to casualty with an offensive brown discharge from his wound, but was systemically well. The mother was anxious, angry that the child had not been seen by a consultant prior to discharge, and argued that he had been discharged too early.

3. Describe to a mother the reasons for an emergency hernia repair in a young child. Explain the method of repair.

4. You have to explain the situation of a urology patient to his anxious father. His son is about to undergo a percutaneous nephrostomy for an infected, obstructed kidney.

5. A young female patient attends clinic for the results of a biopsy of a lump in her breast. The results indicate a cancer. Tell what she has and what to do next.

6. A patient had a left thyroid lobectomy 10 years ago for a multinodular goitre. Since then her voice has never been as strong as it was previously. Now the same patient needs a right thyroid lobectomy for a cold nodule and is worried about her voice. Talk to her.

7. Consent a 50-year-old with rectal bleeding for a flexible sigmoidoscopy. The patient is anxious, and during the discussion a history of a change in bowel habit and a concern about the possibility of cancer emerges. The patient asks about the possible management afterwards depending on the results.

8. A lady has a myocardial infarction five days after repair of her abdominal aortic aneurysm and is transferred to CCU. Explain the situation to her husband.

9. Consent a man for TURP explaining the procedure and outlining the risks. The actor was a kind intelligent man with no inappropriate reactions.

10. A patient is arriving in clinic for the results of a previous FNA of a lymph node. The results show atypical cells. Discuss this and consent for a lymph node biopsy in the neck.

11. A healthy male competitive swimmer in his thirties presents with unilateral gynaecomastia. Discuss possible causes, diagnosis and treatment options.

12. You are a casualty officer when a ten-year-old boy is brought in who has been knocked off his bike by a car. He has a closed, displaced, angulated fracture of the left femoral shaft but is cardiovascularly stable with no other injuries. His mother has just arrived in the hospital and knows only that her son was in a serious road accident and is going to the operating theatre. You have been asked to go to the relatives' room and tell her what is going on.

13. A patient has just been diagnosed with a low cancer of the rectum, and you have been asked to counsel his relative about the diagnosis, abdominoperineal resection, radiotherapy and chemotherapy.

14. Speak to the husband of a RTA victim before emergency surgery for a ruptured spleen.

15. A 70-year-old patient develops a haematoma and MRSA two weeks after a dynamic hip screw for a fractured neck of femur. Talk to his son about prognosis and management.

16. You are a Urology SHO when a 65-year-old man comes in with acute urinary retention. The surgical houseman has told him he may need an operation. The prostate is smooth and symmetrical. The patient is catheterised and a residual of 1,200 ml of urine is drained. Try to allay the patient's concerns about future holidays and sex life.

17. Talk to the parent of a 17-year-old girl diagnosed by her GP to have thyrotoxicosis with eye signs, weight loss and fatigue.

18. A 15-month-old boy is booked to have a herniotomy for a reduced right inguinal hernia. The parents have already discussed the case with the consultant, but have asked to see you, the SHO.

19. A retired man, recently married is due to have a cystectomy due to G2 pT2 transitional cell carcinoma of the bladder. He is concerned about the implications of ileal diversion. He had a myocardial infarction four years ago and would like to know about the risks of surgery. Counsel him and discuss alternative treatments.

20. An elderly patient is ten days post an abdominoperineal resection. His stoma has not worked and his abdomen is distended. His electrolytes show an increased urea and creatinine. An angry son would like to know why his father is confused, unshaven and smells of urine. He also thinks the ward is a disgrace! Talk to him.

21. A 15-year-old boy is due to go to theatre with a probable perforated appendix. Talk to his father, whose wife died under a general anaesthetic.

22. Speak to this HDU nurse whose father is under the care of the general surgeons. She has concerns about his postoperative care, including his fluid replacement and general nursing care.

23. A young boy has had a normal appendicectomy after a colleague made the incorrect diagnosis. Talk to his disgruntled parents.

24. A patient requires re-exploration for a possible anastomotic leak ten days after a large bowel resection. Obtain consent for re-exploration.

25. A young man is due for a Whipple's procedure but a drug overdose patient has taken the last ITU bed. The consultant is playing golf and the registrar cannot be contacted. Explain to the patient about the cancellation.
26. You are in the Endoscopy department and your consultant has been called away for 20 minutes. The next patient has been referred by his GP for an upper endoscopy following a suspicious barium swallow performed for dysphagia. The patient needs consenting but wants to know why they are doing another test. Speak to him.
27. You are the Orthopaedic SHO and have been asked to discuss the risks and procedure of a dynamic hip screw insertion in a 76-year-old with ischaemic heart disease with his concerned relatives.
28. Your patient is a 66-year-old demented lady in Accident and Emergency with extensive burns from a house fire. Explain her treatment and prognosis to her son, who is planning to sue the GP for not getting her into residential care sooner.
29. Discuss a planned hernia repair with this patient, who is keen to know the cause of hernias, what the operation entails and the postoperative course, all in non-medical language.

GLOSSARY

AAA	Abdominal aortic aneurysm
ABPI	Ankle-brachial pressure index
AF	Atrial fibrillation
AFP	Serum alpha fetoprotein
AJCC	American Joint Committee on Cancer
AKA	Above knee amputation
ASA	American Society of Anaesthesiologists
AV	Arteriovenous
BCC	Basal cell carcinoma
BKA	Below knee amputation
CCU	Coronary Care Unit
COAD	Chronic obstructive airways disease
CVA	Cerebrovascular accident
DVT	Deep vein thrombosis
EMD	Electromechanical dissociation
ESR	Erythrocyte sedimentation rate
FBC	Full blood count
FCU	Flexor carpi ulnaris
FDP	Flexor digitorum profundus
FNA	Fine needle aspiration
GA	General anaesthetic
GI	Gastrointestinal
HCG	Human chorionic gonadotrophin
HDU	High dependency unit
JVP	Jugular venous pressure
LA	Local anaesthetic
MEN	Multiple Endocrine Neoplasia

MESS	Mangled extremity severity score
MRA	Magnetic Resonance Angiography
MRSA	Methecillin-resistant *Staphylococcus aureus*
MSSUs	Mid-stream specimen of urine
MUA	Manipulation under anaesthetic
NASCENT	North American Symptomatic Carotid Endarterectomy Trial
NSAIDs	Non-steroidal anti-inflammatory drugs
OA	Osteoarthritis
ORIF	Open reduction, internal fixation
PE	Pulmonary embolism
PEG	Percutaneous endoscopic gastrostomy
Pr	Per rectum
PUVA	Psoralen drugs and u.v. light
RA	Rheumatoid arthritis
RIND	Reversible ischaemic neurological deficit
RTA	Road traffic accident
SFA	Superficial femoral artery
SHO	Senior House Officer
SOB	Shortness of breath
SVC	Superior Vena Cava
TEDs	Thrombo-embolic disease stockings
TIA	Transient ischaemic attack
TMB	Transient monocular blindness
TPA	Tissue plasminogen activator
TPN	Total parenteral nutrition
TURP	Transurethral resection of the prostate
UC	Ulcerative colitis
UICC	Union Internationale Contre le Cancer
UTI	Urinary tract infection

BIBLIOGRAPHY

ABC of Breast Disease: Dixon, 1st edition, BMJ Books, 1997.

ABC of Colorectal Disease: Jones D J, Irving MJ, 2nd edition, BMJ Books, 1999.

ABC of Urology: Dawson C, Whitfield H, 1st edition, BMJ Books, 1997.

An Aid to the MRCP Short Cases: Ryder, REJ et al., 1st edition, Blackwell Scientific Publications, 1992.

An Introduction to the Symptoms and Signs of Surgical Disease: Browse N, 3rd edition, Arnold Publishing (Hodder Headline), 1997.

Cash's Textbook of Orthopaedics and Rheumatology for Physiotherapists: Tidswell, ME, Downie PA et al (editors) Mosby Year Book Europe Ltd., 1992.

Clinical Anatomy for Medical Students: Snell RS, 6th edition, Lippincott Williams & Williams, 2000.

Clinical Orthopaedic Examination: McRae R, 3rd edition, Churchill Livingstone, 1996.

Clinical Signs: Hayes C and Bell D, new edition, Churchill Livingstone, 1996.

Concise System of Orthopaedics and Fractures: Apley A G, and Solomon, L. 2nd edition Butterworth Heinemann, 1998.

Operative Surgery: Calne R and Pollard, S, Gower Medical Publishing, 1991.

Oxford textbook of Medicine: Weatherall, D.J. et al. 3rd edition, Oxford University Press, 1996.

Picture Tests in Surgery: Stiff et al, 1st edition, Churchill Livingstone, 1996.

Practice Exercise Therapy: Hollis M, Blackwell Scientific Publications, 1998.

Practical Fracture Treatment: McRae R, 2nd edition, Churchill Livingstone, 1989.

Spot diagnosis in General Surgery: Ellis H, 2nd edition, Blackwell Science Ltd., 1993.

The New Aird's Companion in Surgical Studies: Burnand K et al, , 2nd edition, Churchill Livingstone, 1998.

INDEX

Page numbers in *italic* refer to illustrations

COURSES

Feeling in need of a helping hand towards success in your exams?

PasTest has been helping doctors to pass postgraduate exams for 30 years. Our extensive experience and network of advisors means that we are always one step ahead of other course providers when it comes to knowledge of the current trends and content of the exam.

Over 4000 candidates attend our courses each year at centres throughout the UK. To give you the most up-to-date information and help you to achieve the best results, we constantly update and improve our courses based on feedback from those who attend.

Clinical and Viva courses

Run in association with various hospitals, our two-day clinical and viva courses offer small teaching groups to provide you with the best help possible.

Maximum candidate to tutor ratio of 6: 1

Over 40 exam-type, high-quality short cases

Viva practice in the three areas tested in the exam

Communication skills session

Valuable feedback from experienced consultants on exam technique and performance

Course places are limited to 36, so early booking is essential

77% of candidates who attended our last clinical courses passed their clinical examination first time.

Anatomy course

The MRCS Anatomy four-day course has been specifically designed to prepare candidates for the viva component of the MRCS Examination.

There will be small group tuition on cadaver material, osteological and radiological material. Ample opportunity is given for hands-on practice, assisted by demonstrators, and using some of the best dissecting facilities in the country.

The course is presented by experienced anatomy and surgical tutors, all of whom have been specially chosen by course directors Professor Harold Ellis and Dr Alistair Hunter.

Our New Anatomy Course for the MRCS Viva is an ideal accompaniment to our MRCS clinical course.

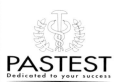

SUMMARY CARDS

Feeling in need of a helping hand towards success in your exams?

The following set of summary cards are to cut out and keep for handy reference

CONTENTS